My Beautiful Detour

An Unthinkable Journey from Gutless to Grateful

Amy Oestreicher

Singing Tree Publishing

New Haven Connecticut

Amy Oestreicher/Singing Tree Publishing
www.amyoes.com

Book Development: Thomas G. Fiffer
Editor: Joshua Stuart
Book Cover: Amy Oestreicher

My Beautiful Detour: An Unthinkable Journey from Gutless to Grateful/ Amy Oestreicher. -- 1st ed.
ISBN 978-1-7331388-1-9

Praise for *My Beautiful Detour*

In her bravely shared memoir, Amy Oestreicher traces her journey of pain, loss, and resilience, bearing witness to and transforming her traumatic experience through narrative. The reader is invited into a determined, poetic representation of life in all its beauty, with a mindful acceptance of the gift of the present moment.
—Nirit Pisano, PhD, author of *Granddaughters of the Holocaust: Never Forgetting What They Didn't Experience*

Amy's book is a gift—a fantastic reminder and an inspirational guide that shows us that painful detours happen in life, and it's up to us to choose to find the beauty in the struggle.
—Joshua Rivedal, author, international speaker The i'Mpossible Project

Thank you, Amy, for this book and teaching us all that when we live in and from gratitude for EVERYTHING life hands us, ANYTHING is possible.
—David Friedman, Broadway Composer, author of *The Thought Exchange*

Amy has a remarkable story of faith, resilience and determination.
—Srinivas Rao, Host/Creator: The Unmistakable Creative

Amy Oestreicher is truly a 'life lover'. As courageous and feisty as they come, this woman has lived gracefully through things that would crumble most of us. She has turned her trauma into her gift and this memoir reminds others that anything is possible.
—Sheri Gaynor, LCSW, Creative Awakenings Int.

Acknowledgements

Many thanks to...
My three brothers, who showed me how to never give up.
Mom for looking up.
Dad for everything.
Grandma and Grandpa for your laughter.
Trees, who've always shown me the way back home.
Stories—mine, yours, and ours.

In memory of Great Uncle Morris, whom I never met, yet showed me all that can bloom from bringing a single story into the light.

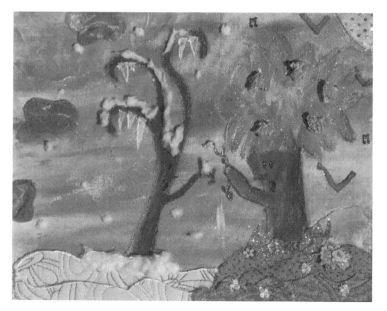

"Winter Meeting"

Contents

Foreword

YES, LIFE IS WHAT HAPPENS WHEN you're doing something else. Amy was on course to be a creative star when a detour emerged.

This is a narrative about the many detours within detours that end up where the author was always destined. It would have surprised no one if the detours went off a cliff and never got back on course. That would have been the story were it not for an indefatigable spirit, grit, determination, vision, and dare I say...guts, in the face of overwhelming odds. That also would not have been the story were it not for an unyielding support cast of tireless advocates made of her parents, brothers, family, and true friends.

This is a template for being accountable and responsible for one's future, never a hapless victim, but a positive force for the possible. There are many stories like this. This is an especially good one.

- Charles J.H. Stolar, MD
    Rudolph N. Schullinger Professor emeritus of Surgery and Pediatrics, Columbia University, College of Physicians and Surgeons

Introduction

WITH ALL OF THE CATASTROPHIC events that cascaded through my life at once, it would be hard for anyone to keep track. Trauma is remembered in a non-linear way. It is the sounds, sights, flashes of memory, and images that write not history, but my story. Trauma memories lie in our felt sensations, and it's hard to assign exact dates to specific events to or sequences.

At this point, I call it "six of the past ten years" unable to eat or drink because, if I have tallied everything correctly, it was three full years at first, until I had my 13th surgery, then 14th, and 15th to put me back together. From then until 2013, the months I was asked to "stop eating and drinking" added up to at least three more years.

So that's my disclaimer for the variable numbers you'll find on Google, in articles about me, and even in slips I make myself. Any way you look at it, who's counting? The idea of instantly shutting down something as human and primal as hunger, over and over again, as casually as turning a light on and off, is incomprehensible. It makes every sip of water still feel like it is my first and my last. I am still overwhelmed with gratitude, and no doubt Costco, Stop & Shop, and every Chinese restaurant in Fairfield County is grateful for me and my restored appetite, too. (More books sold = more food for the stomach-less girl. Thanks!)

This book is about energy in all of its forms—in rolling ocean waves, in bursts of creative sketching sprees, in dance, in belly laughter, in brainstorms, and in spirit. My many references to God and spirituality throughout this book can be interpreted as whatever that magical, kaleidoscopic swirl of energy is to you. It's the grand energy of the universe we inhabit and the blue sky that sweeps over us all. It's something to look to and someone to hear you. Feel free to personalize that "energy" as you read along.

P.S. Some names have been changed.

CHAPTER 1

My Life Exploded

ON PASSOVER, DURING MY SENIOR year in high school, all my dreams exploded in one big bang.

As a teenager growing up in Fairfield, Connecticut, I had the normal high school worries—boys, grades, keeping up with the latest fads. My sense of self was filled with loving family and friends and lit up by the bright future spread out before me. Life felt full of heart, possibility, and spirit. I've always looked at spirituality as a childlike, wondrous mindset that made my world come alive. Life felt magical when I pretended everything around me was holy, enchanted, and filled with an inner spirit I could sense, but not see. This pretending felt real to me. Even as a young girl I was never satisfied just walking through life, doing my homework and extracurriculars, and going out with friends. I never outgrew my early days of discovering endless wonders playing with a simple cardboard box. Daydreaming was an aspect of my homemade spirituality—it made managing work and life a thrilling process of discovery.

Spirituality also meant connection. I couldn't wait to find the "spirit" in everything from ancient Greek myths to the newest food layout at the grocery store. Finding spirit in everything meant that I belonged to a world I was fascinated by but knew so little about.

My sense of spirituality was rooted in a lovingly overbearing family bound together by the culture, traditions, and legacy of Judaism. I was raised loving my Jewish faith, family, and traditions, and growing up around Jewish folktales and storytelling. I was inspired as a young girl by a classic Hasidic story. In this branch of Judaism, the ordinary is hallowed, because it is thought that holy fragments of God are trapped in everything from kitchen chores to the sun's daily rising. It is the responsibility of all humans to set these shattered pieces free by using them, and in doing so releasing beauty into the world. Anything that is useful is thus beautiful by definition because it grounds us in our purpose on Earth.

Hearing this story as a child gave me a powerful tool—the power to elevate the everyday and find joy in in my surroundings—a resourcefulness-based resilience and happiness. The idea is we can take advantage of the usefulness of practical things that assist us in our everyday lives and use them to find meaning. As a teenager, this idea sounded cooler to me than the latest cell-phone feature.

The philosophy that we're responsible for healing the world, known as Tikkun Olam, also set the stage for my life as a teenager. When my friends were throwing big parties for their sweet sixteens, my dream was to spend my birthday weekend at Kutsher's resort in the Catskills celebrating Passover, eating dense, flourless matzoh-meal birthday cake, then walking among my beloved trees, stuffed with cake, and heart hungry for life.

My Early Faith

I first read *The Diary of Anne Frank* in middle school and was struck by Anne's spirit and how closely her mindset and vivacity resembled mine. I too would journal like crazy about the beauty of nature and the hidden blessings in life, and I realize now my Jewish identity has always overlapped with my creative practice and life now as an artist. I shared her infectious childlike wonder and a burgeoning curiosity. I'd read her journal and repeatedly be awed by her appreciation of life, faith, hope, belief. Playing Anne in two local productions, I truly felt alive—grounded in my heritage and my endless love for life.

I always felt I had a close relationship with God. When I was in third grade, every night I would tightly press my fingertips together before I drifted off to sleep—it was my special language I had with God. Every night, I would perform this ritual, like a grasshopper rubbing its legs together, and chant the same words: *Dear God, thank you for a beautiful day today. Please let me live a long, happy, and healthy life. Please visit me in my dreams.* And then I'd slowly feel my eyelids fall, and I would be transported into the world of dreams.

As I grew older, I rubbed my fingers together more fervently—all the way until I was eighteen. I never gave up my search for God. I saw Him in all of nature, but I wanted my own message in my dreams. Outside my window, there were so many different trees; each stretching its branches to God in its own heartfelt way. These trees reached out towards each other, too. They all knew that God was everywhere—including in themselves. This was the lesson I was to learn myself: that no matter where I went in life, or what I went through, God would always be in me. More importantly, I always had myself.

Trees were the sacred symbols I would daydream about in between my high school classes. I would take nature walks and fantasize about trees having faces and moving like people—much like the animatronics at Disney World—a favorite (if not our only) family vacation spot. At a young age, trees were my mentors. I turned to trees for advice, humor, and inspiration, but I had no idea how much I would need them on my journey.

Trees inspired me to create—but so did everything else in my world. My high school assignment notepads were feverishly scribbled with the five lines of a staff as I made them into makeshift music composition paper, along with words, images, and thoughts that the trees from my morning walk had inspired. I remember once being distracted for an entire Biology period because I was tensely awaiting one lingering leaf to fall from a slender, shaking branch. You might have thought I was watching a baseball game, from how I was cheering on that leaf. "You can do it!" Everything around me was stimulation for a poem, song, or story.

Theatre was My World

I grew up thinking my life was a musical. Call it the "theatre bug," or call me a great big ham—I lived for the stage. I was the kid who got sent to the principal's office because when the teacher left the room, I would jump on her desk and start tap-dancing. I'd write songs in my assignment notebook as I waited for the school bell to ring, then hop on the train to the next open call audition I'd read about in *Backstage*. I was the girl who forced every unwilling classmate to join me in a *Les Misérables* medley, assigning them their designated parts to pass the thirty-minute bus ride. When I fought with my brothers, I could only debate with them if we could do it in the spirit of a musical theatre duet. They weren't so keen on that.

Throughout my childhood, I wanted to create something extraordinary for the stage, and to be on stage to perform it. The passion felt like a wild flame inside me—a raw burgeoning single flame straining its tip as far as it could in search of more dry wood, more fuel it could consume to burn more brightly. My dream both distracted me and accelerated me in my schoolwork. It was the silkscreen that shielded my eyes from the fun my school friends were enjoying, yet it was also the lens that intensified my focus and pushed me to dig deeper into every task given to me. I yearned to create a grand-scale musical for the Great White Way. I'd be the world's youngest playwright, composer, and lyricist. Then I'd be the youngest person ever to receive a Tony for best score, best book, best musical, and best actress in a musical.

Sometimes I would be so taken by the conjured stories and soaring melodies in my head that in the middle of class I'd pull my chair away from my desk and scoot it into the far back corner in an inspired daze. It all felt so real. I would ride my fantasies like a wave and follow wherever they chose to take me. My visions were my best friends. And when I transferred them onto paper, it was like investing in a newly solid friendship to take with me into the rest of my boundless life.

"Ms. Oestreicher," a familiar voice would startle me from across the room. "Would you care to join the rest of the class?"

"Sorry, Mrs. Olsen. I'm having important daydreams right now."

I was a girl very much guided by her values: family, theatre, and nature, with "learning" filling in the cracks. I loved life, learning about it, living in it, doing leaps in the rain after school, raising my arms in the air, and relishing the stimulation of the lucky life I led. Firmly rooted in the world around me, I would identify my values based on what I could observe in my surroundings. This way, I could never lose myself, even if life should change overnight.

I also learned to tap into my five "superhero" senses—touch, taste, smell, sound, sight—which put the magic in my life as a child, and, would become my survival mentors later in life. But as a child, they were the kindest of friends, like the birds that flitted around Cinderella's dress in the enchanted Disney movie. I was a young girl who lived in an enchanted castle where everything was magical.

Inspiration was everywhere, and simply going outside after school gave me a lift. My assignment books were filled with random notes of poetry. Here's part of a journal entry from my fifteen-year-old self:

I respect and admire and love the trees for shamelessly shedding their lovely leaves! The world is lit in a new sparkling radiance!

My three brothers, who range between eleven and thirteen years older than I am, were my tribe of wise men, and trees were the magic guardians that made my world an enchanted place. At fifteen, I had a firm identity and anchor in my world. I always felt fortunate to be the "baby girl" of the family—even though I yearned to be treated as a grown-up, though I had the best childhood I could have asked for. Though at the same time, I had overwhelming anxiety I would miss something, and felt I needed to learn everything there was about life.

Jeff

Jeff was the baby boy of the family—a mama's boy, affectionately known to my dad as Pesto Sauce. A drummer, he has always been loud, outgoing, charismatic, the life of the party. Jeff may seem like your stereotypical jock, and yes, I was dragged to many of his high school soccer games. But my favorite memory of Jeff is getting to be an "extra" in *Forensic Assassinations*, a documentary shoot he was running when he was the head writer for *This Week in History* on the History Channel. He loved learning, and I loved learning from him.

Adam

Adam is the oldest of my three brothers. Caring to the point of neurotic, he holds most of our family's third generation Holocaust guilt. His heart is filled with nothing but love and protectiveness, and in a family of loud, opinionated thinkers and creators, Adam was always the one who made sure I was heard—even if I didn't have much to say.

Matt

Matt, sandwiched between Jeff and Adam, is your typical middle child—quiet and lost in the world of his music. I admired him for his radical (to me, at least) ideas, passion for creativity, and sheer talent. Matt has always been a freakishly gifted musician—playing with everyone from Lady Gaga to Stevie Wonder to Michael Bolton—contrasted by a passion for Eastern thought and philosophy.

Matt was the soundtrack to our home, and I remember coming home from school to hear him playing jazz from the front window. For us, music is a way of life that comes as naturally as breathing.

Matt's viewpoint on life inspired me to believe that seeing the world through creativity was the key to happiness.

Family Dynamics

My family kept a lot of secrets. In a household with three older brothers romping around, someone was always looking to stir up some good-natured sibling rivalry or pull a harmless prank. Some secrets were more serious, I'm sure, but as the youngest and only girl, there were probably many things I didn't know about, although I was always curious. I remember feeling exasperated as a child because I had a hard time relating to everyone in my family because of the huge age gap between us.

My father was never overly emotional growing up and around the dinner table we always felt loved, but none of us talked about "feelings." My mother's habit of not sharing what was happening in the family was passed on from her mother. My father's stoicism and thick-skinned mentality was a remnant from his tough upbringing in the Bronx. My three brothers, I learned later had been coached by my dad to "not talk about anything serious" with me, because I was "too young to understand." My brothers felt more like fun, interesting idols in my life, rather than a best friend I could really confide in or express any feelings to. My family could celebrate, but any feeling that was not "joy" or holiday-related, was kept under the table.

So, I managed to vent any stigmatized feelings I needed to get out, by slamming my bedroom door, blasting "Epiphany" from Sondheim's *Sweeney Todd* and belting my rage at the top of my lungs. Lonelier days were saved for "On My Own" from *Les Misérables*, and the days I worried if I would ever really belong anywhere I saved for my favorite ballad, Mira from *Carnival*.

I have to find a place |Where everything can be the same... | A street that I can go | And places I can go | Where everybody knows my name...

Finally, a Friend

The biggest hurdle I went through having much older brothers was trying to get them to see me as an adult as I matured. For a long time, I felt left out by my family, as though I wasn't being "taken seriously." But what I ultimately learned is that the most serious way to be taken is through love—something my family has no shortage of, regardless of circumstance. I finally found that someone, in the oddest of places. I was referred to a New York voice instructor after I overwhelmed my local voice teacher with a long list (five pages, typed, single-spaced) of vocal concerns. Wanting the best for me and seeing how determined I was, he told me he didn't have all the answers for me and suggested that I see *his* voice teacher in New York.

Upon meeting Blaine, my world was changed. I was inducted into the world of real Broadway-style teaching, meeting stars before and after my lessons, and learning the ins and outs of theatre craft and professionalism. He was kind, personable, and connected musical theatre to poetry, nature, philosophy, and everything I was passionate about, too. I had finally found a friend in someone four times my age, and I took to him immediately. Before I knew it, I was staying after lessons, showing him my poetry, music, and journals. We'd talk about philosophy, art, songs, life, nature, my family, and soon I couldn't wait for my father to drive me to the city after school every Friday for that inspiration-packed hour, which eventually turned to two hours after I learned he was an acting coach as well. At a time when I felt my family didn't always get me, I felt Blaine really understood me.

On top of that, he soon became part of the family. We were blown away by his knowledge, creativity, and warmth. Most of all, my mother was so touched by someone who could care so much for her daughter. He was my mentor, and I could talk to him about everything. My entire family adored Blaine. We couldn't believe this Buddha-like figure had come into our home and had recognized me as having star potential. After we had spent so many hours together, Blaine wrote a two-page typed letter to my parents asking to be my godfather, which thrilled all of us.

Besides Blaine's charm and sophistication, and the fact that he treated me like an important person and a grownup, he seemed to understand me in a way no one else did. I knew I felt this intricate connection to nature, but no one *got* it. I loved nature, but I also loved people and really wanted to connect to others in a way I hadn't before. I also wanted a best friend. I never kept one best friend for long because my life in theatre was so hectic with constantly changing casts of characters. In my daily nature walks, I took joy in discovering this whole beautiful world, then immediately felt the frustration of having no one to share it with. I was always surrounded by people, so my friends didn't get my intense loneliness. All week I looked forward to sharing my thoughts and feelings with Blaine, with *someone*, just as I want to share with someone now.

My high school scrapbook traces the exact evolution of my relationship with Blaine and captures the magic I felt in that season, that whole inspired year. There are pages crammed with photographs I took that year on the mornings of both Thanksgiving and Passover.

Passover is a holiday of remembrance when the Jewish people gather to symbolically relive and commemorate our escape from slavery in Egypt. For my family, holidays, celebration, and of course, food, was how you showed appreciation and expressed love. Our Seder on April 25, 2005 was true to form. It also turned out to be the last meal I would eat before my stomach exploded, sending me into years of "medical exile," and "slavery" to IV nutrition; a decade of wandering in the "desert of uncertainty" of whether I'd ever eat or drink again.

So, what do you do when you've invested everything into your passion, and you can't follow it anymore? What do you when you suddenly find your dreams out of reach? I've always thought about what a world-concert pianist would do if he injured his hand, or a dancer broke a leg. But I never dreamed that anything like that would or even could happen to me. Until it did.

CHAPTER 2

Me, A Survivor?

"SURVIVOR" IS A WORD that belongs with plane crashes and armed robberies and Dateline specials. In suburban Connecticut, we faced stress for final exams or a spat with a best friend. I almost laughed and was about to put the book, *The Courage to Heal,* back on the shelf...but I couldn't. The subtitle read loud and clear: "For survivors of sexual abuse."

I opened the book up and read through the symptoms in the first chapter... One word that stuck with me. *Numb.* The soft "b" felt tingly on my lips as I swallowed up that word in terrifying secrecy. Numb. That is how I felt. Like my body was physically going through the motions of everyday life, but the me I had known my entire life was not a part of it. It was as though I determined to remain in denial. I didn't mean to keep Blaine a secret, but I had no idea I was being molested and couldn't fathom the idea of such a tremendous betrayal. I was confused. Something felt dreadfully wrong, but I couldn't put my finger on it. For months I kept that secret inside. I had an instinct that something within me had changed, but I wasn't exactly sure what. It wasn't yet real to me that someone within my circle of trust could do something like that to me. Such a thing didn't happen to someone like me. And our family just didn't talk about things like this.

Courage, I remembered learning, meant to share who you are with your whole heart. But I had a secret I felt I couldn't share with anyone. A secret that was eating me alive. Wasn't I being courageous by keeping what happened with Blaine to myself? By dealing with it—or not dealing with it through denial?

Was there something I was scared to face that I needed to find the strength to confront? Was it possible to restore yourself to a sound state by sharing what's happened to you and who you've become after trauma? I reached for the thick yellow binding—as though someone else was leading me. Now I was face to face with the cover, glancing over my shoulder to make sure no one was looking. *Me, a survivor.*

When I met Blaine, my abuser, I was an innocent fifteen-year-old, and my journals were swelling with the inspiration he'd give me at voice lessons, poetry I thought he'd like, pictures of trees I'd save to show him, and thoughts I was certain only he could understand. I didn't yet know you weren't supposed to put people on pedestals. Blaine appreciated the beauty of the world as I did and became a god-like figure in my mind. He made everything feel special, alive, real. I told myself, if the only person I ever could talk about deep things with were Blaine, I would be okay. You only need one person.

When Blaine started to abuse me, it became harder to keep up my scrapbook. I was shutting down inside and could no longer share my deepest, conflicted feelings. I felt there was no point in documenting things, and the days seemed to pass endlessly until I actually developed a fear, a hatred, for waking up every day. I soon stopped chronicling altogether. I didn't wish to think about anything at all—or feel. I just wanted to stay numb.

The morning after Blaine first took advantage of me, I was wearing a yellow knitted tank top from the Gap and my hair was down and sitting perfectly around my face. I was wearing pearl earrings and I felt like a precious pearl, who had been ruined. I was afraid he would get scared right away, like *God, what have I just done, I'm a pedophile!* I even expected him to come to his senses the morning after! But no, he was in his sex-crazed trance, and part of me was scared out of my mind. But part of me was also numb, dazed, and confused, as I remember unemotionally going to his kitchen cabinet like a zombie and lifelessly pouring muesli and milk into a bowl. It was bright out—we ate outside on his porch, and I felt dirty coming into the light. I was squinting and my shoulders were hunched.

I didn't know what to talk about. Loud Amy just wanted to come out and say, *"Well, Blaine, what the hell was that?"* and just laugh about how crazy it was, but quiet Amy was scared of him kicking me out. I needed him now. So, I thought, *okay, maybe I do belong here.* But it was more like I was trying to tell myself that just to settle my uneasy stomach—a large part of me was nervous, uneasy, and confused. An awkward, shy little girl who needed her parents back in Fairfield.

But I accepted that this was the mess I was now a part of. And thinking back on it, the idea I made myself believe, that Blaine and I could really run off together to la-la-land and live a life together as "soul-mates," whatever that means, was as much of a lie as the lie I made myself believe every day for so long, thinking that my automatic-pilot routine was a better way of life than actually living. But they were both ways to cope with disturbing situations.

Before I understood trauma, I was ashamed of how gullible and naïve I was. How taken under his spell I was at a point before I started to really hate him, because Blaine had cut me off from my real, feeling soul. And I think I knew at that point, I was living a lie, but I couldn't bear to face it. Not Blaine. Anyone but Blaine. It just couldn't be.

How, after two years of a seemingly healthy, paternal relationship, could my voice teacher have molested me? (Later, I would learn he had been grooming me.) Now I didn't know who to trust and was keeping this horrible secret inside, burning in my gut, hidden from my family.

Once Blaine had invaded the "sacred trust" he had called our relationship—even going as far as to call it a "covenant," I was completely out of touch with my feelings. I was so numb that I was still going back months later for lessons, figuring there was something wrong with me to account for why I was being tortured by negative emotions. I was losing my inspiration, my faith, the magic I saw in the world. I thought maybe I was just getting older and losing the wonder and open mind that came from childhood creativity and imagination.

Eventually, I learned that our secrets do make us sick. We lock emotions, memories—any terrible things we might try to suppress—in our fragile, mortal frames.

By age seventeen this trusted mentor transformed into a complete stranger. One night I had come to his studio for a voice lesson. When he started to molest me, I went into shock and coped by leaving my body and staying numb. By the end of that night, I couldn't remember a thing that happened. I blocked it from my mind. But when I woke up, my voice teacher did not go back to the man I thought he was. And I didn't go back to the girl I had been. I stayed numb. For months and months. After a while, all I could feel were my feet pacing back and forth over the endless passing of days.

My family didn't recognize that I had become a virtual space-cadet. My parents were concerned that I was suddenly not laughing, not singing, not showing signs of any human emotion. My brothers were angry, confused, and worried that I had transformed, seemingly overnight. Matt, whom I had always felt closest to, glared through my vacant stare with, "You've been pretty unlikable lately." That sharp comment stung me with hurt, yet resonated deeply, because even I didn't like myself anymore. The more upset my family became, the less able I felt to turn to them. Tension mounted, and I felt trapped in a situation I did not understand.

And then there I was in Barnes & Noble somehow holding an impossible book—one not meant for me. *The Courage to Heal.*

Nervousness rushed over my body, as though I'd just been caught shoplifting. The warmth that filled my cheeks was a peculiar heat I hadn't felt since I had last laughed or smiled. Words had the power to pierce through my skin with more potency than my fingernails, and my body was rattling now with uncontrollable energy.

It suddenly became clear that I had to fix something I couldn't yet name. That I had to find the courage to heal the unspeakable.

Mom: Amy and I went for a weekend retreat. Amy saw a sign advertising a psychic reading for $25 at a diner. Amy assertively said, "We must meet with her!" I responded, "I don't see psychics." But after pleading, we walked in and Amy went behind a curtain, and I heard this woman telling Amy that her life would get difficult and challenging. But she would be alright in the end. That she would not graduate high school in the usual way, and that she was meant to be a wounded healer.

In the wake of my abuse, school had become hell for me. Just a few months before, my bouncy outgoingness had annoyed my classmates. Some thought I was too loud and wild. Some found me intimidating. So, when I got to the point where I went inside myself and froze, I glared at everyone with eyes that said, "Are you happy now that this is what I have become instead? Would you rather have me like this?" Now my classmates were throwing crumpled up bits of paper at me in physics class because I was in such a daze. My spaciness had become a source of humor for them, and I couldn't wait to escape the daily torture of being treated like the walking dead. At the same time, my compulsive thoughts and behaviors were eating away at my soul more ferociously every day, and I feared I would lose myself completely if I didn't take time for myself to heal. I desperately needed a break. Using my old proactive instincts, I took charge and typed up a proposal to my principal to see what liberties he would give me.

To both my mom's and my surprise, Fairfield High School gave me the time off, no questions asked. As soon as I had been granted permission to stay home for two months, my mother looked at me as if to say, "okay, Amy, so what's your plan now?" The truth was, I didn't know. I just knew I needed safety. And I needed an escape.

Starting to Unfreeze

During those two months at home, sounds, thoughts, triggers, memories, senses, and images began to thaw from the permafrost in the back of my mind. Ever so slowly I was reconnecting with my soul and I longed to feel again.

Finding *The Courage to Heal* was the catalyst. I must have had that courage inside myself, as I was somehow instinctively led to the book. Sometimes all it takes is the transformative power of words to signal to us that we need something profound.

But courage came slowly and in layers. Before I spoke my secret, it consumed my body with fire, and I expressed that fire through movement that felt out of my control, like a force coursing through me, needing to release something from my system. The healthy way this energy expressed itself was dancing out the desperation. I remember losing myself in the world of music as an escape, dancing my way out of this mess. Through leaps and twirls, I could escape from everything yet be centered in what really mattered. Years later, my mother told me a woman came up to her at a dance workshop I was attending and said, "Please watch your daughter dance. If you look closely, you'll see she is struggling with a very big issue. She's calling out for help. Find out why she is suffering."

At the time, my mom didn't think much of that woman's ominous observation. Somehow, subconsciously, I was trying to send a message to my mother through dance, before I could find the courage to share it openly with words. The courage to heal starts with an individual and spreads throughout the family; words can act like viruses in this way.

It was difficult for me to say that Blaine had molested me. I was young, innocent for my age, and I had been seeking validation of all the inspiration I felt flowing through my veins. To have that affirmed by a wiser, older mentor who taught Broadway stars and celebrities was surreal to me, and to my family as well. How could abuse be a part of that picture?

Finding that book, *The Courage to Heal*, forced me to face my own denial. Eventually, I spoke the truth. And wrote it. And expressed it through art. I realized the value of my story once I was able to write it, and ultimately read it for myself. Ironically, my abuser, the sociopath who demanded my silence, was a voice coach. Truth is stranger than fiction. My life had become so miserable and difficult to endure and I couldn't figure out why I would not let myself be happy anymore, why life was always a panic. My childhood had been spent wrapped up in self-love and compassion. Now I hated life and myself with every shallow breath of my tormented body.

I also felt ashamed that I was no longer living up to my reputation as an active, outgoing student at Fairfield High. No one at school had any concept of what I was going through right under their nose. I wanted to open up so badly, to just joke about what an asshole Blaine was and what my hell was like, but here my friends were sharing the latest gossip about this boy or that party, and I had all of these secrets weighing down on me. I felt like an alien.

After taking my break from school, I heard whispers and rumors about what had happened to me. I wished I could go back to my high school and see some of the people who drew their own conclusions and tell them what I actually went through. I needed their respect—not their ridicule.

My Secret Comes Out

My world became spiritless and directionless—a big black hole. I lost my sense of safety in the outside world—I didn't know *who* I could lean on. I thought Blaine was my everything, and I didn't know *what* my family was now. Beyond that, I felt no safety in *myself*. Here I had relied on myself as my own anchor in the wide-open sea. I had thought I was an adult; that I could handle this. Eventually, I couldn't take it anymore. I opened up to my mother. Although part of her already knew.

> Mom: Amy was not herself the past few months. One day she and I took a walk at Penfield Beach and it was a clear day. I began asking her what was bothering her, why couldn't she tell me. And then for some reason, I looked her in the eyes and asked if her fifty-nine-year-old voice teacher was touching her. I don't know why those words came out of my mouth; call it God's voice inside of me pushing me to ask. The moment I asked that question, she said "yes"—and then began to give me a litany of the many things he had done. I began getting hysterical and frantic (although I blocked this out from my memory).

I remember holding my hysterical mother's hands, trying to ground her, insisting, "Mom. Tell me something good." She looked up exasperatedly, and said, "the sky is blue." Repeating this mantra back and forth to one another gave us enough strength to carry forward. Just like me, my mother had been traumatized, and she had not realized how much of her memory she had repressed. And like me, she was able to move forward and heal only after she was able to let herself remember and speak of these things.

I had dissociated because the confusion had torn me in two. First Blaine was a teacher, then he wasn't. The suddenness with which his being in that role was taken away from me left me in total disbelief. But in time, I came to accept it. I had been searching for that golden statue, but it was forever gone. I wanted to slap myself for having been so silly. I hated myself for being so gullible. And I lamented the loss of my friends, the trees, where all my child-like innocence was invested. After my mom told my family about Blaine—first my dad and then my brothers—it freed me more completely of my secret and freed us as a family to process what had happened. After everyone knew, we were all trying to come to terms with what Blaine had done. Each family member dealt with their shock and anger differently and wondered if they had seen signs before.

The Passover Table and the Meaning of Family

The day after our Passover dinner, I was rushed to the emergency room, where my journey through a whirlwind I came to know as the trauma vortex would begin. But first, a few words about who was with me on that fateful night. As we sat down to our Seder that night, my beloved grandmother was seated to my left. At eighteen, she was already a Holocaust survivor. A talented seamstress, she survived because the Nazis forced her to sew uniforms. My Grandma was never bitter—she sang, found blessings and gratitude, and savored life. Her creativity and determined spirit enabled her to survive, along with her unwavering faith. When I was growing up, she and I would take nature walks (hence my love of trees), she would sew buttons on my coat, make her delicious noodle kugel, yell at me for not wearing socks on the cold tile, and although she never liked to discuss the pain of what she went through, I could always see the suffering deep in her eyes. But I never expected my grandmother to start recounting the entire events of her horrific past to me. Instead, she always filled our house with joy, love, and food. She always exclaimed that she "was going to dance at my wedding," which would be the greatest moment of her life.

A Jew in Czechoslovakia during World War II, my grandmother had been married just six months when she was taken by the Nazis to Auschwitz. She and her husband had been hiding on a tobacco farm, and they were sent to separate camps when someone turned them in. My grandmother survived the war (her husband did not) and eventually made it to Manhattan, where she met a tailor—my grandfather—and married him. She and others like her never talked about what they had experienced. They had endured more pain and felt more fear in those few years than most people experience in a lifetime. Her generation raised children while trying to keep so much bottled up inside. She did her best to keep this fear and pain from her daughter— my mother—and while my mother remembers her as the most loving mom, she also remembers feeling a real sadness and fear in her home. We all grew up understanding that some things had to be kept quiet.

After the war, my grandmother moved to Brooklyn and worked independently as a seamstress while my grandfather built up a tailoring corporation with his brother. My mother often recounts how my grandparents would sew all of her clothes and Halloween costumes. I do remember my grandparents sewing pinstriped wool suits and old-fashioned dress pants that I courteously accepted.

My grandmother's anxiety—anxiety about the possibility of losing the people she loved at any moment, and about the presence of evil in the world—was unconsciously passed down to my mother, along with her grand sense of love, kindness, and family values.

My three older brothers, who spent most of their time with our mother, because my dad was a medical resident and frequently in the hospital, bore the brunt of this inherited anxiety because by the time I was born my mother was more comfortable with having children in the world. Still, I remember feeling certain fears when I was young; in fact, I have vivid memories of my dad tucking me in and allaying my fears of nuclear war.

But this pattern also brought a richness to our lives. My favorite quote, simple and profound, was originally my grandmother's, then my mother's: "You must celebrate when times are good." My house felt like summer camp—that place where every kid in the neighborhood always was. It's where there was a party thrown on every possible occasion, where we cleaned out the garage on President's Day to have a neighborhood donut eating contest. It was as loving and warm a home as I could ever have hoped for.

On my grandmother's left at the Seder table was my grandfather, a big, happy child of a man. I always remember him sitting at our kitchen table in Fairfield, sorting socks. He was a tailor who used to sew for all the big department stores and designers. My grandfather had fought in the resistance in Poland and had been sent to Siberia. My grandmother loved my grandfather, but she lost her first husband in the war and always spoke of *him* as the love of her life, even in my grandfather's presence. No one in my family learned much about this man, except for my grandmother's doting on how handsome he was. She always thought he would make it through the war because he was so strong. She was shocked she was the one who survived.

My grandfather, who grew up in the woods of Poland after his mother died in childbirth, had this childlike wonder—he was like a little kid with an enormous grin. One day he was sitting at the kitchen table with a cereal bowl and a carton of milk and this big silly smile on his face. He also had a bag of Chex Mix. Regular Chex Mix. With his grin widening, he poured the whole bag of salty Chex Mix into his paper cereal bowl, poured the milk over it, then dug his spoon into it and started chomping away.

"Grandpa, you can't do that," I explained.

But he never responded when he had that silly smile. We often felt he didn't hear anything we said because he was so far off in his own world. But he was listening at the times he wanted to—like when my grandma was telling him what was for dinner, or when he decided to sew us a pair of pants. But when my grandma would nag in her thick, accented sing-songy voice, "Oy-ving (Irving), you have to take your medication before you eat. Your medication..." That silly smile would go right back on, and he would retreat into his own little world.

For me, the Chex Mix moment epitomized my grandfather's happy oblivion. He didn't even know what he was putting in his mouth. He was just so darn happy all the time and madly in love with my grandma. Our family would joke, when we lost track of Grandma and Grandpa on our Disney vacations, that they were probably off on "Pleasure Island." My grandfather, the tailor, was also obsessed with pockets. He even sewed my three brothers and me our own wallets, each with a handwritten note that said, "Good health" in it—but at seven years old, I didn't have much use for a wallet. He always wore his thin white undershirts around the house, and each one had a mismatched breast pocket he sewed onto it from his scraps of old fabric—an adorable variation on upcycling or repurposing material.

My mother felt close to her parents and ended up clearing out our entire basement to make a home for them to live in, complete with its own kitchen space. That meant our huge holiday gatherings of thirty people with music, food, and fun were always spearheaded by my grandparents, in *their* kitchen, cooking and entertaining, which made my mother so proud.

Despite their struggles, both my grandma and grandpa had put their faith and trust back in the world again, even after it was shattered. I believe their combination of hope and resilience is what drove me to make them the spiritual mascots of my life.

Seated across from me was my mom, who has always been the glue of the family—the overly emotional heart, and with an overabundance of optimism. She inspired my passion for learning, creativity, and play by breaking every traditional parenting rule. She'd help me plan elaborate birthdays—roller-skating in our basement, or a beach-themed party with tons of sand on the basement floor. We hosted book clubs, cooking parties, and paint nights. She would drag me to my brothers' sports games armed with crafts, markers, and workbooks.

My mom's greatest excitement was seeing her children thrive. She would sign us up for every mommy and me class and activity, as long as it was inspired by creativity. I'll never forget how I talked her into running a mother-daughter Thanksgiving race at eight years old—which became the story she told the entire congregation at my bat mitzvah ceremony. We had arrived at the big event in our mother-daughter colorful outfits, in our dress up shoes and frilly socks, not knowing it was an actual race...that you run. Despite all the stares and the five-mile trek, we made it to the finish line together, and she's always thanked me for pushing her.

By the time my mom was thirty, she had three little boys. A Brooklyn-born, Barbra Streisand-adoring music-lover, once she had the first little girl of the family, she loved taking me to Broadway shows and auditions.

That brings me to my father—the best father you could find. In our thousands of family pictures and home movies, my dad is always absent, because he was always the one behind the camera, and despite my brothers' cries of "c'mon Dad, not now," they thanked him later for capturing and chronicling our childhood. My dad is known for his sarcasm, politics, corny jokes, and Yankees obsession (a byproduct of being born and bred in the Bronx). I didn't care much for sports, but I often indulged my father by going with him to Yankees games—mostly for the giveaways on special game days, Derek Jeter, and the fun animation on the jumbotron.

He was also a loved dermatologist in the area, and growing up, as soon as I'd say my name, the next expected question would be, "Oh, are you the daughter of Dr. Oestreicher? I love him! He took care of my..." So of course, I never forgave him when I ended up with a huge pimple on the morning of my bat mitzvah, which at the time I thought was the worst thing that had ever happened to me.

By the time Passover arrived, we were each beginning to heal in our own way and all moving towards liberation. Spring was in the air, and the big round tables were set up in our basement to accommodate our extended clan. But this time, the holiday had special meaning. After a year of confusing chaos, we were finally taking ownership of our lives, finally becoming free. This made the holiday's timeless message personally symbolic.

I loved Passover's quirky rituals—dipping your finger in a goblet of wine for each of the ten plagues, or my dad's favorite dermatology joke as we recited each one: "Thank you to the boils for paying for our Seder..." My dad and I had put together our own Haggadah after years of collecting excerpts from various texts, integrating the themes of the holiday—persecution, escape, wandering, and fulfillment of promises—into our customized guide. I led our Seder and was starting to burgeon into my old, bubbly self as I expelled Blaine from memory.

After dinner, I went upstairs and crawled into bed. Something didn't feel right. I was used to getting stomachaches from trying to drink so many smoothies to gain back the weight I had lost, so I waited it out. But the next morning, I was still hurting. This had never happened before. So, I waited and finally complained. My mom started looking up natural remedies, calling the neighbors and asking for advice. Of all things, they told her to buy Coke syrup. I lay on the patio all afternoon, in the bright sunshine, clutching my stomach and taking sips of sticky dark brown liquid. It was such a beautiful day, and I was in such intense pain. By that night, the pain was unbearable. I was up all night in the shower, sitting on the floor, letting the scalding stream run down my back. Morning came, and I was still in agony.

When my dad came home from work that afternoon, April 25, 2005, he was surprised to see that my stomach was distended—the first time I had ever heard that word—and I was starting to get worried. But I still managed to have a drawn-out debate with my brothers about which college I should go to, after being accepted into some of the top musical theatre programs in the country. I couldn't believe I had gotten into the musical theatre program at the University of Michigan! All my life, I had dreamed of pursuing a career in theatre, on Broadway, in every musical possible—and this was my golden ticket! After all my hard work, everything had come together. I would train for Broadway, win my Tony Award, and conquer the world.

By early evening, the pain was excruciating, and my memories are a fiery haze of images. I was in the car, screaming "I'm in pain!" I got to the ER—didn't even know we were going there—where I was yelling, "I'm in pain" to everyone. Passover was not supposed to turn out this way.

Stream of Unconsciousness

April is the cruelest month
—*The Wasteland*, T. S. Eliot

AFTER I AWOKE FROM THE long coma, I went into at the hospital and healing became my full-time job, journaling would become a daily, even hourly practice and a critical aspect of my journey. But it would be my brother, Jeff—the sentimental one who recorded my first life-or-death days in the ICU. Because I was unconscious, unable to write, move, or speak, having dreams of being underwater, and blissfully unaware of what lay ahead.

Night one in the ICU

What goes through your head when your baby sister is suddenly rushed to the ER in the middle of the night, and you're not sure if she'll live or die? You fear the worst and hope for the best, but you probably don't imagine the ICU will become your sister's home for the next five months. Somehow, Jeff had the presence of mind to open his laptop and write an account of that first terrifying night in the hospital. My dad, my mom, and my other brothers, Adam and Matt also captured their reactions. Since I lost consciousness for quite some time soon after arriving at the hospital, these fragmented passages have become my "memories" of this time. I nearly left the world, and until I came back and awoke from my coma, I had to rely on my family to document, each in their own way, not only the surreal series of events that followed but also to capture how it felt. I am grateful to all of them for taking the time to do this. Without their journal entries, from which I quote liberally below, an entire section of my life would be lost.

Jeff: You went to the ER at about 8:30. You were there twenty minutes before you saw doctor. They put IV in to draw blood. Took three times. Wheeled you to x-ray. Told Dad you'd need surgery. Pain kept getting worse. Air pockets formed on neck and face. Then you collapsed. They stabilized you with IVs.

The details of what happened when they got me into surgery are like something out of a horror movie. Only I lived it.

Jeff: When they cut into abdomen, blood hit ceiling because of so much pressure from ab blowing up. You went into septic shock which precipitates DIC (life-threatening blood clots). Bacteria so overwhelmed your defenses that you couldn't clot, and everything started leaking. You blew up to three times your normal size.
First night took part of stomach out because of 4.5-inch tear. Most of it was dead. Blood supply not enough. Some of your colon. Pain intense. Stomach crushed blood supply to intestines. Stomach and intestines perforated.

My dad also wrote about those frightful first hours, during which he and my mom were told I would die. A guy with a ton of heart, but not one to express much emotion, he had the tremendous responsibility of keeping it together while communicating to his colleagues, as a doctor himself, and trying to understand what measures would have to be taken to keep me alive. I would not be here were it not for my father, watching every move, catching every little thing that could have gone wrong.

Dad: Got to E.R. twenty-five minutes before your stomach exploded. Everybody mobilized to whisk you away to the operating room. Dr. Garvey came in about 1 a.m. and told us you were out of surgery, but it was critical. We waited till you came upstairs and were settled in the surgical ICU bed. About 2 a.m. the nurses said we should get some rest and we went to the waiting area which was now empty and laid down on the floor. About 4:30 a.m. a resident woke us and said you were failing and would die. We rushed into your room and looked down at you in the bed. Mom and I hugged each other and cried. I faced the small window, looked out and said, "Take me instead, God."

Matt: Jeff called and told me to go to the hospital. He said to hurry up. He said, "This could be bad." He was preparing me for the possibility that Amy wouldn't make it through the night. Before this, our way of dealing with problems was avoiding them. Now we had to face them head-on.

Adam: When I got the call, Matt said you were sick, and I needed to come home. I arrived at the hospital, and some friends and family were there. Every once in a while, I'd go to the bathroom to compose myself and process. I even snapped a photo of my face (a selfie) to show myself later that I "did okay." It helped me feel stronger.

Mom: You looked so beautiful—it didn't make sense to me—you couldn't possibly die! I ran to your side and shook you gently, crying, "You can't leave us Amy, you promised." Mark stared straight ahead, like a robotic machine, and said, "If she dies, I will never believe in God again!" I grabbed his shirt so hard, looked him in the eyes and said, "Don't you dare say that again— don't tell me there is no God and my daughter goes into a box to be put in the ground full of dirt!" He backed off and cried and said okay. I kept whispering into your ear, "Fight Amy. Fight to live; we all need you. You are my warrior." Two physician's assistants stood up all night past their shifts giving you blood all night, refusing to leave your sight until they tried their best to stabilize you with what turned out to be 123 pints of blood.

Because my grandparents were Holocaust survivors and had been through so much tragedy in their lives, my mom decided to protect them. She called her brother to pick them up in the middle of the night from our house, where the Passover table remained as we had left it when I was rushed to the hospital and take them back to their home in Queens. He was instructed to tell them that I was just a bit "dehydrated," and needed to stay in the hospital for a few days. To this day, my parents aren't sure they did the right thing in sending my grandparents away. For a while, they distanced them from my life and death situation; neither they nor I had any idea that I would be the only family member never to see my grandparents again. Both my grandmother and grandfather passed within months of each other after I was discharged from the ICU.

Miraculously, I survived the night, but it became clear that I would not be leaving the hospital or even the ICU any time soon. My condition was beyond critical, and since the doctors had never seen anything quite like it before, they couldn't make any predictions. The Bridgeport Hospital ICU became my family's second home, camping out to support me as I lay unconscious and monitor my situation, which was changing minute by minute.

Week One—a New Neighborhood: The Bridgeport ICU

The ICU is a place with a single purpose—keeping critical patients alive until their condition stabilizes, so they can then be moved to a regular hospital room for recovery. It's not a hotel designed for a large family to live in for months. But that's what my family did. My ever-present dad put his private dermatology practice in Connecticut on hold. He didn't sleep and watched the nurses' every move. We took over the ICU and made it our new neighborhood.

Dad: Back at the ICU, Mom and I read you *A Walk in the Woods*, played Janis Ian nonstop and rubbed your legs which were terribly swollen. Days were long, but at night, the waiting room became a happening place. Routinely, 30-40 people would visit and sit with us. We had a catered dinner almost every night with hot plates, coffee makers, a microwave, and music. We even commandeered the janitor's closet for our bedroom and installed night lights, a radio, and a stereo.

While my amazing family was there for me every moment, I also had an incredible team of hospital staff who saw to my care. At the helm was Dr. Garvey, a quiet, soft-spoken man, reserved but efficient, with a clear understanding that he had to do whatever possible to keep me alive. His words were gentle but real as he explained the severity of my situation. He was also a forceful man of action whose tireless dedication and team of nurses kept me alive.

Meanwhile, our actual home in Fairfield had been abandoned when I was rushed to the ER. With my parents by my side 24/7, my brothers took turns staying at the house to take care of our dog, Gabby, who had no idea why my parents and I were suddenly missing from her life.

Dad: After a week, I finally got to go home and get new clothes. When I went down to the basement, I saw all the Passover tables still set. Each table had a bottle of Kedem grape juice on it along with a plate of matzoh. Tears welled up and over and over I repeated, "I want my Passover back, I want my Passover back!"

Everything during that first week at Bridgeport was minute to minute, and my dad recalls the medical procedures Dr. Garvey had to perform again and again to finally stabilize my condition.

Dad: Dr. Garvey was in the OR till about 1:30 a.m. when he came to talk to us. He knew things were not good but remained professional giving us the facts. Every day he took Amy back to the OR to try and save a little more tissue until the last of the gangrenous tissue was removed. Then it was like a faucet had been turned off. She stopped bleeding, started clotting, and Garvey was able to smile at us for the first time in days.

Jeff managed to pay a visit to our Fairfield house, to make sure my Hamster, who I had just gotten before my coma, was taken care of too.

Jeff: I have made leaps and bounds with one Mr. Hamster who shall (and does!) remain nameless. He loves me. You would be jealous. We speak about you every night, and he now lets me pick him up without fighting back. I dare say he waits for me to come home each night to take him out of his cage. (Last night, we got home around 11ish, and he was standing on the top floor looking out into the kitchen.)

When you are as sick as I was, you need all the help you can get on every front—medical and spiritual. As doctors did their share, my family looked to any way they could help and gathered all the prayers we could find from anyone and everywhere. What my mom remembers are the many heroes who helped keep me alive during those first critical and chaotic days in the Bridgeport ICU. In addition to receiving top-notch care from the medical personnel, I was surrounded with love by our family's friends, prayed for by countless others, and helped by a wide variety of healers. From gospel church choirs to naturopaths to the melting pot of faiths, races, and backgrounds, these diverse individuals who had been brought together in one space shared a common purpose: that I should live. The ICU was the great equalizer, and we were all humbled by the reality of our mortality and the lives of those we loved.

The many friends who came to visit me in the hospital formed a support system for my family, just as my family was the support system for me.

Jeff: For as long as I can remember, Dad has said that he needs only his family; no friends. He certainly no longer thinks this. Something of this magnitude is not possible to deal with without all of these people we've been surrounded by. I cannot overstate how amazing this community has been. Mom said, "After this, everyone is going to feel like Amy is their child." It's so true. Everyone adores you, and everyone is thinking about you and praying for you.

Visitors continued to stream in, and we became the old guard as a new family took our original seats in the hospital waiting room.

Mom: Amy required at least nine surgeries at once. The doctors were unsure about her recovery from this devastating assault on her body. But the prayers began to flow from everywhere. When you were "asleep" in your hospital bed, I brought in this reiki person (massage) to Bridgeport hospital so she would massage you and lay hands on you. Jane paid for a psychic to come to see you. This woman walked all around your ICU bed, who then nonchalantly said to me, "Angels are all around your daughter, and she is close to death, deciding whether to live or die."

Living in the ICU was exhausting for everyone, but it took perhaps the greatest toll on my father.

Jeff: I see how tired Mom and Dad are. Mom fell asleep on the waiting room couch yesterday and Dad, defying explanation, doesn't seem to sleep. If he's not talking to doctors, he's on one of the nurses' computers looking at your stats and examining your chemistry numbers. When not doing that, Dad's standing beside you, reading A Walk in the Woods to you and rubbing your left hand. He is tireless. It's a beautiful thing to see. We have often said that Dad is not very passionate. He is passionate about saving you and bringing you home. I can't not cry thinking about what he's done here for you.

Week Two—Big Changes

Jeff: You've been sleeping for a week now, and we know your body is strong enough to be awake. They even want you to start breathing on your own, which I know you will be doing soon.

My condition seemed to have stabilized, at least enough for Jeff and Matt to get out of the hospital for a quick jog. The ICU can make anyone crazy if you stay there for too long, and even the most dedicated family members needed to get out once in a while for their own sanity. Being trapped with forty-eight of the sickest kids in the country was a solemn existence. ICU psychosis was a real and present threat for anyone who stayed within those four walls for too long. While I was there, four kids died.

Jeff was always investigating everything and used to grill me like a detective when we were kids. Now he turned his forensic skills on the hospital staff to solve one of my medical mysteries, maintaining his sense of humor even in the face of crisis.

Jeff: May I be annoyingly boastful for just a minute? Airess, the ICU's most aptly named respiratory therapist, came in yesterday to clean your ventilator. After she left you looked more labored, not less. I noticed that you were having a harder time breathing the moment she disconnected one of the vent tubes and connected it to something else. I knew that she had made your breathing worse, but I wasn't sure how. Your nurse checked everything and dismissed it as nothing. I told her that it started with Airess. Then I noticed that your O2 number on the monitor had decreased from 100% to 92% and spoke up. Finally, Airess came back in, a little peeved but still sweet, checked what I was pointing to, and discovered that she had not turned the vent hard enough, causing the tube to leak. What's up now?!

It should have been the first sign that years later Jeff would drop out of politics and become a doctor.

Though I was not fully conscious, I did begin to emerge from my coma while still in the Bridgeport ICU.

As the day wore on, my condition and energy level began to deteriorate, as I was burning so many calories trying to move and speak. Once again, my outrageously heroic father came to the rescue. The nurses were going to leave me on my own, but my dad was worried about how hard it was for me to breathe. So, he left and found the chief of cardiology at the hospital.

During this time, I was in and out of consciousness. It also became clear to Jeff early on that I would need all the encouragement I could get to succeed on my healing journey.

Jeff: I was reading A Walk in the Woods to you, and I came to a sentence that contained the word "convivial." I love when, and you do this often, you raise your hands for us to hold them. That's what you were doing every little while as I was reading. It is indescribably cute. So, after reading "convivial," I asked you if you knew what it meant. Your eyes were closed, so I wasn't sure if you were listening, But, with closed eyes, you nodded your head to say "yes."

That night, one of the nurses, Sarah, told Jeff I would be fine, though it would be a long road ahead. It was a welcome departure from some of the predictions we'd been hearing.

On Mother's Day, Jeff remained convinced I would heal completely and imagined taking a trip with me when I got out of the hospital. A common line in Jeff's journal was "I want you to wake up today."

But Jeff's journaling was interrupted as the sharp pain of the memory of Blaine's abuse pierced through my semi-conscious state and came out in the first coherent words I spoke after falling ill.

Jeff: You were talking today with the help of the trach device that Sara, your favorite nurse, gave you. What you said over and over again made us all cry, "It was him! It was him! It was him!"

Week Three—New Digs

To say my progress went two steps forward and one step back would be an understatement. I was missing large parts of my digestive system and undergoing numerous surgeries to keep me alive. When a procedure went well, it was cause for celebration even though it represented only a small step on the long road ahead. When things went badly, a new plan had to be formulated, and a new map of my radically reduced insides had to be drawn.

Jeff: Weds., May 11: Bad surgery. Leaks in small intestine. Knew things were wrong. Mom called, had been crying. Found many holes in your small intestine. Held your left hand the way I always did. Had to walk out and just started crying. It's so sad. You're so beautiful and young.

The brilliant staff at Bridgeport Hospital were doing all they could to keep me stable and begin to address my multiple medical issues, but despite their best efforts, my condition continued to grow worse, and my vitals kept dropping. Soon it was clear I would have to be transferred to a facility better equipped to deal with patients like me who required longer-term critical care. One advantage of Bridgeport was my father's position there as chief of dermatology, which enabled my family to use his badge to get access to me more easily. But I was slipping away, and we couldn't stay. After considering options, including Yale New Haven Hospital, my dad ultimately chose the state-of-the-art ICU at Columbia in New York City. Now the challenge was to orchestrate my transfer, a delicate move given the constant care and interventions I required.

Interestingly, it turned out that my doctor at Bridgeport, Dr. Garvey, had gone to medical school with the man who would become my new primary physician at Columbia, Dr. Stolar, a connection that both Dr. Garvey and my dad found comforting. In addition to the superior facilities at Columbia, I would benefit from having a complete medical team that included specialists for all my conditions. My body had suffered so much trauma that it was well more than one doctor could manage. Before I left, the entire staff at Bridgeport that had been caring for me came in to say goodbye.

Jeff: It seemed that the entire nursing staff was crowded around your room to wish you well. Truly a sight to behold. This will be my happiest moment: taking you back to Bridgeport Hospital, when you return to perfect health, to meet all the amazing Bridgeport Hospital people who saved your life and absolutely adored you in the process.

Dad: By the time I left, a wall had collapsed on the Henry Hudson Parkway and shut it down. When the wall collapsed, a mudslide ensued and closed the highway. With all the detours, it took me over three hours to get to Columbia. Then it was welcome to the biggest and sickest ICU in the country.

I had always dreamed of moving to New York, but I never thought it would be like this. When we arrived at Columbia, my mom was impressed with the size of the ICU and all the sophisticated equipment, but she also found herself finally beginning to process how sick I truly was as she realized this was where, for now, I belonged. The first sign of her distress was a sudden dislike for food—completely out of character for her.

Mom: When the ambulance rushed you to Columbia, they wheeled you upstairs to the ICU, which reminded me of what a station in space would look like. They told me to leave and get a bite for a while so they could examine you. I went down to the lobby in a bit of a stupor.

I had many new doctors, nurses, and helpers on my team at Columbia. The team leader was Dr. Stolar, whom we quickly came to know as Dr. Doom—the title he actually gave himself. He was a mix of spunk and logic. He had a dry wit and lightning fast sense of humor, but he was never optimistic, always serious and urgent when it came to the job that needed to be done. He soon told my parents, "You are now entering a world that the outside world knew nothing about." He was right. The ICU was a vortex that no one could ever understand unless you were there.

For the first couple of days in Columbia, everything still was touch and go, but my family remained cautiously optimistic and tried to find humor and lightness in what was still a desperately dark situation.

Jeff: You told me you loved me today. And you hugged me. I kissed you goodnight and said to you that I love you the most.

By Sunday, my condition was finally beginning to improve, and family members were able to take a little time off to attend to their own needs, which they'd been ignoring for the past three weeks. Jeff got a haircut and a new shirt—he had only brought one change of clothes for the Passover weekend in Fairfield. And my parents got a little time to themselves. Jeff also got a medical lesson from Dad.

Jeff: When your body goes through this kind of trauma, your kidneys are the first things to go. No urine is an indication that the kidneys are not working. Dangerous and hard to correct. I was talking to Dad about this last night, and he said it was probably your very strong kidneys that kept you alive that terrible first night.

The news on me was finally good.

Jeff: The surgeons told us that the area they operated on looks great. Mom is praying that these sutures hold.

Week four—first signs of progress

Jeff: 1:17 a.m. Today marked three weeks. Yesterday, was your greatest day thus far. They tested you off the ventilator for an hour and you did fine. I came in to see you breathing on your own. I welled up. You were working very hard and breathing quickly. And, you were talking!

CHAPTER 4

Words of My Own

THROUGH MY FAMILY'S MEMORIES I've been able to pull together a somewhat coherent account of the first month after my stomach exploded and I nearly died—time I lay mostly unconscious in first the Bridgeport and then the Columbia ICU. At eighteen, my near-death experience ultimately transported me into the deepest gratitude for life and daily celebration of its blessings. This gratitude wasn't felt once I had to first grapple with these truths of all the bodily trauma I was going through, but there was a sense of calm and rest in my coma, rest that I badly needed.

The ordeal my family was going through, being there 24/7 as I lay in a coma and then woke up to begin my agonizingly slow recovery, continued through the spring of 2005, past May and into June. Long before I awoke, my mother was planting the seeds of gratitude.

Mom: Step by step, we move towards finding God's way of giving you your life back the way it needs to be. Yesterday, I left the hospital for the first time to exercise, take a shower, do some laundry in the apartment, and breathe new life so I could come back refreshed and ready to provide whatever my very unique, beautiful daughter needs from me on this journey. In reality, Amy, you have made the best of all the difficulties life has thrown your way. What an amazing woman! As I was leaving the building, on the elevator was Deepak Chopra, and I thanked him for praying for you. He gave me a big hug and looked deeply into my eyes and told me to list what I had gratitude for before I went to sleep last night. He also told me you would be fine.

I only have vague memories of my coma, as though I was looking up at the sun from under the sea. The fact that my airway was clogged with phlegm probably contributed to this feeling of breathing underwater. My coma dreams were surreal, mismatching times, places, and alternate realities. Dreams and reality faded into each other. I had pleasant dreams of fantastical places, occasionally interrupted with muffled words that were said over my bedside. These dreams had a spiritual quality, and I remember searching for "God" in them, only to be interrupted by the sound of suctioning. My life may have changed, but my search for Him carried on.

I began to experience waking moments, but I preferred to remain asleep. I remember looking forward to my naps a lot because I used to love my dreams when I was on so much medication. They were all dreamy, serene fantasies—with me living in an underwater sea-kingdom, floating around effortlessly. I enjoyed this altered state of consciousness, and I had no idea yet of the realities my altered body faced. Suctioning was a regularly occurring memory—the shrill sound of a pump and the gagging feeling of having a long, licorice-shaped tube plunging into my throat. Everything felt larger than life. I recall the sounds of booming voices over my heads offering me this magic wand that would clear this constant feeling of choking. I really did think it was licorice or a magical device that was alive. Imagine my disappointment when I learned it was just a little piece of plastic tubing.

I always remembered "Twizzlers" going down my throat. And a fish pointing at me and singing, "Under the Sea, Under the Sea! Down here is better, down where it's wetter..."

The Miracles Begin: Beauty at its Best

For weeks, I had been breathing with the help of a ventilator. As my body grew stronger, I was finally able to draw my own air. As I returned to more sustained periods of consciousness, I would soon realize what a blessing being asleep twenty-four hours a day had been—both for my body, seemingly damaged beyond repair, and my mind, which could avoid learning about my condition and processing its impact on my future. I was sleeping through a reality that no one would want to face.

> Mom: First movement of her hand, a squeeze of our hand, and as she woke up, she began to take notice of the changes in her body—tubes everywhere, drains up and down her chest, a bag on her neck.

The World Returns

I have fuzzy memories of awakening from my coma, seeing the world from my back, untangling confusion as I dealt with tubes, bags, and medical appliances stuck to me that I had never heard of before, and grappling with comments that I was "doing much better" now. I was hungry, and at one point I tried to take bites of my brothers because I thought they were fruit. But I still couldn't speak. To communicate, I invented my own sign language, which was mostly just the thumbs up sign and pointing to words on a board my mom made.

> Jeff: We are starting to see you exhibit some signs of the ICU psychosis that the psychologists told us about. Today, you saw fruit and spinach, and the

sea. You tried to bite mom thinking she was fruit. "I don't know which part to bite," as you pulled her head toward your mouth. Best line of the night, though (said very solemnly and declaratory): "I don't want to be scared just to take a little bite out of Adam."

I expected to feel more normal as I woke up, but I found that I was further and further from being a person, and real people felt like aliens to me. I forgot what it felt like to not be connected to any tubes or equipment, to speak, to walk, and especially to eat and drink freely.

Trouble in Paradise

I was still there, but what was left of my digestive system was barely held together with sutures and staples and prone to leaks and tears, which could become life-threatening.

Jeff: The rest of Thurs was pretty terrible because surgeons found some other leaks that Garvey had sutured. I walked into your room after this, and saw mom crying a bit. There is a little tear in your esophagus as well that they are hoping heals. They tried to staple it, but it didn't hold, and, apparently, they don't want to do it again as the esophagus is especially fragile. Scary.

In addition to the problems with my esophagus, my belly was still a giant open wound. The surgeons couldn't stitch me up, due to my body's extreme swelling. As the swelling began to go down, the doctors were able to close first 25%, then 50% of my belly. But I would need to be 100% stitched before I could sit up.

Slowly but surely, the doctors were trying to repair the damage to my body, working with what was left of my digestive system. Sometimes their work was successful, and sometimes it created new problems that needed to be addressed. A surgical procedure going well seemed like a miracle to my family, and any indication of optimism and hope was practically cause for celebration.

> Jeff: You had another surgery today. I've since lost count. Today they wanted to wash you out again and check your esophagus in which they found a slight tear. Hopefully, that tear was responsible for all the phlegmy stuff in your throat that's been making breathing a little more difficult for you. Mom told me that the surgeon did say that one day you would dance at your own wedding.

I came back to life in stages of awareness. The memory stage was particularly painful. The first few days of being alert were very difficult. The more alert I became, the more I remembered of my old life P.C. (*pre-coma*). Things like water—I missed water so *much*—drinking it, touching it. The first time they let me splash water on my face, I cried. It reminded me of washing my face in my old bathroom, in my old body, and I didn't know if it would ever feel the same way again. In the hospital, the highlight of my day was finally being *allowed* to brush my teeth, just for that soothing gargle of ice-cold water that would kill me if I ever dared swallow it. Those basic human needs I couldn't fulfill reminded me of other primal needs I couldn't fulfill, like being outside, feeling the cool air on my skin. It's funny how we take the little things for granted.

> Jeff: Around 4, you would not stop moving, and I kept asking you to go to bed. You kept mouthing to me, "I have so much to say to you." I found your nurse and asked her if she could deflate your trach and put the collar on to let you speak. As soon as she did, you adorably started yelling, "I can talk! I

can talk!" Then you thanked her, told her how nice it was to speak to her, and proceeded to ask her to draw a picture of a horse with "many hooves."

Going to sleep took on an entirely different meaning in the ICU. The lights were constantly on, and lying in bed all day, I was restless, uncomfortable no matter what I did, and lost my sense of day and night. But when the day shift started to do their final rounds of vitals at 6 p.m., I knew that night was approaching, and I anxiously started thinking about how on Earth I would ever get to sleep.

At night, my ICU unit was dead quiet. All you could hear was the occasional sound of a nurse receiving medication from the pharmacy downstairs, which sounded like a vending machine. I remember feeling so paralyzed at night trying to get comfortable in that narrow, still hospital bed in the lonely night. I would stretch my arms as far over my head as I could manage and stuff my shaky hands behind my pillow. Quarantined to a hospital bed all day, I felt so closed in that it was soothing to open up my chest when I could manage to reach my arms over my head, on the rare occasion it didn't disrupt my constantly running IV's. I'd tumble around in bed for hours, eager for day to arrive with some kind of distraction—even an x-ray—anything to take my mind off the impossible quest to find one comfortable resting position, all the while looking out my sliding door to see people, walking back and forth, uncontained by wires. Freedom felt so...surreal.

When I started to come out of my coma and was just very sedated, my memories actually become more surreal. I heard music throughout, especially my beloved Janis Ian, which my mother played ad nauseum. All three of my brothers also played their guitars and serenaded the nurses and staff.

The oldest living Holocaust survivor, Alice Herz Sommer, once spoke of music's role in survival. Indeed, it was ours too.

Mom: She began to cry fearing that she could no longer sing. Her voice was one of the ways she communicated best in her daily life—it came from the deepest part of her soul. As she got stronger, each of her brothers came to her room with their guitar, encouraging her to sing each day as she began to sing the Muppet song, "Rainbow Connection," and each day her voice got a little stronger. She sang for anyone who walked in the room. To all of us who knew how sick she had been, we were watching beauty at its best.

The Comfort of the Berkshires

While I was stuck in the hell of the ICU, unable to eat, drink, talk, or sit up, I found solace in being elsewhere in my mind. I had always been active, and I couldn't believe that I couldn't get out of bed. Matt helped me travel to my beloved Berkshires by talking about my trip there.

Jeff also took me on a virtual camping trip, and we gazed at the moon and stars together.

Saving My Voice

There was a lot of talk about my future. No one really knew what it held. The problem with my esophagus was serious because the tube they had put in to drain it wasn't working. So, I was headed back to the OR for yet another surgery—my eighth. This procedure would reroute my esophagus through my neck.

It turned out the surgery to reroute my esophagus was necessary to save my life. Surgery number eight would take six hours. It was also intensely risky. Not because there was a chance that I wouldn't survive it, but because it would mean working close to the nerves of my vocal cords. My parents were in tears when Dr. Stolar warned them that I could lose my ability to sing or even talk at all if my nerves were damaged. My mom, always the caretaker, tried to reassure the family. "It's okay if she loses her voice in this operation. She'll learn sign language."

In an ironic twist, the voice teacher who abused me had stolen my voice on another level, causing me to remain silent for months about what was happening until my body literally exploded. Now the stakes were raised to a completely different level, and my life was determined with a whole new range of factors. As a teen, I kept a little notebook with me to ensure I'd be on vocal rest, so I'd have a voice by opening night of my performances. I counted the number of words I spoke and tried to emit no sound whatsoever, if possible. Would silence now become a stark reality?

Fortunately, Dr. Stolar had another idea about how to perform the surgery to avoid my vocal nerves. It was music to our ears. When we found out, Jeff described the whole room as brightening in mood and color and that Dad's expression was beautiful. Mom sat at the edge of her chair, waiting to hear Stolar's idea. He said he might be able to reroute the esophagus through my hip (or right above) instead of through the side of my neck as originally proposed. This would avoid the vocal cords altogether. He wouldn't know if it was possible until he was in the OR. If successful, this also meant I would need to have a bag collecting saliva on my body, possibly permanently, but we would cross that bridge if we came to it. How nice it would have been if they could figure out how to reconnect my insides inside of me instead of doing it on the outside.

Things were much easier for me when I was sleeping, and the night before my esophagus surgery, Jeff and I had an ICU sleepover. Nicole, his favorite nurse, said Jeff was actually more agitated than I was. I had been given pentobarbital which put me out for the entire night. Sleep is when the physical body heals. But my full healing wouldn't start until I woke up and could begin to understand all the things that had happened and were continuing to happen to me.

Jeff: Finally, around 8:30, Dr. Stolar, still clad in face mask, walked through the door. Instead of slicing your esophagus, he elected to use just one tube, which meant he didn't have to cut your esophagus, meaning that you could probably use it to reconnect in the future.

Fortunately, Dr. Stolar was able to reroute my esophagus without damaging my vocal nerves. The bag for collecting saliva ended up on my neck. My "esophagostomy" was an amazing idea that allowed me to eventually drink long before I was surgically connected.

Jeff: Good news! Dad got the good waiting room couch tonight! And by good, I mean the one that is not directly under the lights you can't turn off. 2:06 a.m., it is so hard to have any perspective on this yet. This is so huge. It's still so hard to digest the magnitude of what is happening to you and our family. I can't even write about this yet.

One of my earliest memories after waking up from a coma is hearing this guy, May, cry in his deep, kind voice, "Oh, Amy, I'm so sorry;" and feeling this burst of pain, and blood going everywhere. He was trying to put a tracheotomy in my throat and by accident, he shoved one in that was a size too big—a messy disaster. I saw the world at that time as though I were at the bottom of a hole looking up at the light coming down from the sky. Because for a long time, life was just lived on my back, so the only things within my view were the doctors over my head and sometimes I would see people brushing by the curtains, peeking their head in to say hello. I could strain my neck and see the television which was very misplaced. And if I looked to my right all the way, I could see my mom lying in her cot, but I couldn't turn my head that way because I would choke from where the esophagostomy was.

Drains, Lines, and Tubes

As I began to understand my condition, I realized how gravely ill I was. My dad explained to Jeff that my condition was so serious because, usually, people lose either their stomach or their colon, but I lost my stomach and two-thirds of my colon. That's why my body was so devastated. On top of that, my small intestine, which you need to live, was so badly inflamed that they couldn't do anything with it. Hopefully, it would survive, but no one had told us what would happen if that died as well. Thankfully, I was out of it for this part.

Jeff: You have 2 drains draining out your lower abdomen, one on each side. These are sizeable tubes going right through your belly. There are two smaller tubes going into your upper belly. Then you have the esophagus pouch on your neck. Also, you have the colostomy bag on your right hip. You have a red laser tied to a toe on your right foot reading your O² saturation. You have like 9 lines connected to a port which is sutured to your right lower shoulder. This delivers all your meds and nutrition through IV. You have 5-6 square patches all over your upper body which read your heart rate. You have your trach. I think that is all. You had double this just weeks ago.

People think that being in a coma might be frightening, especially coming out of one; facing a world that changed overnight. But on the contrary, there was a sheer fascination and wonder, like I was appreciating life for the first time. There was also a sense of peace, as though I had been saved from a scary situation with Blaine, and a sense of release. I was not depressed. It was almost like I had a new appreciation and fascination with life.

The longer my parents were in the ICU, the more normal life became for them, and then, everything was back to normal. As I started speaking (although incoherently), as usual, my brothers wanted me to "shut up already" and started to lovingly pick on me again. I remember Jeff hiding my "talking piece" because he was tired of me talking. It was those normal sibling fights in the midst of a near-death situation that almost made us laugh—it made life seem bearable, or any bit encouraging that things could go back to normal. It reminded me that my brother still loved me.

I was becoming more alert, but not enough to catch the many medical mishaps made during the involved care I still required. Thankfully, my family never left my side, and only with their careful watch could they catch the small errors that decided between life and death.

Wars with Psychiatry: Who's Really the Crazy One Here?

Besides the teams of doctors attending to my body, we had a team of psychiatrists treating my mind. My family felt these head doctors were the crazy ones and fought their diagnoses and recommendations tooth and nail. The "psychos," as my brothers fondly called them, were not the biggest help to me in the hospital. They insisted on having me repeat the date and time when I had just been in a coma for months. If I wasn't correct, they thought I was delirious. This was clearly aggravating, considering, my parents couldn't even say what date it was anymore. The most frustrating misconception was that because I was not "depressed," I was in denial. My childlikeness made my family laugh and think I was very cute during such a scary time. There was an odd wonder to being a child again.

I did, however, say a lot of "crazy" things. Jeff told me I said things like: "I don't have bread or meat," "keep blanket on land," and "we're in Hollywood!"

In my head, I had just gotten my college acceptance letters. I remember, half-sedated, dialing contacts from my phone—students who were going to be my future classmates at the University of Michigan! This was where I was going in the fall! I had just visited the campus that April break and had gotten to know theatre kids like me, eager to launch a professional performing arts career at one of the most prestigious musical theatre schools in the country.

Jeff: You took two, one-hour naps today, which was new for you. You also made Mom write down a letter that you dictated to her, addressed to Mr. Wagner of Michigan. You were declaring your intention to attend their program.

Some psychiatrists created more commotion than resolutions, but then there were also the silent heroes, compassionate caregivers, family members, and advocates who gave us the most important medicine: smiles, understanding, and hope.

One day my heart rate was elevated, and Jeff sat watching the monitor, trying to will it back down. It was stressful for my family. Food, something we all loved, offered some relief.

Jeff: Your nurse turned your bed around so that you could face the window and peer outside. All of us watched the sunset together. A preview to that camping trip you and I have talked so much about. Tomorrow they say you will sit up in a chair. That is truly exciting.

We could only see the progress of how far I had come when those who had worked so hard to save my life came to see me. Day to day, the minute progress was painfully slow, but in the scope of things at Bridgeport Hospital that first night, I wasn't even supposed to make it at all. Now, we marked my progress by how many appliances could be removed from me, how much I could speak, and how much I could sit up. And as always, progress meant two steps forward and at least one step back.

Unable to fully talk, I craved the ability to communicate the questions, thoughts, and feelings stewing in my bandage-covered body. My mom even tried to create a poster board of words, so I could point to what I wanted to say. When I finally got the tracheotomy taken out, Jeff told me this was the first real milestone in my journey. I thought to myself, *This is going to be a really long journey.*

I could finally start speaking, through a talking piece, and so one part of me that had been stifled—my voice—was back. But I still felt stifled by lack of movement. Each time I got something back, I wanted more. I remember being soothed to bed by Matt playing "Trip to Pooh's Corner." Matt would play it for me every time he came to visit, and although I was discouraged that at first, I couldn't even emit a sound, slowly I got the smallest ounce of voice out. How would I ever be able to belt again? But each day, I was able to sing a bit more, although even taking a breath exhausted me. But what invigorated me was the power of music. We were family unlike any other, with our guitars, and our spirits—that was all we had and all we needed.

Jeff: 1:11 a.m. I am close to screaming. You will not sleep, and you insist on pulling tubes. I am losing it.

CHAPTER 5

My Secret is Out

WHILE I WAS STILL IN A COMA, my family leaked my secret to other people, including doctors. In my sedated trance, it was too late for my disclosed secret to heal me. When I awoke months later, and my ventilator was finally removed, the first words I breathlessly shouted were, "It was him!" However, this radical realization was overshadowed by the surgeon's subsequent disclosure. I had no stomach anymore, I couldn't eat or drink, and he didn't know when or if I'd ever be able to again. They had kept this secret from me as long as they could but decided to tell me when I appeared "healthy enough" to hear it. But I was too afflicted by my secrets to be saved at that point. The "secret" that everyone now knew; one that had made me sick. All that anger, guilt and confusion, I felt in my stomach. And two weeks after I turned eighteen years old, my stomach exploded. Coincidence?

Mom: I wanted to kill him then and there. But she made me remember— the sky is always blue, something she reminded me of often before she got sick. I saw the world lift off her shoulders when she told me. I thought, now she's back! She was finally opening up, and we were going to heal together after this man had wrecked our home.

Some doctors credit my stomach bursting to the top of the operating room to my rapid weight loss. Others say that it was the bursting of a band that had formed around my stomach. Some said it was genetic. But a few insightful officials speculated that a stress ulcer had developed, which then caused a blood clot. The secrets I kept weighed in me like large red bricks. The tension just gathered until my system couldn't take it anymore. Blaine had left large, poisonous seeds in me that were festering because I had not yet dealt with their full ugliness.

I was in a coma, and my mother had to do the dirty work, while my family worried for my life.

Mom: When I eventually die, Amy, the first question I will ask God, is how He could let this happen to such a beautiful person and at such a young age. Hopefully, by then I will already have known some of the answers because you have evolved into the woman you want to be.

A few weeks before my stomach exploded, my mom had told my dad about what happened to me. Then she had told my brothers. Just before I became ill, she had told my pediatrician. While I remained in a coma, my mom told my teachers and the principal at my school about Blaine, and I'm thankful I didn't have to be awake for any of it.

Jeff: Mom is on the phone with your old voice teacher. Mom told him about Blaine. He can't even respond: "Oh, my God, Oh, my God..."

Mom: A friend of ours remembered that when he was auditioning for the part of the Phantom in *Phantom of the Opera* on Broadway, Blaine coached him saying, "You are in love with Christine, and as her mentor, you have the power to get her to do anything. All you have to do is 'gain her trust.'" He is a mastermind, a manipulator, and a predator of mother and child.

Once Blaine traumatized me, I was living life constantly in fear, always running from invisible monsters, ugly secrets, running from myself, a self who had suddenly become so dirty with truths and scariness I was not ready or prepared to handle.

My teachers had attributed my distress to Type A perfectionism or an eating disorder, but when they got my mom's calls, that all changed. I had given my guidance counselor a garbled account while the abuse was happening, but he hadn't put two and two together. Later, he would call my mom in the hospital, devastated. Now my family was beginning to process Blaine's role in triggering my illness. Even Jeff now understood.

Jeff: You will pay for this, Blaine. For the foreseeable future we will be completely focused on Amy. And then, when she is safe and out of danger, my family and our attorneys will spend as much time as we need to send you to jail. You almost killed her. And to think that you sat me down and told me Adam was "raping" her by scribbling notes in her poetry books while you were actually raping her.

Now all of these realizations were hitting my family at once. Was our world to be forever changed now? That small, safe world—Thanksgivings, going from audition to audition, fun little sibling arguments?

If there were two words to describe our family and the life that I had, they were loud and bright. Now the secret overtook our small ICU, and in this small space, each member had space to individually reflect.

Now that I had a voice, and even music in my voice, I was taken back to a song I had written at thirteen, "Circles"—the first song I had ever composed as a wide-eyed, innocent adolescent. I had no idea that these lyrics would prove to be powerful at a time like this, a time when we all seemed to be going around in circles.

We're turning, turning in circles and circles

And turning and turning away
From living our fates
Is that what they try to change?
Something awaits
It's already been arranged
We hide with facades though we search for faith and trust
We have to look inside, where we don't explore much

But with this discovery of the emotional recovery I would have to undertake, at least I was making physical progress. Time was passing, and I was gaining strength.

The Double-Edged Sword of Truth

"It was him." As soon as the trach was inserted into my throat and I was granted the power of speech, these three words spewed from my mouth like paintballs, faster than I could plan for or predict. Trying to recall any events of my past life, which I was slowly trying to untangle from a post-coma blur, allowed my memories to wander to Blaine, and how a trusted relationship had gone terribly awry. I imagined myself like Little Red Riding Hood who strayed from the path because a seemingly-friendly wolf tricked her. Why had I trusted so blindly? And how had I wandered so far down a path that led to such unpredictable destruction? Was I supposed to have lived through this, and if so, why did God make me go through all this crap in the first place? This was a lot of trouble all for a stupid sixty-year-old voice teacher. I prayed that I would eventually get the most glorious prize out of all this, this long-winded journey.

I became numb to the innocent things in life, like the beauty of a flower. I also became numb to physical pleasures. It should feel good to be fondled, kissed, embraced. But it didn't. It couldn't—he was a disgusting sixty-year-old who was supposed to be my mentor. To cope with that, I shut off my sensors to physical pleasure. My life was a gray haze, and it was safe that way because it protected me from the emotional hurt I was feeling. I was grieving the loss of beauty in the world, my teacher, spiritual things. I felt betrayed. The haze protected me from mourning.

How do you deal with all that staying in your body? Your soul is special and delicate. It doesn't like screaming at the top of its lungs in pain. In that stiff hospital bed, I told myself the story of Little Red to come to terms with my wounded self, so betrayed and taken apart. I made up lullabies as I lay there.

Dear Little One,
I know all that you've been through
They cut through your skin and you
Were silent and dazed
Turned from the sun
They prodded and stung so deep
And when they put you to sleep
It's all just a haze
I flow with dusty memories
Safe sensations—cozy and kind
Then I am told the safety I know
Only is survived through my mind

Searching for Blaine

Blaine was the last thing I could remember in my old life that reminded me of the innocence I wanted to rediscover, and his sudden transformation still perplexed me. When my mom handed me a mirror (I couldn't get out of bed to go look in one), I saw that she was right; I still did look beautiful underneath all the scars and wires. I saw the broken innocence still in my eyes. As numb as I tried to be, as strong and robotic as I tried to stay when I caught a glimpse of myself, I ended up staring into the tear-stained eyes of my precious wounded bird. Even in my numb state, I could not overlook who I was now.

I allowed myself to feel that I didn't deserve my innocence to be taken away from me. I gave myself permission to grieve the trivial days of high school. I thought about my teenage handwriting—it was big, bubbly, and full. The dots on my i's were little hearts, my letters were big and round and went over the lines. I would write "teehee" in notes I'd get in trouble for passing to friends in class. I would always get caught because I would start laughing and couldn't get a hold of myself. Even thinking the most serious thought couldn't stop the laughter explosion, to the point where everyone in the class was just like, "Amy, shut up already!" I needed that "trouble" back. I needed a few more slow dances with my school crush, where I got nervous just having his hands on my hips as we would stand nearly two feet apart. Those were the kind of harmless men in my life who were okay to idolize.

In the ICU there was plenty of time for soul searching. What had changed? Had Blaine? Or had I? How had I let myself be abused? And why had Blaine changed himself? Why did it take me so long to tell someone? Why did it take me so long to realize myself? Did I see signs and decidedly not acknowledge them? Had I pushed away help and concern from friend and family who perhaps were more alert? For some reason, with Blaine, I unabashedly surrendered myself to him. How had he worked his way into me? And how had he worked his way into my family?

Now I was remembering flashes of my physics classroom: a crumpled up ball of foil thrown at my shoulder, me feeling tension in my legs and glaring around and all the kids who thought I was a circus freak, adding up numbers in my assignment notebook to keep my mind off the tension growing in my chest like spiders, the urgent need to forget the whole world, and shame. I remembered how my formerly enchanted nature walks were now out-stomped by my pacing feet, turning every lyrical aspect of life into mechanical marching. Trying to act like everything was fine as I lifted thirty-pound weights above my head while I met an old teacher—"How are you doing Amy? Wow, you're strong!" And I would force a smile, which is actually very hard when your face is frozen. It really took more muscles than it did to lift the actual weights. "I'm good. Nice to see you!" and just try not to look like I was sweating to purposely torture myself, which felt a lot better than the shame of sexual assault.

Stages of Recovery

As painful as the secret of abuse was, it was that much easier out in the light. And it was amazing how I was treated differently. My body began to treat me differently too. I felt more liberated than I had ever before, even while hooked up to nutritional IVs twenty-four hours a day. I was gaining strength, and now my life was out in the open. The bad guy was gone. My family cared for me. I was going to be okay. I was back to an innocent child, healing with my mother through arts and crafts. Over crayons and computer paper in my ICU bed, we created a new routine.

Mom and I had a nurturing relationship in the ICU, and I vaguely re-membered her before screaming at me in our Fairfield garage calling me an exercise anorexic after she chased me up a hill with her car. "I don't recog-nize you anymore. Your eyes are hollow," always stuck with me, along with fighting and tension months before, as my anxiety built to a grand climax, with a secret pitting my family members against one another, while we were all secretly grieving some hidden loss in ourselves—the thing Blaine had taken away. All we could feel was the rumbling of the earth that something had changed.

On that last Passover in 2005, I remember feeling that we were finally leading ourselves to freedom just like our ancestors in Exodus. But instead of the Red Sea parting, it closed in on us halfway and sent us tumbling around in the wild waves, and down a black hole into a whole alternate universe, the universe of trauma.

The Central Park Jogger's memoir was the first book my mom read to me while I was lying in bed. I think she felt I needed to hear someone's account of losing everything and building themselves back up because I felt so weak and inhuman, I didn't think it was possible to ever become human. My feet shook every time I tried to stand. How would I be able to get everything back? Would I even be able to exist again in the real world without having to be connected to a monstrous pole? While I grew bitter, angry, and depressed, my mother, the ever-eternal optimist, tried to find the momentous events, the heroic comeback stories, and the courageous heroes of these "inspirational" autobiographies. I was not ready to hear that people could get better. That was someone else's reality, far from my own story.

The Jogger's story was mom's attempt to get me to see some sort of light at the end of the tunnel. With every line, I could hear my mother's voice pleading, "She was in a coma too, and now look at her, she's on top, she's strong, she's running again, and that will be you!" And all I thought was, *are you kidding? I can't even walk, and I'm starving, and no one is sure when I will be let out of here, when I'll stop leaking out of fifty different openings in my body, or when I'll be able to have more than one cherry Lifesaver a day!*

As long as I couldn't eat, I lacked the concentration to focus on reading a book myself, so my mother's inspiration-of-the-day books were my only choice. On the occasion I was allowed to suck on a hard candy, I would savor every bit of sugar I could feel on my tongue and let that sweet taste infuse me with a passing jolt of mental energy, and somehow get my mind to concentrate on a few lines of a book.

My mother didn't give up. After the Jogger, she tried to read me Lance Armstrong's book, because he had also been knocked down to nothing and was now stronger than ever. It was impossible for me to believe I would ever get to that point. Would I really be able to run again? Or just walk without limping? I used to do leaps across my basement to get to the door on the other side, and I just wanted to feel lightness again. Now I was out of breath standing up, and my hands were so shaky from all the medication that I couldn't even string beads together like the occupational therapist was trying to get me to do.

The stories my mother was reading of marathons and joggers were not the level my body (or mind) was ready to accept yet. One day, after my mother had finished an exceptionally heroic chapter in the Jogger's memoir, I asked my occupational therapist as my hand trembled during our beading session, "Do you think I'll ever be able to dance again?"

She excitedly responded, "You'd be amazed at what miracles can happen. I worked with one patient who was pretty bad like you, and when he was discharged, he even walked out of the hospital!"

I didn't ask about dance again. This frustrating uncertainty was something I had to wrestle with on my own. I needed realistic hope.

As I gained more control of my motor skills, I was able to write without a tremor in my fingers. Soon, I started to find expressive ways of feeling through my doodling beyond, "I wanna go home." I made comic strips of my days in the hospital. I cartooned myself hooked up to a potassium pump and drew the faceless swarms of doctors as evil scissors plugging me up with lots of sticky patches, declaring, "Don't move, don't breathe, don't live, and play dead!"

I was somehow accumulating hope to get me from each day to the next, all the while breaking up my thoughts which were not so hopeful. My "healing army" was gaining strength in numbers as I passed day to day in the ICU. Now that my numbers were stabilizing, we were hardly visited at all by doctors. It was a double-edged sword: there was less to be concerned about, yet more cause for boredom and a feeling of purposelessness. After all, as a theatre ham, I thrived on attention. What do you do all day in an ICU, restless, bored, with no CAT scans or men in lab coats to prod you?

You do whatever you can. And now I had watercolors, too. I had music on my iPod, from Matt's guitar, and a raspy sound coming through my own throat. I had my dad reading to me. I had my mom sitting by my side. I had support.

Cartooning these doctors as numbers and scissors were not too far from the truth. I felt more like the machines I was hooked up to than a flesh and blood person, and I started to become as numb to the doctors as they seemed to me. Do you know what you would say in high school if you were sitting alone in a classroom for detention or something and you saw a group of kids huddled around looking in at you and discussing you? *Stop talking about me behind my back!* What makes the rounds with doctors any different? They don't care if you are in a diaper or your legs aren't shaved, or your hair isn't combed or even if you're trying to sleep. It's embarrassing, but it doesn't have to be because if you turn into a machine, you don't have to feel any of that shame or helplessness. And how do you become a machine? Act like one. Go brain dead. Do dead-like things. Stop caring about anyone or anything, including yourself. But numbness is a double-edged sword—you protect yourself by destroying yourself. Still, what other way is there to go?

As much as I was tempted to let my mind wander back into memories of Blaine, of the pain of abuse, of the joy of food, and my pre-coma life, too much thinking, and feeling, was dangerous. Becoming numb was not only how I survived the hospital, but also how I protected what faith I had left, knowing that deep down, a small part of me wished to surface and start believing again.

I grew up thinking an "illness" was either a fever or croup. Illness was a stuffy nose, a sick-day, an excuse to miss a day of school. Now at eighteen years old, "illness" meant waking up from a coma, learning that my stomach exploded, I had no digestive system, and I was to be stabilized with IV nutrition until surgeons could figure out how to put me back together again. Illness meant a life forever out of my control and a body I didn't recognize. Doctors were fighting to keep me alive, but I had no chronic or terminal illness. Suddenly, I was just "ill."

For me, Passover symbolizes a time of exile, redemption, and rebirth. The more I thought about it, the more I looked to the Moses story to guide my shapeless journey in the ICU. I saw my soul as Baby Moses, and I couldn't think of a more appropriate story as the framework for my own catharsis. I left my baby soul by the river, the way Moses' mother sailed him down the river in a basket to protect him. Do you think Moses' mother wanted to lose her son? Of course not, but it was better than death. Miriam, Moses' sister, took the risk of abandoning her precious baby brother, trusting that he would find safety. Like Miriam, I gave away my soul to shield it from the sharp pangs of trauma, leaving it to float down a river, somewhere far off from the hospital and a terrorizing situation. But first, I had to survive. Get through now, form identity later. *Survival trumps meaning.*

Hope is never something that magically appears in a puff of smoke. You have to believe in magic and miracles for them to be present in your life. You have to see those dragons and sorcerers and believe that fairy tales are on-going occurrences to feel that you're living for some higher, noble cause. Hope and faith are grown from our own intuition and our insistence that our intuition is as tangible as the rain. In the hospital, I strained to use my imagination to blend me like a big juicy smoothie into the world where I used to roam free. My imagination helped me connect the soul deeply buried in me to the stories I heard and bring my soul into the light.

In the words of Muhammad: *"Every raindrop that falls is accompanied by an Angel, for even a raindrop is a manifestation of being."*

Just as my family was starting to process my abuse, we were reminded of the day-to-day severity of our environment. I was still in a place where others were fighting for their lives while I was fighting for my voice. Sickness did not discriminate, and in the ICU, everything felt like a crapshoot. Who would live and who would die? What curtains would finally close? When they reopened, what child and shell-shocked family would now be in their place?

Jeff: Vinny's kid died at 4. Matt talked to him, and then the father came to say blood pressure dropping. Died 5 minutes later. Dad walked over to hug brother, sister, Vinny. Then, Vin and wife came over to say bye and told them Gabriella would be an angel for Amy.

By June, I had gained enough strength to even celebrate Jeff's birthday, no cake, of course. I was gaining enough strength to go down to the Child Life Center and give back to the brother who I was starting to remember how much I loved and how much he loved me.

Jeff: I heard plans you might be painting a watercolor picture for my birthday, but with brush in hand, and halfway through what appeared to be a tree, you fell asleep. So instead, you sang me happy b-day.

Reconnecting with the Outside World

Slowly but surely, my numbers were improving. And as I gained strength, I also gained a little bit of freedom. I hadn't been outside or even seen outside in months. My whole world had been confined to the walls of the ICU.

Jeff: Your trach came out today, replaced with one that is capped. If things go okay tonight, it will come out tomorrow. Nurses talking about moving to floor, out of ICU.

Eventually, I didn't need to be plugged into as many machines, so my family started taking me on high-speed rides in my wheelchair, racing through the halls of Columbia Hospital. We'd explore all of the hidden nooks and crannies of every floor. I'm sure we weren't supposed to be in half the places we went, until one day, we found a beautiful spot outside. I remember seeing the sunset for the first time. I felt like a child being born all over again. Even the mundane became glorious—seeing people having lunch outside, the roaring of traffic, birds overhead, the more I wanted to be a part of it.

The hardest thing was not being able to drink. My throat was also especially dry because of my medication to dry secretions in my throat. I basically felt like I was choking all of the time. The thrill of my day or at least a break from the monotony was getting to take a walk outside. We broke all the rules. My brothers would sneak my wheelchair into the garden, and we stayed there for what seemed like hours.

Being chained to an IV is what sustained me for years without food or water. I was on TPN: Total Parenteral Nutrition. TPN could go directly into my veins to sustain me while bypassing my abdominal cavity and my unfed hunger. It was saving my life, but it also meant I was chained to a pole all day, until my chemistry was stable enough that the doctors could start cycling the feeds, meaning they could run it at a faster rate for a shorter amount of time.

How was I supposed to live like that...and for how long?

CHAPTER 6

The Surreal Setting of the ICU

AS DISMAL AS A SURGICAL ICU may seem, the Columbia Pediatric SICU was vibrant, colorful, and oddly cheerful. The curtains were covered in bright, neon animal prints, and I vaguely remember zebra-striped wallpaper. I was fascinated and perplexed by what I couldn't see. I knew there were various plugs and machines behind me, connected to the bed, but I was unable to tilt my head far enough to see that monstrous collection of equipment making the loud puffing noises, the shrill beeping, or the frightening alarms. I only knew what I was told; that I was dependent on these machines for my survival. I was particularly confused by the large vials of green liquid I was connected to, resembling a bubble machine. Were they replacing my blood with this mysterious green potion?

My family made up names for everything. It turned out the whimsical imaginary "friends" from my coma dreams were actually wimpy little medical accessories. "Freddy the Fish," with whom I had swum through igloos and oceans, was just a plastic little stick with a green sponge attached to it. In my dreams, I possessed this magic wand that could quench my thirst, until I learned it was just something my mom would dip in a cup of water to wet my lips. The "Twizzler" I remember dangling in my throat, causing me to gag with a sharp vacuuming noise was "Ralph." It was a name I had come up with myself, along with Freddy, and the name stuck. Now even the nurses referred to the thing as "Ralph." Jeff was officially known as the "Ralpher," armed with this magic suctioning wand whenever I choked, which was frequently.

Jeff: You and I have learned how to make the suctioning as bearable as possible. I hold both of your hands and tell you to close your eyes and take long, slow, deep breaths. You oblige. Then they squirt some water down your trach to make you cough. Then they stick that tube down. Your body convulses a bit because you, temporarily, are unable to breathe, and it is very hard to see.

I was awakening to Jeff's touch, to Matt's voice, to Adam's concern—all three siblings whom I had shut out to keep Blaine in my life. These were the people who really mattered. This was my family.

By the time I started to wake up from my coma, my parents and three brothers had already adjusted to their new normal day-to-day life in the anything-but-normal ICU. I, however, was just getting acquainted with this "alternative universe," not only the place itself, which resembled my idea of the international space station, but also the way I was plugged and tubed and wired into it. My memories of those first few months in intensive care are hazy. I was in and out of consciousness and under heavy sedation. Jeff devotedly stayed by my side, fluctuating between the overprotective brother who almost lost his baby sister and the mischievous pesky brat I had known growing up. This tragedy-induced bonding was the closest we had felt in a long time. Before I got sick, I had lost Jeff's trust with my unintentionally destructive behavior. My numbness and erratic moods both confused and angered him, and my anxiety put an ocean between us. Waking up in the

ICU to Jeff kissing me on the cheek, calling me "Amala," and giving me tender sibling affection, I had turned away was the first medicine I needed. I hadn't known I was so close to death, but even more, I didn't realize how much Jeff really loved me.

My family took over the ICU and made it as normal as possible, made it home with enough of our belongings to have moved in for a year. It wasn't long before they knew which cafeteria had the best salads, which nurses told the funniest jokes, and which psychiatrists to avoid. The ICU had a language all its own and in this alternate universe time and space don't exist, let alone school assignments and news headlines.

Would I have ever been able to believe this as a happy-go-lucky teenager scribbling in my assignment notebooks? Could I ever guess I'd be used to taping a big bag of green discharge to the side of my neuropathied leg any time I wanted to go for a walk? Or that re-inflating a bag taped to my neck would become as routine as going to the bathroom? And forget about going to the bathroom. I didn't know if I would ever be able to go on my own again. I couldn't sit up or stand. I was so overwhelmed with being connected to so many wires that I didn't even realize I was also connected to a catheter. I quickly had to accept that in "this life" I was always attached to something— a pole, a drain, a tube—and I forgot what an unappreciated pleasure it once was to walk freely from place to place. Although I ached to walk around, I hardly had the energy, even if I was able. Lifting my neck left me winded. I was back in diapers, back to being a baby, wide-eyed, innocent, and unable to manage in the real world.

Waking up in the ICU, seeing the ceiling and hearing the beeping of IV pumps, I thought I had lost everything.

At the very beginning, I used to be so frightened of my stoma and ostomy bag. It seemed like this big alien head bulging out of my stomach, and all of the sutures made me feel like Frankenstein. Within a few months, I seemed to handle any kind of grossness without thought. Having intestinal fluid leaking all over me felt as normal as washing my hands. I crossed a certain threshold of tolerance where inner and outer body fluid was all the same to me. I wanted my childhood fear of pain back, even those raw, authentic fearful feelings that came from horror movies or haunted houses.

In the hospital, as these monstrous tubes invaded my body and leaks were spurting mysteriously everywhere like toxic geysers, I could barely understand my lonely medical entanglement. I wracked my brain to search for any warm, familiar connection to myself that would make me feel safe. I was so hungry for any emotions that sometimes I would even think about Blaine to feel a familiar comfort. It made me feel less alone, and it made me feel. I would take anything to pretend I was a person in that bed, rather than a frail piece of machinery with a tracheotomy sticking out of my throat. Feeling any type of emotion reminded me of myself, my pre-coma self. I needed her here to keep me company in that lonely ICU. But with no nourishment or freedom, there were no recognizable signs left of the Amy I knew.

As I became more and more alert, I slowly rediscovered the world I had been away from for so long. As my family sat by my bedside, I noticed things about their demeanor and our dynamics I had never taken the time to see before. I realized that these quiet, intimate moments could speak volumes. Being snatched from the hustle and bustle of everyday life provided an opportunity to connect more deeply with my loved ones. We had been given the precious gifts of quiet time; no distractions. Things I hadn't noticed before—my mother's smile, a friend's laughter, the love and support all around me—now evoked feelings of profound gratitude.

The familial support was a powerful antidote to my medical circumstances. As uncomfortable as I was, seeing my family members constantly by my bedside felt like much-needed protection like I'd escaped the nightmare with my abuser. From what I could strain my neck to see from my bed, my family had moved in. There were my mom's magazines, my brother's guitars, my father's audiotapes, and enough fluffy throw pillows to fill three HomeGoods stores. There was a hominess and a strange peacefulness to our new setup. My brothers, now the SICU troubadours, would pass the days strumming their guitars every day and make up songs about every nurse on the unit. We were forced to slow and scale down, to be honest with each other, and with ourselves. We were now healing together. After harboring secrets from my family, I felt safe, protected, and understood.

I started to feel myself materialize back into the girl I knew before my coma. This time, however, I was equipped with a deeper wisdom and a renewed desire to discover the world. "Minute to minute" had turned into "day to day" and now we were living "days to days." I could go stretches at a time without having a crisis or emergency procedure. Sometimes, I could even go a full day without doctors examining me, and eventually, four chest pressers went down to two, five IVs went down to three, and with less machines plugged into me, I was able to enjoy my first breath of fresh air in months.

The more alert I became, the more I realized how much there was to be grateful for. Things like water—drinking it or even just touching it. The first time the doctors gave me permission to splash water on my face from a hospital basin, I cried, "I miss my sink!"

Wheelchair rides took the manpower of my entire family and were no easy task. My drains and wires had to be untangled, unplugged, rewired, rethreaded, and re-snapped into place. Two oxygen tanks had to be attached to the back, and an oxygen mask and one family member (the "caboose") had to be in charge of wheeling the connected IV pole behind my chair. Just getting from my bed to the chair was an ordeal in itself, but that didn't stop us from exploring any square foot we could sneak into.

The grounds outside of Columbia were lush, green, and majestically landscaped. Parched and delirious with thirst, my eye would always go straight to the sprinklers on the majestic surrounding lawns, or the staff watering nearby plants. *Water!* I'd stretch my lips out and exaggeratedly mouth to them, as I talked my family into pushing my chair and IV pole outside. All I wanted to do was run in the sprinklers, and when they let me push my pole towards those fountains of luscious, wet, goodness, I would get my hospital gown absolutely soaked. The first time I re-experienced rain, I was outside on the stairs of the lobby, and I felt the raindrops start tapping me drop by drop. Was this God speaking to me, whispering in every pure, cleansing drop? It had been so long. But then Jeff made me go back in because he said it wasn't a good idea to get the TPN pole so wet. When you are part-machinery, you can't run around in the rain like a real human being.

Once I was lying in bed on a super-hot day, depressed, and helplessly watching TV. A Taco Bell commercial came on for a spicy "limited edition" burrito. To show just how hot and spicy it was the actor took a bite and then reached for a gigantic aquarium overflowing with water. He proceeded to pour it over his head and tried to drink in the gallons of water that were pouring down on him. I couldn't look away from the screen.

My only dim glimmer of hope was, "One day, you'll be able to drink." I fantasized about an entire buffet table set up for me, decked out with every drink I could imagine of any flavor that ever existed: ginger ale, Kool-Aid, fruit punch, seltzer. And me just going back in line over and over again all day, drinking and drinking, throwing cups up into the air like dollar bills, and the liquid, fizzy happiness would never end.

In the meantime, dry, ICU time crawled by. When all you can do is lie there, and your day isn't broken up with meals, you can go crazy from boredom. I would eagerly look forward to "field trips," like when they took me downstairs for a CAT scan. At least I got to go somewhere and break up the monotony of the 9th floor ICU. I even started to like the clowns that came in and played the ukulele. Any distraction to divert my mind from the agony of feeling thirst was a welcome one however irritating the clowns were for a frustrated eighteen-year-old.

The Joy of Disconnection

Because the nurses had left me turned on my right side for months, all of the nerves of my right leg became compressed, giving me severe neuropathy. I had no working muscle to even stand on it. Eventually, I managed to walk on it with a severe limp. I worked tirelessly to regain my strength and spent the endless non-eating hours by going from one exercise to the next.

Every day I did little things: flexing my toes in bed, rotating my wrists. Soon enough, the physical therapist was giving me Thera-Bands (stretchable exercise bands), and before I knew it, I was able to stand for more than a minute at a time without falling into exhaustion. One morning I was finally able to stand in place on my own as my nurses changed my sheets. I beamed with pride like I had crossed the finish line for the New York Marathon. Small victories like these were frustrating. I tried to not let myself think about what I was able to do just months before. I had to start all over again, relearning muscle memory, which, with open wounds and leaking parts, was not quite as simple as learning to ride a bike again. Feeling the freedom in my arms, I felt that I could deviate a bit to the side and not have to instruct Dad to move along with me, though I think he still needed to hold my hand because I couldn't walk entirely steadily and stable yet.

I tested myself standing for seconds longer. Soon I could stand without bracing myself on my bed rail and could move one foot just a step in front of the other.

One day, I took two steps. Then a third. I could walk!

The first thing I sang when they unhooked me from TPN for the first time in the Columbia ICU for just an hour or so was "I Got No Strings" from *Pinocchio*. I stumbled from pole to pole exhilarated from being able to zigzag back and forth down the hallways, proudly exclaiming "I own this hospital!" I relished the new feeling of freedom in my arms, proud that I could deviate a bit to the side and not have to instruct Dad to move along with me, though I think he still needed to hold my hand because I couldn't walk entirely steadily yet.

Dad: The first time you got out of bed. You rose on wobbly legs like a deer getting up for the first time, and I walked you to a pole and back. We were amazed, and I took you down the hall and then back to bed. After that, you would go for a walk each day, sometimes multiple times a day.

Soon enough I was the "runaway patient" constantly pacing the ICU. My family trailed behind me as Dad took me for my five laps a day around the unit in my giant Ugg boots, serenading every patient in their cubicle as we passed them. When Adam got a hold of a few extra cups from the nurses' station, we even set them up like bowling pins in the aisle of the unit. As unconventional as we were, we managed to make some acutely ill patients and their grief-stricken parents laugh. Sometimes humor was the most practical medicine. And leave it to Jeff to start dating my night nurse. Now, I knew things were getting back to normal.

I created a schedule for myself—walk a lap, do a Thera-Band exercise, which winded me enough to collapse back into bed, close my eyes for a good twenty minutes, and get right back up again, passing yet another unnumbered day. I created intricate choreography. Even the simplest of motion left me winded. But I was determined to repeat my exercises every day, even if my eyes were half-closed, to finally get my strength back. When I was hardly able to sit up, I created exercises raising the band over my head, sticking my feet in loops I'd made, attaching the bands to my bedpost and pulling with all of my might, like a baby playing with their cradle mobile. It was still confusing to me that months before I had been lifting twenty-five-pound weights and now I could hardly stretch a flimsy yellow band or reach behind my head. I could feel every muscle straining with each minuscule gesture.

My day consisted of going back and forth from one miserable thing to the other, and the only way I could get through was thinking, "Doing this is miserable, but at least I'll feel better once this thing is over." Each day was an endless cycle of pushing myself in and out of bed, feeling tired and empty, with nothing to count on to rescue me out of this, with no sign that anything would change. I was guided by the sole mantra: "Just get through. Don't Think. Get Through."

Eventually, I started to get my old spunk back, which made the doctors happy, and not so happy. I was restless, antsy, and feeling like a prisoner. My parents slept in the ICU every night with me, so they were feeling cooped up too. We had to get out. We decided one day to make a break for it and go shopping. It was 3:35 p.m. on a Tuesday. The doctors had rounded, the nurses were filling their meds. The coast was finally clear to make our escape. Dad kept a lookout while Mom and I headed towards the service elevators, down to the lobby, out the back entrance, onto 166th and Broadway. And we were free! I felt like I had broken loose, into the "real world," but now I was filled with envy as I watched people who came and went freely, by choice, their bodies running on natural fuel, filling them with the vitality of living.

Still, I was having a great time, finally free of my IV pole for an hour, dancing in the middle of the street. I was thrilled to walk on actual pavement, to hear the beeping of taxi cabs, and to breathe in the city smog. My mother bought me a cow-printed purse from a street vendor. I felt so proud to be carrying a purse, even with nothing if was in it, wearing a purse, rather than an IV pole. I felt almost like a real person. With my beautiful new purse, I didn't understand why everyone was staring at me until my mother reminded me that I was still in my hospital gown. I didn't care! I raced down the street, turned the corner, and found myself face to face with Gila, the social worker. Someone must have tipped her off. We were escorted back. Busted. When my parents finally settled me back into bed, (with their heads hung low in embarrassment) and the nurses had cleaned up all of my bandages, Dr. Stolar came in, leaned over and whispered in my ear, "I would've done the same thing."

I eventually learned from doctors that I would be in the ICU for an indefinite amount of time. I could hear these words, but my "self" was still frozen as a high school student. The first thing I asked, in the most endearingly clueless way was, "What about college?" And then I remember the terribly sobering day that a doctor finally told me that a sip of water or a bite of pizza would be suicide. Suddenly, my childhood dreams of one day finding God shattered. Now, it seemed as though there was no God or anyone to protect me anymore. I felt betrayed, as though the promises made to me as a child were all lies and that fervently rubbing my fingers together day after day for eighteen years was all for nothing.

As a child, I was told to give all of my troubles to God. So, every night in the hospital, I would pray to God. I would pray that he still existed for me. I would pray that he would let me at least drink a sip of water "next week." And I prayed for "next week" every day for three years. If I did not keep God and my Jewish faith alive throughout all of the uncertainty, I felt like a part of me would be lost forever. I thought of myself as a museum, trying to preserve my soul. It was my job, mission, no matter what.

CHAPTER 7

Losing Your Faith

LOSING YOUR FAITH IS A SCARY thing especially in the midst of dangerous uncertainty because you don't have anything substantial to stand on. Here I was, a teenager, completely displaced out of the life I felt belonged to me, suddenly a medical marionette with a new body, woken to a different reality that I could never have anticipated. I refused to rub my fingers together, as I had done as a child. I wasn't sure what it was for anymore. Most importantly, I wanted to know the simple luxury of taking a sip of water again. But I could only hope.

That hope is what allowed me to move on. I did not drink two weeks later. Or a month later.

"Jeff, I wanna walk," I croaked.

"Again?" he asked ever so patiently. "We just hooked everything back up..."

And walk I did. However painful it was to get in and out of my surgical hospital bed, taking walks was the only way I could seem to make time pass, without feeling like time was passing me by. My father would carefully unplug the dozens of medical apparatuses from the wall, which took almost a half hour, carefully help me out of bed, watching to make sure I didn't step on any drains as I winced from the pain that came from standing upright with sutures pulling all over my body. In my clunky boots, we'd try to smile at the nurses, who cheered us on with "There she goes again! Our unit marathon runner!"

It was near impossible to keep generating the strength (physical and mental) to get back up when constantly knocked down, with no set endpoint in mind. But the scarier idea was just lying there. My biggest fear was that at eighteen, I was to live the rest of my life in bed, as a patient, a has-been, weak, forgotten, and never to make that mark on the world that I had dreamed of just months before in that "other" life.

The only marking of time and sign of hope were the small triumphs— being able to sit upright in a chair for the first time and my vital signs getting a little bit better. After months of not being able to talk, they finally took me off the ventilator. But within an hour, I talked so much that I used up all of my oxygen, so they had to put me right back on. Patience was impossible but our only choice. No promises could be made about even the most immediate of futures. I would always ask doctors as they came in, as a ritual, just to hear myself say it, "When can I start drinking?" Every time, I would be met with the same, long and apologetic sigh, "We can't say yet." Until numbers told them otherwise, no doctor could give me the answer I needed to hear.

Outside, there was a small garden on the hospital grounds, Olivia's Garden, with twisting paths my brothers would walk me down as I pushed my pole along. Some kids used their IV poles as scooters, pushing off the concrete to glide effortlessly down the wheelchair ramps. I told myself that even if this meant the rest of my life would be confined to hospitals as a surgically incomplete patient, dependent on machinery to survive, at least I had a good childhood and happy memories that no one could ever take away from me.

But the more time passed, the harder it became to remember that old world which I wanted back so desperately. Through the gates surrounding Olivia's Garden, I would see the awnings of corner stores, of streetlights, of

Starbucks. Even the golden arches of McDonald's looked tempting, if deadly. What would it be like to walk into a store unattached to anything, to sway my arms back and forth without anticipating the screeching sirens that would go off with the slightest twist in direction? I could not recall the unburdened feeling of being able to go wherever I wanted, unconcerned with how long I was unplugged for before my battery ran out.

As life became less "minute to minute," even my parents felt more comfortable leaving our ICU "nest" and venturing out into the real world. When my parents left, one of my brothers was always keeping me company. Once my mom started going out, she grew to love the surrounding streets, or "her Columbia hood" as she called it. She knew where to get her hair done and score the best chicken salad and even found a spinning studio where she could let off some endorphins. Determined to find any kind of distraction to bring to me upon her return she'd buy children's crafts kits, books, and games so I would have something to do. Her feeling of helplessness often materialized in piles of toys stacked in each corner of our increasingly cluttered cubicle, much to the nurses' chagrin as they inched their way to me hourly for vitals.

One of her more misguided shopping trips and while I was still in and out of sedation, I demanded to my mother over and over, "bring beans!" It sounded like I was saying beads, so my mother proceeded to go to every store down 166th street and buy every packet of beads she could, in every color, shape, and size. Exhausted, my mom came back hours later with two enormous shopping bags filled with beads and costume jewelry for me to break apart and string. I blankly looked at the bags, and said, "Now cook 'em."

As my health started to stabilize, my dad could start going back to work. Not even for a second would he consider not coming to be with me daily. Instead, he would come to New York straight from his private practice in

Connecticut, stay overnight with us to check on the night staff, and head back to his office in Connecticut at 5 a.m. the next morning. When my dad started to go back to work during the day, my mother and I struggled to both pass the time and find closure after the chaotic months that had threatened to tear us apart before this.

My mom sat beside me as I helplessly stretched myself across that stiff bed, pressing every button on the remote control to try to adjust the stiff frame to sit up higher or make the feet go lower, experimenting with what positions would most effectively alleviate the discomfort I constantly felt. It was impossible to find any comfort from such a clumsy piece of furniture. The remote was covered with random buttons controlling the bed, the light switch, and the TV, which never went to the channel you wanted. Frustrated with the clumsy remote's lack of cooperation, my mother and I would always press the nurse or emergency button by accident, which didn't do any good because they never came when you wanted them to. With no good TV channels, I was subjected to hours and hours of my mom's *Everybody Loves Raymond* DVDs. By the time we were discharged from the ICU, she had watched every season at least once.

There were a variety of ways my mother and I tried to pass the endless expanse of day shifts. In pre-hospital life we had purchased every kind of crayon and artistic self-help book we could back then, and our days were spent either at the beach or coloring together at Barnes & Noble bookstore. Then, I colored with secrets I couldn't get out. Now, I colored with longings I couldn't fulfill.

With no more secrets of abuse, I was truly a kid, filled with the innocence that comes from a new start. I had woken up from living life as a total blur. Not only did I have no idea what had been going on since I was in a coma, but I also didn't even remember what the hell was going on in the months leading up to it. Maybe this was my chance to escape (or try to erase) trauma. Whatever it was though, I felt I had been rescued.

Mom took a makeup kit out of her purse so I could see my reflection for the first time in that tiny mirror. My lips looked very pink. "You've gotten your beauty rest," she told me. "You look more beautiful than you have in a year." It was true. There was a peaceful, almost angelic quality to my face. The worry lines had had relaxed and retreated. No pre-coma anxiety mattered now. Blaine had caused an intense amount of stress that not only showed up in my body, but my face, my voice, and the world around me. Now, life and death was a more pressing matter, and in a way, it felt healing to only be worried about things of true importance. Maybe my agonizing memories of Blaine had all dried up in the wake of the coma. Without realizing, my world had become filled with colorfully illustrated scenes from children's books that lined the hospital hallways on the way to radiology procedures and enchanted wheelchair rides under the sunset.

When I was watercoloring with my trembling hands, I wrote "I want to go home" over and over on a single sheet of paper, feeling like a child writing from summer camp. I missed my dog, and I missed my room, where Dad said the light was still on for when I got back. Of course, I never did go back.

Growing up as the only girl with three much older brothers, I sensed there were adult secrets that were kept from me. My family also believed in the power of denial: if we didn't talk about something, it was as if it didn't happen. Perhaps that's why when I had my own terrible secret—that my mentor had abused me—I kept it to myself. The sicker I got, the stranger things got between my mother and me; she knew something was wrong but couldn't get the truth out of me. When I finally did tell her about Blaine, we were still concealing it from the rest of the family, enmeshing us in an unhealthy way. Now I was free to be honest, and my mother could focus her full nurturing power on helping me heal. As we colored, crafted, and played games to pass the endless hours in the hospital, we grew closer and closer, sharing our hopes, dreams, fears, and frustrations with each other.

But no amount of distraction could take my mind off food. I was envious of the stale trail mix I knew my mom was hiding in her purse. But what I really wanted was her human freedom. Every moment she would simply get up from her chair was a deeper reminder of the prison I was in.

When I was wheeled outside with my IV pole, I longed to be free like the visitors casually strolling beyond the hospital gate sipping from their water bottles. I'll never forget how a foresty green glass Pellegrino bottle sparkled in the sunlight. How had I ever taken a simple glass bottle for granted before?

I saw children skip along, fall down and pick themselves back up with such innocent, bubbly ease, and I wondered if I would ever feel that lightness in my feet again. I knew this would be a long road and didn't know how I would ever start, or if I *could* ever start again. At this point, there wasn't even a road to be intimidated by. I was just stalled, waiting for something to give.

Graduating High School in the Hospital

On the outside, I was an ICU patient trapped in the hospital. But on the inside, I was a stir-crazy teenager, a teenager who was supposed to be enjoying her last summer before college. My friends had all graduated, and I wondered what their commencement ceremony was like. They were all getting ready to go off to their first year of college, and I, who had applied to seventeen schools and gotten into my top choices, was eons away from being ready for college, much less any semblance of independent living. Life was moving on, and I felt forgotten by my school, my friends, and my life. I was still unable to mark times with meals or any kind of nourishment. To say I was "surprised" when my headmaster surprised me at the hospital with my own private ceremony right in the middle of the ICU—cap, gown, diploma, everything—was a massive understatement.

When I was in a coma, my mom was looking through my scrapbook and found a fan note I wrote to Broadway composer William Finn who actually called me back. I was so thrilled to get a phone call from my musical theatre hero, that I took a picture of my caller ID and glued it into my scrapbook. Flipping through more pages, my mother found the picture, called his number and told him what had happened to me. Besides writing wonderful music, William Finn had also dealt with medical battles of his own, almost losing his own life in a coma when doctors unexpectedly discovered a tumor in his brain. After his complete recovery, aided by the healing power of "Heart and Music" (also the title of one of his songs), he was inspired to write his off-Broadway musical, *A New Brain*.

My mother is usually the one with the far-fetched and bordering-on-impractical ideas for healing. She had already brought in a Reiki specialist, a psychic, a ballet teacher, a rabbi, Bernie Siegel, a dance therapist, aromatherapist—anyone who might possibly find answers that doctors wouldn't necessarily. My mom has always been a persistent researcher. She always reminds us that she got her master's in history and spent her entire graduate school career in the research archives of the New York Public Library. When everyone else wanted to give up, my mom did research that felt pretty whimsical and almost silly. But, in a realm where no one had *any* immediate cure, these wild, far-fetched ideas were the most effective medicine to nurture my spirit. With hope, the biggest miracle is possible: being able to persevere from one day to the next in the midst of uncertainty.

Suddenly, the curtains were pulled open, and I was, receiving my high school diploma in the middle of the ICU. In attendance were my parents, my six best friends, *and* William Finn, my personal commencement speaker, the same mentor who I had adored as a fifteen-year-old musical theatre geek. I was shocked and started crying hysterically. It was the first time I cried since the doctors told me I had lost my stomach, but this was a different kind of overwhelming emotion. This was a feeling of connection I had not yet felt in this post-coma life, and it flooded me with forgotten life and bittersweet memories. The last person to emerge from the curtain, much like the Wizard of Oz, was my headmaster. Now, I had a whole entourage following me as I walked down the aisles of the ICU and downstairs to the main lobby to have my ceremony.

With William Finn there, I couldn't have cared less about my high school graduation. This was my musical theatre kid dream! Tony-Award winning Mr. Finn was chatting with my brothers and my nurses! I was so excited and really wanted to impress him, so I tried to start tap dancing. Having just learned to walk again, this was probably not the smartest move. In the middle of my routine, I clumsily stepped on one of my wound-drains that was suctioning bile from my intestines and ripped it out, causing a "minor" interruption to my graduation festivities. The ceremony was put on hold while my nurse frantically paged Dr. Stolar, who proceeded to come in and perform some emergency stitching, asking me, "Don't you ever sit still?"

My mom had also invited all of her college, neighborhood, and gym friends to attend. As we walked outside to Olivia's Garden for the "official ceremony," my entourage had grown to nearly thirty people! Jeff had mysteriously and very uncharacteristically disappeared for most of the day. Now he proudly appeared holding a large rolled-up scroll of butcher paper behind his back. It turned out he had spent the day in the Child Life Center making arts and crafts with all of the hospital kids. Now he revealed the "masterpiece" he worked on there with one of my nurses: a huge banner in my honor that read, in lopsided, colorful painted capital letters: HAPPY GRADUATION AMY!

After the ceremony, I eagerly took my friends back through Olivia's Garden to show them my "hood" and my usual ICU route I'd walk five times a day with my father. Imagine seven teen girls, one IV pole, and three guys on guitars all doing the Macarena dance, singing along and jumping around under starlight in the Columbia Hospital garden. My high school senior year dance, at last! Life finally felt as if it might move forward, even if my IV pole was coming along with me into my new, uncertain future.

Back to Surreality

As quickly as my friends had entered the realm of the ICU on graduation day, they had vanished. My dad drove them back to Connecticut, and I was stuck in my hospital room, due for another round of the usual vitals. As I bit my lip for the poking and prodding, I imagined my beloved friends going back to their bedrooms, washing up for bed, perhaps getting up, unchained by wires, for a satisfying midnight snack, then rising with the next, life-filled day, going through a human routine, interacting with and actually *affecting* the living, breathing world.

As constant as the monotonous ICU days were, my family always tried to drum up some excitement. As the "regulars" in the ICU, the Floor Nine staff was used to the Oestreicher antics, but they did their best to make our stay as "life-like" as they could, recognizing my burgeoning energy that seemed to triple by the day. The doctors would often coordinate their "rounding" schedules to ensure I had my five walks a day (I was their only patient who could get out of bed, let alone maintain a "daily agenda"), and sometimes I'd talk them into just giving me a quick check-in as they accompanied me for a stroll outside, so I didn't even have to be on the unit.

During walks with my dad, he and I finally had the bonding time that a year of running from the terrifying memories of abuse had stolen from us. My idolization of Blaine had caused me to push my father away, especially when I sensed my father's (accurate) distrust of him. Combine that with your typical teenage girl moodiness, and you had a strained pre-coma relationship. Now, with both us of starting from the ground up, we managed to laugh, talk about favorite family moments, color or sing songs. This was a new love, appreciation, and admiration I hadn't yet felt, something that had to be built. Learned. It was a safe, protected trust. During our walks, occasionally I could fool myself into thinking, as I felt my hand in his, "Maybe this isn't so bad."

As burdened as my father was with handling my entire medical situation, checking on my meds, and discussing every little detail with the attending staff, he still put on a smile with me, made conscious efforts to laugh, distract me, talk about current events, and even save me Michael Riedel's *NY Post* Theatre Column every Wednesday and Friday, which he used to do for me when I was a kid so we could laugh at the snarky headlines together. My father didn't seem to sleep, and I was worried about how naturally and eagerly he seemed to handle everything at once. He was our rock for reassurance, and also the only one who could translate the data the doctors would spit out every morning at 6:30 a.m. Without his careful attention, I would have died.

Eventually, I got to a point where I was physically healthy and okay, I just couldn't be reconstructed to eat yet. Not only was I not "healthy enough" yet, but doctors hadn't figured out exactly how to make that happen. The doctors seemed to expect me to just be happy that I was alive. I, on the other hand, wanted a timetable for how long it would take to get my real life back again.

People kept telling me that I would be surgically reconnected at some point, that I would eventually eat and drink. My question was, "When?"

One night, the unit was dead quiet, so quiet I could hear a light rain start to tap on my window. The rain quickly gained momentum, and soon it seemed to be a downpour from what I could hear over beeping medical machinery. I was thankful for some kind of sound—anything but that awful silence. For the first time since I had come to, I felt at peace and sleepy. I still couldn't fall asleep, but I knew what I could do. I could talk to God. Nervous to bring this idea of childlike faith back into my life, I softly held my fingertips together, and I started to shift them back and forth. It felt odd to feel my fingertips again after so much had happened. They felt wrinkly, thin, and dry. Not like the baby-soft, stubby fingers I remembered. I took a breath as deeply as I could from my groggy, mucus-filled lungs and strained my neck to look up at the ceiling as far as I could.

Please, God, grant me a miracle and let me be back in Fairfield eating and drinking again sooner than the doctors think, like maybe even in two weeks or so. Please God, give me a miracle.

I did not drink two weeks later. But a miracle did happen when I started to pray. I fell asleep. And in my sleep, I found God. I didn't see Him, as I always thought I would as that old man watching over me in an oak tree. I found something far greater. I found my faith. And once I found faith again, I saw God everywhere. He was the one giving me the strength to hold on and the hope that things would get better.

Most miraculously, I had the realization that God was in my dreams all along, and even better, with me day and night, everywhere and anywhere. Once I could dream, I had a spark to last me through from day to day. Dreams, hope, and faith filled my soul with a warmth I needed to sustain myself. This was a medicine that gave me much more vitality than any antibiotics and relieved any agony better than any pain patch from the dreaded pain team. This replaced the feelings that I looked to in my memories with Blaine. I had me, and that was the best memory of all.

But even with gradual improvements, no surgeon could give me an answer, a deadline, or a guarantee, which is all that I wanted. I was stable (essentially not dying), but by no means ready to be operated on, or in any shape to even talk about surgical reconstruction. My family and I were simply playing the waiting game at this point. Not sick, not infected, no sepsis, no fever—just no digestive system, and a gaping open wound down my entire abdomen. I still walked around with a fear that my guts might spill open any minute, but I was getting used to the idea of my insides being on my outside. Life wasn't a new "normal," but at least I was easing into what was now a new reality, whether I wanted it to be or not.

Still no progress felt like progress as long as I was denied water. I had my mom fill large basins with cool water from the sink, so I could just dip my nose into it and pretend like I was swimming. After reassuring my mom that I wouldn't try to swallow any of it, I'd dunk my face in the water, letting the fragile, liquidy surface stroke my nose, my cheeks and my forehead in the water, blowing bubbles, and feeling my eyelids splash the wetness. This could entertain me for a good hour.

I was told by my doctors that "water was lethal" but "lollipops were okay." However puzzling this was, I took what I could get. I would get so excited when we would take wheelchair rides around the hospital and the time of day would come when I would be allowed to have one lollipop or sucking candy. I was told to be cautious with that because even a bit too much saliva could contribute to the yellow drainage that came out of the big orange tube in my left side, clumsily stitched in with big ugly black sutures that scared me because these stitches resembled big daddy long legs. I glanced at my reflection as I passed the service elevators and cringed at my mustard-yellow face, huge half-circles under my eyes, and that strange plastic bag hanging off of my neck like a puppy dog's ear that would choke me sometimes when the plastic adhered to my throat. Then I would have to open the cap at the end of the bag and let in some air so it would puff up like a balloon which finally allowed me to breathe. Lollipops, unfortunately, dried up my throat even more. With no water to clear out my airways, the secretions in my throat thickened enough to send me into a choking fit.

I hated candy, but I'd look forward to that one lollipop I could have like it was caviar. I didn't have an extensive range of options. I tried everything—lemon glycerin swabs over my bleeding lips, gargling some water in my mouth and spitting it out, sucking on empty water bottles. It was the most amazing feeling to be able to hold some of that cold water in my mouth for even just a second and feel it shooting back into the cup through my lips like a sperm whale blowing a stream of water through its spout. A worker at Child Life told me that all the kids who can't eat end up playing mostly in the toy kitchen because that is where they can't help but focus their attention on it. I was the same way—fantasizing about what certain foods would taste like, reading cooking magazines, watching the food channel from my bed. I would call out through the curtains of the ICU when I'd see a nurse drinking and make her come in my room and drink it so I could watch her. I loved seeing someone hold a clear plastic water bottle in their hands and tilt it over their mouth as they chugged it down so carefree. I envied how they didn't even seem to notice the casual tilt of a cup towards their lips. What's a sip here or there? *To me, everything.*

In the middle of one night I tried to get out of my bed, which was an impossible task considering I was hooked up from every side, and crawl into Mom's hospital recliner, which she positioned next to me, just to feel like times as a child when I would run into her bed in the middle of the night. Attached to three wires and two poles, I somehow made my way to her with no blaring alarm being set off.

My mom and I silently held each other in the dark room, experiencing how these months in the ICU had shaped us both, and nervously expecting the machines to start beeping because I had occluded the line, wishing for those old moments of freedom and lightness that we never used to think twice about.

CHAPTER 8

Moving Out of Columbia

AFTER MANY MONTHS, Columbia was now home, and the staff was family—except the night nurse who now officially was no longer dating my brother. I was once the sickest patient; the one doctors were worried wouldn't make it to the next day. Now, I had more sass than Gloria, the head nurse who would join in on my duets with Matt. I was barely in my room anymore and frequently seen gossiping at the nurses' station, and after my mother had tried every salon on the surrounding streets, the doctors decided to transfer us back to Bridgeport Hospital. Whether they liked it or not this time, I could talk back.

> Dad: In Columbia, when you got antsy enough and disappeared for most of the day, that's when they decided to transfer us back to Bridgeport. They were very happy to get rid of us. I think going shopping on Broadway was the last straw. We went back to Bridgeport where they were happy to let me do all the bandage changes.

The day we had to be transported from Columbia to Bridgeport, Jeff jokingly put a garbage bag over his head and asked the nurses if we really had to leave because, in a twisted way, the staff had become our family, the hospital our home. We had even written a song about Josephine the PA. My dad bought chocolates for the nurses every week on his way from work, and Jeff had become the floor's eligible bachelor. I was the five-walks-a-day patient with her trademark yellow Ugg boots. We had already adjusted and made a new home there. If we couldn't stay in this new world, where would we go?

Wherever we went, the Oestreichers were vocal, spunky, and made our presence known—whether it was a Disney family vacation, Thanksgiving dinner, or the Columbia ICU. But the hospital didn't always find our antics cute or entertaining.

I was now back to where it had all started but much, much better. Being transferred to Bridgeport Hospital was a big deal. It meant I was stable enough to be taken care of in a smaller, local hospital that was closer to home. It was strange adjusting to a different environment, especially since I knew it was minutes from my old house but not allowed to venture beyond the surgical recovery unit. The staff at Bridgeport never really went for, "Well, my Columbia nurses let me do this *all* the time!"

I had grown accustomed to the alternate universe of the Columbia ICU, and now here I was in a more familiar setting where some of my old high school classmates were even in other rooms recovering from minor injuries or stopping by to visit an older relative. I was embarrassed at how inhuman and different I felt from them. I was jealous because they were real people recovering from normal things, or just coming to spend time with a grandparent. And here I was, chained continuously to an IV pole, covered in bags to capture my leaking fluids, and in my eyes, not a person. I overheard one patient next door routinely getting her peripheral IV out before being discharged. When the nurse came to take my vitals, I asked her, "Will mine come out when I'm discharged, too?" She replied with a friendly smile, "No sweetie, you'll have yours for a *long* time."

It was a strange feeling being so close to my childhood home but unable to access it. Talking about current events, anything that placed life in real time, here and now, was unsettling after having been in the Columbia vortex for so long. After waking up from a coma, how do you just "go back" to life as it was? *Can* you? In a way, it was easier to be oblivious to the outside, safe in our nest, and protected from reality, which might make me miss life too much. Even a straw I'd spot by a nurse's station would bring me to tears.

Mom: During the second time at Bridgeport Hospital, you and I were walking in the lobby with the IV pole when a doctor abruptly stopped us. He looked at you and spoke only to you. He said he was there when you first came to Bridgeport Hospital in the ER, and how so many doctors and nurses worked to save your life, and what a miracle it was, and how you should do great things in your future life and realize your life was meant to do important things. For a moment, he freaked me out when he spoke.

The summer in Bridgeport Hospital was an encouraging phase of recovery. Eventually, my parents felt I was ready to test the waters. "Amy," my dad said to me during one of our usual strolls past the NICU, "How would you feel about leaving for an afternoon?"

Since I was the lowest maintenance patient on the floor, my parents had the nerve to ask the doctors for a "field trip,"—not a CAT scan field trip, but a real one. It was a request for a three-hour "pass" (I'm not even sure if that was an official thing). My parents asked if they could take me out, in the car, and back home, or wherever else I wanted to go for three hours, disconnected from IVs. So where does a teenager go when she's finally been let loose from hospital grounds for the first time since she was in high school? To the mall, of course.

On the day of the field trip, Mom and I were so excited. She helped me into a flowery old-lady dress she'd bought for me in the gift shop. Then, with my IV capped, my bandage changed, and my drains safety-pinned to my dress so they wouldn't pull, we made our way to Trumbull Mall. This mall had been my old stomping grounds in high school. It had the same name and address but it now seemed foreign, and instead of the exciting distractions I hoped to experience, being there was depressing. I had taken pride in walking around the hospital unit in short spurts every day, but here I grew tired and rapidly discouraged. I lacked the stamina to make it through one floor. I wasn't sure, however, if it was the act of walking that fatigued me or the fact that I was fiercely trying to block out any clues of food or drink, which, in a mall, is not the easiest thing to do.

We felt so out of place, so insecure leaving the safe nest of the hospital, that Mom and I were both relieved when it was time to go back. It was frightening how difficult it would be to readjust to the real world again. We only stayed at the mall for thirty minutes, and driving away, we passed old neighborhood faces walking with shopping bags or Starbucks cups. I was so ashamed to see them that I hid in my seat.

After my exhausting walk in the mall, my parents wanted to stop at our old house, minutes away to pick up a few things since they were sleeping in Bridgeport Hospital with me every night. *Home.* I hadn't been there for so long. I approached the house like I had with every other old memory encountered thus far: too scared to look, too curious to look away. I insisted on staying in the car, parked in the driveway, as my parents went in. I didn't want to face my old dog, my old room. I felt like a perpetrator, an intruder in my old life. I couldn't even look at my own reflection without facing the pain of the life I knew I could never get back. Mostly, I did not want to see my old fridge or my old kitchen table. Even though months had passed, I was terrified that some of my old favorite snacks might still be in the pantry.

My mom brought back some old clothes to the hospital. With bags, tubes, and drains all over me, it was unlikely anything would fit over my waist. But she still brought my old velvet stretch pants, hoping they might work. I had dressed for comfort in high school—stretch pants and sweatshirts. I cried just touching my old stretch pants, knowing they once touched the legs of a swifter, sprightlier, more innocent self. I sat on the bed and tried desperately to pull them over my bags and drains, but it proved impossible, especially hooked up to a pole. I didn't realize the emotional impact of anything from my high school life. It was the same situation with begging for cooking magazines. Out of sheer hunger, I couldn't think of anything else to do, but I always felt helpless after the last page.

Soon, being in Bridgeport Hospital felt more like babysitting. The floor knew us all by now and didn't need to pay attention to me, which I guess was a good thing. We all felt more like a nuisance. We just wanted to walk around the unit and entertain ourselves, and the nurses were eager to replace my bed with sicker patients, and for good reason. It was a sign of things improving, but it left me confused, helpless and nervous about what was to come. Who was I now? Not quite sick enough to be in the hospital, but not quite functional enough to be in the outside world. It was an awful state of flux.

We had known it was nearing time to leave Bridgeport, but we needed to hear the actual news. One morning in August, the doctors had my parents and me in a conference room for an official "meeting." My vitals were stable. I was steadily on TPN, and there was "nothing else they could do for me." I was too stable for Columbia, so they had sent me back to Bridgeport. Now I was too "healthy" for Bridgeport, and doctors felt I was "functional" enough to start adjusting at home. What was I supposed to do at home without a stomach? I imagined me pushing my giant IV pole down the cement street. Somehow I didn't think my parents would be so crazy about that.

I was just supposed to "heal" for the next few months. When I asked if there was anything I could do to help, they just said, "Keep staying strong."

Really? I was learning that healing is filled with transitions nobody wants to be up for. As I initially said, being in a coma was the easy part. It was the gradual changes, so gradual you didn't even know if any changes were actually happening, that were the most excruciating. The phrase, "Wake me up when it's over" had never rung truer.

The meeting was so simple, I felt angry. That's all I get for being here for months? It felt unfair to leave without a cure.

As I left that conference room, feeling anger I didn't even know how to handle because I was so used to staying numb, Laurie, a young, sympathetic blonde nutritionist who managed my TPN touched my shoulder and said to me, "It's really admirable of you to be willing to go home with TPN and take all this crap you have to deal with. Any other person in your shoes would hate it and complain about it."

I numbly nodded my head and muttered, "It's okay." Really? Did I have a choice?

The decision was made, and my only option was to cope through stoicism, a quality that was quickly becoming my best friend, and clearly something I would need more than ever once I stepped beyond the hospital doors and into the real world again. My heart was pounding already. They gave my dad bandage kits to change my wounds daily and said to follow up every now and then. "Reconstruction" surgery would be in my future, but not by their staff, and not for a while. I was still an unresolved mess.

Dad: When I found out we were leaving Bridgeport, I called Columbia to start seeing us as an outpatient. At Columbia, we had begun discussions about reconstructing her GI tract. One night Dr. Stolar took me aside and told me that Columbia could not handle this job. I appreciated his honesty and started making calls elsewhere.

No more hospital. This was the worst news of my life. To be discharged with no guide or roadmap was a death sentence into uncertainty. What was I supposed to do? I couldn't go to college or get a job. What could I do to get better? Doctors told me to just "heal." What the heck does that mean if you can't actively do anything to help speed it along? The idea of just "waiting" made me anxious, and kind of sick. Was I just supposed to wait and have life pass me by? At least in the hospital, I could tell myself doctors were brainstorming— even if that was a lie. But how could I make progress now? I was petrified to leave the hospital and be left with the day to day monotony of being stuck at home, on IVs, my father changing my bandages, any friends I had away at college. What was I supposed to do? But more importantly, how on Earth was I supposed to get my mind off water?

CHAPTER 9

Transitions

IN MY FANTASY, on the day I would finally be discharged from the ICU, I would get all dressed up, skip out the handicapped door, grab a burger on the way home, and waltz back into my old life. The second I walked out into the sunshine, all my bags and tubes would disappear, I'd be able to eat and drink and even dance again! Except my waltz partner was my IV pole, and burgers don't go down so well without a digestive system.

In my fantasy, leaving the hospital would take me right back to my former life and right back home. But what is home without its comforts? Or the home itself that you grew up in? Now I learned my parents had moved us! They felt we all needed a "new beginning," so they bought a new house, in a different town! A quaint little beach house in Westport that was still under construction. By the time I was ready to leave the hospital, the new house was finished, although completely devoid of furniture, memories, or life. Yet, to my parents, the move made perfect sense. In a small house, I wouldn't have to walk as far, we could all be close together if I needed them, and I could heal by the beach. We moved in the day I was discharged, and my old life was gone forever.

Instead of dancing into freedom, I left Bridgeport with my hospital band snipped off but still chained to my IV pole, wearing one of my dreaded "old lady" dresses from the hospital gift shop. After rising from my wheelchair, I nervously tiptoed (or, rather, limped) into the new world that awaited me, the next chapter. My supposedly normal life. But what *was* normal now?

Our new home quickly transitioned from a family residence to a residential hospital unit. Since IVs were my only source of nutrition, it was imperative that the feeds be running constantly. If we didn't want a nurse living with us day and night, my parents would need to learn how to administer my "food" themselves.

Our first night in our beach house was a night that would never end, as I watched my family bring in boxes from the car and robotically pile them on top of each other in the center of what I assumed to be our "living room." Then, Jerold, a friend of the family, came over to bring us a bag of bagels as a housewarming present. "They're still warm," he said, smiling. I hated him for being so thoughtless, but he meant well, and food was always the perfect gift for my family who systematically devoured the assortment of plain, sesame, onion, poppy, and everything after my mother arranged them on a tray. Before the last bagel was gone, I remember grabbing it—a poppy seed—and standing at the kitchen counter mindlessly picking off the seeds, then playing with its doughy insides, carving it out with my fingernails, making its delicious crust as hollow as I felt as a human being.

I was ready to reboot my life and hungry for a purpose, but mostly I craved food. Staring blankly at the mess I had made, I left the mangled bagel on the counter and hobbled upstairs to what was to become my room, now empty just as my heart and this "new beginning" felt. I didn't know what else to do but lie on my bed, confused, staring out the window and waiting for the night to pass. Then my father set up a small TV, put on a movie, and I fell asleep—in an empty, sheet-less bed.

The next morning, two different nurses arrived bright and early to teach my dad how to administer my fluids and keep everything sterile. These visiting nurses converted our beautiful new home on Compo Beach into a hospital room. They gave my father extensive directions for the TPN fluid I was to be connected to at all times. Now Dr. Dad was nurse Dad, and I was dependent on him for my daily care.

My dad mixed my TPN every week and would fondly call this "making the donuts." Our shopping lists had changed overnight, and staples such as "cartons of eggs" were now replaced by "boxes of alcohol wipes," "milk" with massive boxes of "latex gloves." A steady stream of boxes arrived at our house filled with medical supplies. Beside every garbage can was now a sharps container to dispose of hazardous materials. We even had a hospital bed shipped to the house so my dad could change my wound dressing three times a day. I had everything the hospital had but none of the freedom. Surprisingly, my new surroundings felt starker and more sterile than the Columbia Bridgeport ICUs. It had been easier to roll my pole around the smooth unit hallways than it was to wheel it in circles on the wooden floor around our tiny kitchen table. And I couldn't exactly head outside with it onto the uneven gravel streets or the inviting sand of the beach. The sudden sense of isolation was depressing and terrifying.

Getting settled in the new house was like putting the pieces of a puzzle together. Everything we had brought with us was laid out on the floor—most of it in boxes—and our job was to pick up the pieces and reassemble them into a new life. My family and I were starting from the ground up in every respect. In the hospital, all I had to worry about was being a patient—the only place I had to be was in a hospital bed. I could fool myself into believing that my "purpose" was to rest, be there when doctors came for rounds, and hold my breath for five seconds during my CAT scans. That was my job, and apparently, I did it well enough to "graduate." But out of the hospital, living in a house, in the real world, hardly able to walk, I was unable to create a true "person" routine, complete with meals, activities, and a direction. My only direction was running from fear to survive. I couldn't open the fridge and look at it the way my own family could. I felt empty, lost, and scared of my own kitchen, which kept hidden jewels that belonged to every other person with a pulse except *me*.

Who was I now, and what did *home* even mean? What was this body covered in adhesive, plugged into machines, leaking out of openings I didn't even know I had? I was no longer the same person, but I didn't yet know who I would become.

It's not easy to stay optimistic. I try to be present; here with the good, and with the bad. I would love to feel sorry for myself, but I don't know what I would be sorry for. I have such an amazing springboard of support, and I know that I am always down deep in there.

The morning after my first night, I was a mess. My mother had to help untangle me from my nightly IVs, which hung from a makeshift pole more cumbersome than the machine we had gotten used to in the hospital. I finally mustered up the emotional strength to sit up and step out of bed. My neuropathy from the hospital was as painful as ever, and any contact with the floor made me shriek in pain. After I struggled with the decision to get up and "start" my day, when all I really wanted to do was stay in bed, my mother helped me settle on the porch stairs to watch the raindrops fall. It was difficult for me to sit on the steps and have to bend my knees in so close to my chest, which was now covered in gauze and wires. Everything I used to do obliviously, I now had to think about with so much more effort. Would life always be this exhausting? Would every day pass as slowly as this one had?

I stared at the row of beach houses across from me. New people in colorful homes with families and children living a life that I used to live. What did they think of me now? Had they heard anything about what our family had been through?

My mouth was a forbidden temple with no trespassing allowed. I did not have permission to fully access my body and breaking the rules would only be at my expense. Besides being unable to address the needs that my body screamed out for; I was frightened of things happening in my body that were out of my control. When had I gotten so used to feeling stitches pull and break, or fluids leaking out of me, or wires pulling out of my arms? I was constantly feeling wet all over my body, everywhere except the one place I wanted to be wet—my mouth. And my soul. I wanted to be wet with my own tears, crying about how miserable all of this was and mourn my displacement. But I couldn't even cry. It was deadly to feel anything because if I dove into my well of emotion, I might feel the deadliest feeling of all—hunger.

I made it through the first day in our new Westport home, and then the next, and the next. But getting through was a decided effort. Every day felt longer than the next. Every stair felt steeper, every stitch felt more fragile, and every smell seemed more potent than the day before. Life felt larger than me like a school bully determined to intimidate me and scare me out of living, sending me running in the other direction.

I had too much time to let my mind wander and imagine the countless times I had thought about food in my life, and how casual and carefree my thoughts had been. I'd stew over the thousands of times I'd grabbed a handful of popcorn on my way out to the kitchen or chugged a quick gulp from my water bottle on a break at dance class, beating myself up for every moment I hadn't truly appreciated each morsel or sip, like someone going through every past interaction with an ex when trying to examine a breakup that went wrong. I laughed (sadistically) at the times I could remember when I was trying to cut dairy out of my diet for my voice, or refused to eat white bread, which according to my mother was poison, opting instead for sprouted wheat ("much healthier.") What did that matter now? I had no choices.

I missed the social aspect of food. Family meals. Pizza with friends. I was reminded that food wasn't just about solving our physical hunger. It was also a means of connecting with people.

I also wanted spiritual fulfillment, to find God again, but I'd give Him up in a heartbeat for a hunk of steak. Instead, I had what my dad would call my nightly "Pina Colada Cocktail," a three-liter bag of milky white IV vein food that I would carry around in a purse for sixteen hours a day, in addition to a feeding tube in a backpack. My parents were heartbroken that I couldn't eat, so they rid the house of food entirely. My mom hid trail mix in her purse, and my dad would come home from work and scarf down his eggplant parmesan in the garage. Trying to spare my feelings was a total parenting fail— my sense of smell was superhuman. (Maybe pick something with less oregano?)

Our fridge had always bulged with food, and suddenly my parents were clearing it out completely. In addition to the weirdness of food being absent, not eating made me feel inhuman. I was in a body I couldn't recognize. My smooth, rosy, pink skin was now tough, painful, covered in stitches and gauze. I was mad at my body for betraying me. When the nurse came to do my dressing change every morning, I shut my eyes as hard as I could. I couldn't look at my stomach covered with bags, scars, and wounds.

What have they done to you? And how on earth did you get this deformed? Only aliens don't have bellybuttons. Aliens and Alfred Hitchcock.

I wanted to at least hold a potato or smell an orange. Except for walks with my dad, I barely left my room and didn't even raise the blinds. I spoke only with my parents and doctors, and spent all day writing in my journal and masochistically watching the Food Network to satisfy my cravings. The hungrier I got, the more I became obsessed. I knew the Food Network lineup by heart, and I read and reread my stash of cooking magazines like trashy romance novels.

Not being able to eat was horrendous, but not being able to drink, especially in the heat of summer, was torture. I'd start and stop water faucets for hours. Sometimes I'd just let the faucet stream tap my wrist over and over again, just to feel like I still had a pulse. I even tried to talk my mother into purchasing one of those water playtime tables for toddlers, but she insisted that at twenty years old, I might be a bit old for that. So, I amassed a secret collection of every possible drink container—flasks, baby bottles, pitchers (thanks to my mother's retail therapy stops at HomeGoods)—and I poured water back and forth from one vessel to another imagining how a sip of ice-cold water would actually feel down my throat. I killed time wrapping my jaundiced fingers around our garden hose as it gushed watery wet liquid to fertilize the green, nourished grass. Or drenching myself in the outdoor shower and daydreaming about gulping down every drop.

I was waiting for doctors to tell me what the next step would be, but at this point, I realized that the next step would not be the magical solution to all of my problems or my happy, healthy, normal ending. My next step would simply be another slow, painful, agonizingly small transition. Transitions are always the hardest.

Leaving the hospital was also difficult because I was suddenly isolated. Now, instead of a large team of nurses and doctors to talk to, I had my "medical" duo of Mom and Dad. It was unbearably difficult being with other people, and I didn't know how I fit into the picture. I felt so different knowing that none of them had any idea what it felt like to have to constantly suppress the basic human need to nourish yourself. My friends who had visited me in the hospital for my "graduation" that summer were concerned about me after news spread that I was home. The first thing they wanted to do was come over, bring something (What? Pizza?) and cheer me up. But they could not comprehend my new circumstances with terrifyingly rigid parameters.

I couldn't ask my friends to starve themselves. How could I explain to them that I had to detach and go into "robot" mode to not get so hungry that I would eat something and die? They could barely process my numb reaction to being sexually abused, and I didn't even know if, how, or what they had heard about that trauma which now seemed too overwhelming to think about. But the loudest question on my mind was, "How could I face my healthy friends without plunging into despair over how my life had been so on track and was now so badly derailed with so very far to go?"

My first visitors were four of my closest high school friends. Nerves overtook me as they rang the doorbell, as I worried what they'd think of me now, or how I was supposed to act. I didn't want to take part in what my life was now, and I certainly didn't want my old friends to either. As soon as they arrived, I wished they would go away.

But I made small talk with them as they insisted on setting up my Facebook account, an entire phenomenon I'd missed while I was in the hospital. As they filled in my profile for me, I wasn't even sure what to say about myself. I had no picture to post of myself except my headshot from when I was seventeen. Interests? How about "getting my digestive system back." Did I even want people knowing what I was doing now? The only feeling stronger than hunger at this point was shame.

As my body adjusted to the new formula of TPN adapted for home, the doctors—who would touch base with my father every week—agreed to start cycling the TPN again, so at least I could feel some sense of freedom at home. To be safe, the TPN was cycled for twenty-three hours, allowing me one precious hour of escape. I determined to use it wisely: I was going to learn to walk by myself on the beach.

My beach walks were a struggle, and the sand quickly left me winded. Then by mid-afternoon, the heat was unbearable. But I had a goal that kept me going. I was motivated by *love*. Even feeling as inhuman and numb as I was, I managed to develop a crush. I would count the steps to the pavilion where I had become acquainted with a guy around my age I came to know as the "Ice Man." And with my neck bag (like a scarlet letter glued to my throat), I'd meekly ask "Can I please have a cup of ice?" He'd smile with an enthusiastic "Sure!" and fill up a big red paper cup with the coolest, meltiest ice for me every day, which I'd hold onto as though it were my soul. I was in love with free ice cubes. I would gaze at those frozen, forbidden treasures, glistening jewels reflecting in the sunlight, yearning to savor each heavenly piece before the sun melted it all to drips. Once I found my "holy grail" each day, I'd stumble across the sand towards the house, checking my watch to make sure I hadn't exceeded my hour, like Cinderella rushing home before midnight. It was a race against time and a race to enjoy each ice cube before it vanished.

At the beach, I could fully indulge my need to be in and around water. If I wasn't going to drink water, I was damn sure going to feel it. On really hot days I would race to the outdoor showers in my clothes and drench myself. As the water ran over my clothes, the beachgoers waiting to use the shower all looked at me like I was crazy, but I couldn't have cared less. Hope is having something to strive for, even if it's completely blind and unfounded. No other unnatural drive would have given me the inhuman energy to trek a mile across the beach every day in ninety-degree weather, in the land of lemonade, laughter, and luscious frozen treats. Water, even though I couldn't drink a drop, was my savior.

My immersion therapy was usually interrupted by my patient father, who was helping me carry my three-liter IV purse.

I'd sadly leave my "makeshift shower" and walk on, trying to retain that feeling of wetness. My father never questioned carrying my IV bag for me, across the beach, through museums, Costco, or anywhere he would take me in the quest to help me feel as normal as I could.

Dad: Summer 2006. At dinner time we were walking on the beach. Unbeknownst to us, crowds of people are grilling tons of food. We pass by, and Amy starts to cry until we pass by down the basketball courts. I felt so bad I started to cry, too, knowing this was our route every day. We had just not done it at dinner time before.

Like impoverished war victims fantasizing about their ideal supper, with every step across the sand, my father and I discussed every meal we could remember. It was useless to try to avoid the topic of food on our beach walks. Compo Beach wasn't exactly the place you'd head for a "sterile" food-free environment. It was hard not to feel sorry for ourselves, and the only comfort we could give ourselves was, "One day, we will."

In the meantime, all promises of the future rested upon the magical *reconstructive surgery*: the magic cure that was going to connect all the pieces of my intestines and glue together the empty missing pieces of our lives, transforming our family back to the way we were and enabling us to partake in the happy get-togethers we witnessed all around us. When that glorious day of reconstructive surgery arrived, the Oestreichers would be casually eating dinner at the beach with a bippity boppity boo and a tap of a fairy god-mother's magic wand!

We did not know then that several summers later, my father and I would still be taking the same walks along the beach as the misfits waiting to get their lives back, still trying to live vicariously through everyone else, inhaling the smells of fries from that old, rickety boardwalk as though we were ingesting them ourselves, and still vehemently holding onto the thought that would be us someday, because it was our God-given right.

As starving as I felt, my doctors did remind me that I was being "fed." My veins devoured 3,000 calories a day from a big IV I lugged around constantly. But my emotional appetite was ravenous. Food was instinctive, emotional, physical, social, psychological, and life-full. When I wasn't out walking, I shut myself out from the world because any outside stimulation might make me feel alive, and that meant craving the satisfaction of basic human needs. With the danger of food everywhere I turned and my desire for it all-consuming, living life was a constant obstacle course, a relay race in avoidance.

After a while, leaving my room, even for my hour of freedom unchained from TPN, was no longer fun. It brought me too close to a tantalizing world in which I was denied basic sustenance. I didn't want to be half in the world, to feel like half a person, a non-person who couldn't engage in the most basic activity of eating. What can you do to pass the endless time of "I don't knows?"

Once I realized the magical powers of exercise to take away all thought and feeling, I was hooked. For this endless summer (and the next, and the next), the days went smoothly for me if I could just stay in my room all day, daze out, and exercise. I'd commend myself for my numb success, just like I'd commend myself after getting stabbed seven times for a PICC line when I felt like nothing more than a pin cushion or a welcome mat for people to stomp their feet on. Now, I just stomped all over my thoughts and feelings through my constant movement to accomplish the same goal—numbness. I had found something I could do now, something I could succeed at besides being a hospital patient. A sad, but necessary way to live.

I exercised when it was too painful to hope, knowing so many hopes of mine had been shattered. But every now and then, between the kicking in place or the pacing in tiny circles, a sliver of Amy-ness, of soul juice from a tiny lifelike part of me, attempted to squirm to the surface of my awareness. These sharp pangs of emotion reminded me I was still human, whether I thought so or not. Underneath the numbness, I could sense the fear I was trying to cover up. I was a scared, wounded bird, tortured and running from the fearful question: What if I could never eat or drink again?

This was a world that felt eerily serene to me. My numbness could be mistaken by others for being fine, and that was fine with me. I had no outside context to know that the life I had created was totally bizarre, not to mention unhealthy. But what constituted healthy? When not eating is healthy, everything is turned upside down. My parents were always proud to know I had survived another day, no matter what lengths I had to go to. Exercise was my drug, my painkiller, but it didn't feel like popping pills. I didn't think to myself, "Oh, I'm really anxious right now, I need to work my body." Rather, I calmly thought to myself, "Okay, time to cope. Let me find my happy place and zone out doing what I usually do." My parents were so numb from all the medical crises that it didn't even faze them that I was slowly killing my mind, body, and spirit every day. I wasn't eating or drinking, and I wasn't dying in the ICU, so I was safe. My job was to stay stuck until given the medical okay to move ahead. Survival was my occupation, and exercise was the only co-worker I had. In isolation, anything feels okay.

Just as my nature walks had turned sour after Blaine molested me, the robotic pacing of my feet to mark time was losing its impact. On days I allowed myself to leave my room, I created a new routine—pacing through Stop & Shop. I would force my mother to drive me and drop me off so I could pace down every aisle for two or three hours. People must have thought I was either crazy or shoplifting.

I'll never forget one of my grocery store pacing sessions, eyeing all the products, enticed by the brightly colored boxes, brands, logos, and packaging. I'd often pretend I was on one of those supermarket sweep reality game shows and imagine I had just won the grand prize. Now I was able to wheel my cart through the entire store and throw in anything I wanted. Anything! I went through my usual aisles: Produce, Ethnic Foods, Freezer Aisle, Dairy, imagining what I would reach for first on that glorious, surgically reconstructed day. But this time was different. Suddenly, the value of my life in the long term blazed into my consciousness. I saw mothers shopping with their daughters, planning what they would have for dinner that night. I saw a little boy biting into a crunchy red apple as he joy-rode in his mother's cart. I ran through the aisles desperately in search of my mother, who was loading her cart with Clorox and Kleenex—about the only things I actually needed from a grocery store. I rushed to her in tears.

"Mom," I sobbed, "what if this operation doesn't work and I'll never be able to eat? What if I am forever like this?" And she reassured me with the confidence that only a mother has when protecting her daughter and keeping her hope alive is the most important thing in the world. She grabbed me by shoulders and stated, with fierce conviction, "Yes, of course, you will eat."

Mothers have a PhD in the science of hope. I felt like the little girl who got her lollipop taken away from her when her head was turned, worried if she would ever get back that sweet sugary high of life making her tongue tingle ever again. Just pace through Stop & Shop, little girl, and keep your feet moving so you don't have to think about the possible reality that shopping here could be a dream you never get to experience the way normal people do. You might spend the rest of your life pacing through Stop & Shop, salivating but never tasting. *Keep your feet moving so your heart stands still!*

I knew my mother's answer was just empty words, but I decided to let them mean something. I needed them to.

CHAPTER 10

Therapeutic Pathways

MY MOTHER PROVIDED ME WITH OPTIMISM, retail therapy field trips, and endless games of Scattergories. My father provided beach walks, bandage changing, and endless DVDs from Redbox. But even this amazing support system was proving not to be enough. In a relatively short period, I had dealt with more trauma than a whole season of *Law and Order*. My mom wanted to put me in therapy to process both my newfound medical reality and the memories of Blaine still tormenting me.

The day of my first appointment, I was nervous. This was my first real appointment of any kind since I was home. I limped up the three mountainous steps to the therapist's office, and I remember cradling a stick of gum in my hands to save for a time I was especially hungry. The therapist was kinder and less prodding than the psychiatrists in the hospital, and we ended up talking about what my favorite holidays were as he took me for a walk on the lawn in front of his office. After about fifteen minutes, he took me back to my mother, who was waiting in the car for me. He told her with great compassion, "She can't eat, she can't drink. I'm not going to torture her by sticking her in a room, talking about her feelings, and making her think about how hungry she is. Please just let her rest at home and heal."

Healing. What did that mean? Now, even my healing was in limbo. Could anything ever start for me, or was I just supposed to passively wait for my magical surgery that might happen who knows when?

With my acting career and life on hold, I created my next distraction—I became a chocolatier. Starting a chocolate business was the first of many activities I discovered as a happy accident on my way to healing. Pacing through Stop & Shop for my daily food-porn marathons, I would always visit the candy aisle and become overwhelmed with memories of Halloween—gathering trick or treat candies in pillowcases and sorting out M&Ms by color. It's amazing how any food can trigger such potent memories. I found myself fascinated by the many colors, bright packages, shapes, textures and names of all the various sucking candies, chocolate bars, and fruit snacks. Then came Hanukkah, and a week we usually celebrated with latkes and applesauce was spent in a barren home—another holiday spoiled again.

But Helen, my mother's faithful college friend, came to our house and brought over her chocolate molds. Helen had a tradition for the holidays where she would get out her chocolate making kits and make us chocolate houses, chocolate dreidels, and her out-of-this-world chocolate peanut butter cups. This year she came over to make chocolate with me, and I allowed myself out of my room for the half hour it took to make Helen's delights. I was surprised at how therapeutic it was to work with her, to smell the chocolate, and to create something. Helen saw me smile for the first time. So, she left the molds with me.

Now I had a new way to spend forty minutes out of each painful twenty-four hours. It involved both movement and creativity, and I was out of my room. I was in the light, making something with my hands, making something happen. After the last commercial break of Emeril's cooking show, at exactly 8:35 p.m., there were eighty minutes before I could tire myself enough for bed. I would leave my room and go down to the kitchen where my mom had started to heat up the double boiler for me with eight different brightly colored chocolate wafers beginning to melt in glass Pyrex containers.

As I worked, I'd savor how the chocolate smelled, how the molten liquid poured, and how the candies felt in my hands. I would treat every chocolate like it was an individual masterpiece. I loved decorating each one, and now going to Stop & Shop took on a whole new purpose. I began to relearn the art of going to the grocery store to buy things—syrups, chocolate, sprinkles, candy, peanut butter (for my peanut butter cup filling!), every kind of tactile sweet confection I could find—instead of using the aisles for my food distraction walking track. In addition to the actual chocolates, I created bright and snazzy pamphlets for my new business, "Amy's Handmade Creations," which my father handed out in his office, and soon, I was getting orders! I had picked up this new hobby just in time for Christmas, and now I was assembling personalized edible packages, made with love—and desperation. Sending these packages out became my life force—forty-minutes of my day that connected me to others and made me feel useful. Soon, I was shipping off chocolates to states all over the country.

Whether it would be a week or seven years before I could eat again, I resolved I would get through, one chocolate cookie at a time and, hopefully, someday return to the world.

On my chocolate cookies, I made autumn decorations, shaping leaves out of sprinkles. I remembered how in the fall I would go to temple and pray to God for the High Holidays. It was a leap of faith, exactly like the leap of faith I needed to take right now.

My life was keeping me (literally) jogging in place, while life for everyone else was moving on. As numb as I tried to stay, I took to life like a bad habit and tried to join in with the flow of the real world in any way I could, even if it hurt. But reality was harsh. Things that should have been celebrated became new traumas: weddings, movies, family occasions, game nights.

That September, Rachel, an old babysitter, asked me to sing at her wedding. Wearing the first real gown after my hospital gown, I felt like a human for the first time, proudly showing my esophagostomy bag over my neckline. I sang *The Greatest Love of All* as Rachel walked down the aisle, even though I had gotten my tracheotomy out only weeks before and could barely speak. Despite this triumphant comeback, I started crying when I saw champagne bubbling in sparkling glasses. It was the most beautiful food porn I had ever seen; a mirage in my desert of deprivation.

I had lost my bouncy vitality and felt purposeless, even after the honor of singing at Rachel's wedding. I stewed, *But I bet all these cheerful dancers don't know I can compulsively exercise like mad!* That was what made me feel strong in the face of people who could click their heels in the air and think nothing of it. Did they know I used to be like that?

During the wedding, I wore my neck-bag proudly as if to intimate a message to the outside world, "See? This is what I deal with every waking hour!" My mother kept trying to tuck the bag into the bosom of my dress. But I kept sneaking it back out and pretending that I did it by accident. I wanted people to see how hurt I had been, and how astounding it was that I had the strength to sing under the hot sun, with no water to quench my thirst! My neck bag was the only kind of warrior badge I could show to the outside world, and someone besides me had to see the absurdity of this situation.

I miss cocktail hours at bat mitzvahs and good old talking with friends as loud music plays in the background. I miss talking in a super loud voice in order to be heard above the buzzing good times all around you, and every so often losing a word as a cocktail waitress moves past you with a tray of pigs in a blanket.

As I locked myself in my room, relieved to rid myself of outside stimulation once again, I tried to praise myself for what I tried to accomplish:

Sometimes you have to take too big of a leap and fall. This way, you know the right stone you should have leaped toward. Next time, you'll know to aim a little closer.

I fell and fell again. But I told myself it was still worth another try. So, I tried to take another risk.

My family tried the best they could to support me in joining the outside world however painful it was. Some risks were harder and more harmful than others. Desperate to recreate old memories, after some prodding from my brother Jeff, I somehow agreed I would go out with my family for my parents' 40th wedding anniversary, at a restaurant, when I still couldn't eat or drink. I sat at the elegantly set table, staring at my empty glass and my untouched silverware until I started crying. To this day, my parents still say, "Did we really make you do that? How awful!" Looking back, I think we were all numb. I even tried to join a choir, take an acting class, and take a dog obedience class. I would start these activities then drop out because, without food, I didn't feel human.

Knowing that an element of social time was important for my well-being, my parents invited old friends over for a game night. We quickly discovered that food and drink are so essential to being human and social that we couldn't have people over without sustenance. Have you ever tried entertaining and socializing while you're trying to get through the day without food and drink on display, or worrying whether your TPN was running properly?

For a family that once opened its doors to everyone, we became reclusive, and I, in turn, became a hermit in my room.

If I had taken not eating or drinking more than a day at a time, I would have given up all hope. Here's the thing: Hope is a job, not a state of mind you turn to. You have to actively create hope in difficult times, and sometimes, we need to lie to ourselves to do so. Living at the beach house with my sink, my chocolates, my constant exercise, and laptop journaling, and my endless countdowns to the day I could eat and drink, all I could do was hope, fantasize, tempt myself, and wonder. I dreamed of the glorious day when I would jump in a gallon of ice-cold water and drink the entire tub.

Abandoning My Old Life

Just as I was adjusting to life in the new house, I was hit with another transition: My parents were selling our Fairfield home. As I was agonizingly rebuilding myself, my childhood foundations were shattering one by one. There was no sense in keeping two houses when I could barely get around one, but thinking of my childhood home being staged, explored at open houses, (just as my body had been explored by doctors and their trailing teams of curious med students), and shopped around was a weight that came crashing down on me.

We had abandoned our Fairfield house on that fateful April night and left everything as though we would come right back the next morning. Our house had been well "lived in" since before I was born—filled with furniture, food, clothing, and stacked and packed with memories, laughter, music, smudges on the counter, scratches on the walls—all signs that our family had made this our home. Nights tiptoeing across the kitchen tiles hearing Matt practice piano till dawn, chasing runaway hamsters down the basement stairs, cleaning exploding smoothies off the kitchen counters—those memories circulated in the air and would soon be gone. My identity was washing away like sidewalk chalk after a storm.

Preparing the house for sale involved an odd blend of melancholy reminiscence and anxious hope that maybe we could have our old life back again. But where? In the hospital, I crooned the line, "I want to go home," like a broken record. Now, I revisited my childhood room with wallpaper with multicolored hearts, and neon stars stuck to the ceiling, and was overcome with grief. I slammed my old bedroom door with the broken knob and exercised myself into oblivion until my parents were ready to drive back to Westport for the night.

My parents spent the following weeks toting me and my pole from house to house, packing and sorting, with me exercising to avoid thinking about any of it. Our round kitchen table where we had enjoyed so many family dinners was now the perfect circumference to pace around for hours. It wasn't long before my pride in numbness turned to secrecy, shame, and guilt. I couldn't even enjoy the happy nostalgia with my family. Who was I now, anyway? A monster who couldn't eat or drink, chained to a bag of liquid nutrition twenty hours a day. I hated myself.

As my energy and frustration mounted, I started to explore the world of dance I had dreamed about getting back to as I strung beads in the hospital. At first, I felt awkward and constrained, but I soon started doing good old pique turns, which felt very unnatural, but the more I got into it, the more my world expanded with the overflowing beauty and vivaciousness it once had. I revisited songs I used to love in my "old life," calling it my "healing playlist." I danced through the uncertainty, danced back my inner and outer strength, danced back my world, and found a sense of release.

One night me and my parents spent the night in Fairfield. I could sleep in my old room—in my childhood bed—albeit with an IV pole attached to my arm, which was positioned inconveniently next to my wall. With the IV tube running across my chest, I kept getting tangled. So much for happy memories.

While I was in the hospital, Gabby, the Bichon we'd had since I was eight, had stayed in our Fairfield house while Adam took care of her. Now I avoided Gabby to shield myself from painful memories. That night, in Fairfield, my father tried to put Gabby in bed with me as a comfort. He positioned her in a ball by my feet, but she kept getting tangled in my IV tubes.

Animals have a deeper knowing, and I feared I had come out of the hospital without a soul and Gabby could sense my shame. Gabby had nipped at my frilly third-grade socks, broken into the Chex Mix in my backpack, tried to torture my guinea pig, and always loved me unconditionally. Her opinion meant the world to me, and I was terrified of her seeing me this way. I felt I was no longer worthy of my old life, and that Gabby lost faith in me. To make matters worse, after thirteen years of good health, Gabby was dying. Now, she was another reminder of my old life slipping away.

The day we were going to put Gabby down, we spent the night in Fairfield to cherish our last moments with her. Jeff, who had been the closest to her, took the train home from New York to say goodbye. A sliver of me was sad, but my priority was constant motion to keep my mind away from food. But the more time we spent at Fairfield, the sicker I was getting of killing each moment exercising, so that day, I dared to explore the remainder of the house.

Timidly, I tiptoed down to the basement where we had enjoyed so many parties and holidays. My parents had finally cleaned up our last, fateful Passover dinner and put away the eight tables and thirty chairs, hopeful that one day we would take them back out again. Like everything else in our lives, the basement was now stark and bare, except for the corner with my old dance floor, which still felt alive. In high school, I would rush there straight after school, blast some Broadway show tunes or a jazz big band record, and tap dance to release the day's emotions. I even earned spending money teaching private tap lessons to friends on that sectioned out corner.

As I walked through the basement, Jeff was lying on the floor, holding Gabby, who had been unable to walk for weeks. I zipped past her into my dance studio, quietly muttering, "I'm sorry. It's too hard." I started dancing, and through some kind of miracle, Gabby got up, nudged the door open, and limped in. I was frightened like I was being visited by an angel to whom I did not wish to bare my soul. I kept dancing, trying to ignore Gabby, but she walked in a circle around me, and we danced—together. Then she left the room, returned to Jeff, and collapsed. This miracle inspired me to keep on dancing into the night, at peace knowing we had a heartfelt farewell. The next day, we put Gabby down. She had left me, but not before saying good-bye.

Eventually, all that was left in our Fairfield house were the large pieces of furniture we couldn't move ourselves. I felt like a phantom as I brushed by our old couches, chairs, and tables, running my fingers along familiar surfaces. It was strange placing myself in that picture of our past as a present part of it. I found myself reminiscing on my relationships with our furniture. There was the wooden table, made from an elephant's saddle, whose cracks I'd squeezed my toes into when I would relax on the couch. And there was the jolly, big, comfy couch I used to sink on, where our whole family watched movies together. And over there, sticking out of a box, the ceramic menorah with all six of us sculpted on it—figures frozen in ceramics. Would we ever get our life back? Would I ever be whole? Would the picture ever be complete?

CHAPTER 11

Theatre to the Rescue:
Oliver

LESS THAN A MONTH AFTER I WAS discharged from the hospital, I read in a local paper that a community theatre in Stamford was holding open auditions for *Oliver*. Despite everything blocking my path to performing, I thought it would be good for me to be part of an ensemble. Theatre would also help me through the hardest transition of all—dealing with my endless, unquenchable thirst. Even numb, I was hungry and thirsty. But I wanted to live life, and I was not one to lie in bed as a "patient." I was still figuring out who I was post-coma, and one thing I knew—I still loved theatre.

Theatre was a bittersweet topic for me. I had felt so on track in high school, and now I saw on my new Facebook feed that high school friends had gone on to national tours. I couldn't bear to think about never acting on stage again. Blaine had penetrated my entire world, and once he started abusing me, even theatre felt violated. Although I had a solid legal case against Blaine, I was in no shape to pursue it. Just as the therapist my mother took me to determined that now was not the time for me to sit and talk about my feelings, the lawyer my parents found advised that I should steer clear of the grueling process of testifying against my abuser and focus instead on my healing. Exercise from morning to night remained the only outlet for my anger.

Somehow, Blaine had convinced my mother that I should have voice lessons with him on Friday nights and sleep over (he had a "second apartment" upstairs that my parents trusted I would stay in) so we could spend Saturdays together—after all, he was my godfather. For months after he started molesting me, I had kept myself numb enough to attend these lessons every week. One morning I was singing *Hello World* at a lesson after a night trapped with him. I tried to put my heart into it, but I felt dead inside and figured something must be wrong with me. I was wearing an old T-shirt and sweatpants and had barely brushed my hair. I didn't care how I looked. It was the first time I hadn't dressed up for a lesson because I wanted to look like a victim, though I didn't know why.

In retrospect, I subconsciously wanted him to see what he was doing to me. I wanted to scream, "Can't you see how you ripped all my inspiration out of me? Look at me, I feel so empty, and confused, and it's all because of you. It's not your stupid reasons or truths or philosophies. It's you acting so weird, so different. You made a joke out of the world I knew! My firm ground, my magical world, you stole it for yourself!"

My sloppy outfit was a cry for help, but of course, a narcissist and sociopath would never pick up on it. I convinced myself I was uninspired. I did my best to carry the soaring melody of *Hello World*, Blaine stopped playing and remarked, "It feels rather empty."

Rather empty? I was devastated. Had I lost all of my talent? The irony is he was right. I felt empty, but I didn't know why.

I panicked, unable to find the beauty in art anymore because something didn't feel right. But I didn't even try to figure it out. I just believed him, and thought, "Yeah, I guess I'm uninspired."

My body knew that it was him, and I felt that fire in my chest as if my body was screaming out to him, "No you idiot! It's you who is leaving me uninspired!"

I needed to audition for *Oliver*, not just to get out and do something while I was healing, but also to prove to myself that my zest for life never came from Blaine and that no one could take it away from me. No one, especially not Blaine, was going to keep me from the stage.

I was still weak, jaundiced, and could hardly walk, let alone sing. It was not exactly rational to jump into a singing, dancing, high energy musical. "I'm just going to try out for the chorus," I told my mother, who was shocked and debating if she could trust me to go to rehearsals and not sneak a deadly sip of water. I reminded her that if I died, I wouldn't be too happy either, (although I still wasn't entirely sure about that) and convinced her to trust that I would maintain my discipline, just as I had solemnly promised her in high school that if she let me audition in New York every week, I would keep up my A average. Now, this was a different kind of A on which my life now depended.

I also made a deal with my dad that no matter what time rehearsal ran to, I would get in my full TPN cycle every night, which was now thankfully down to eighteen hours a day. That meant he would have to come to rehearsal to hook me up to a three-liter bag of nutritional IV fluids in a backpack at 10 p.m., and I wouldn't be unhooked until 4 p.m. the next day. Six hours of freedom was better than nothing.

Walking into that audition, with my parents nervously waiting in the car for me with my TPN ready, I felt like an outcast returning to society after a period of exile. It was odd seeing people I had worked with in my old life. I was embarrassed and ashamed of what they could be thinking. I had never been one to worry about what others thought of me, but these were people in whose world I once truly belonged. I hadn't always felt comfortable in my school classes, but community theatre—especially this one—was a place I could always call home.

It was a nervy move to audition in a body plastered with tubes and bags, but I went, and I belted out the song, "As Long as He Needs Me," as if my life depended on it (and in a sense, it did). The heartfelt desperation I put into those sixteen bars exhausted me, but I had shaken something free inside. I stumbled out, overwhelmed by my own strength, and couldn't help thinking, "Wow, that was good."

To my surprise, I made it to the dance call. I was nervous—I hadn't known there would be a dance call—and I couldn't jump like everyone else. I got winded just walking up the steps to the stage. But somehow, I harnessed the power I had used to force myself to hop around back when I was doing the Macarena at my Columbia ICU high school graduation, and miraculously I didn't fall over. My body might have been a mess, but my mind still worked like a dancer. I could remember all of the steps!

Imagine my shock the next week when I received a phone call from the theatre owner offering me the female lead, Nancy! My dad, a theatre ham in his free time, got a part, too. Of course, of all the musicals I could star in when unable to eat or drink, I had to pick the one with the song "Food Glorious Food" in it! Not being able to touch food or beverages during rehearsal, combined with lacking the full strength of all the other performers, still proved discouraging, lead or not. I remember watching the young kids in the cast running around playing tag. I was jealous, and more than that, scared those days were long gone for me, as I ran out of breath any time I tried to walk faster than a stroll.

To top it off, the director kept me overtime and made me rehearse a number after 10 p.m. Now, I had to sing and dance like everyone else in the cast—

with a three-liter bag on my shoulder! I felt so much anger in my empty belly that I wanted to scream, then cry. It wasn't fair. I would never be like everyone else. Being in the outside world helped me feel normal, but it also reminded me bleakly of how far from normal I still was.

As Nancy took her journey through *Oliver*, and I worked to memorize her lines while learning a cockney accent, I was going through a journey of my own. Because my esophagus had been diverted so the leak in my abdominal cavity could dry up and heal, it was explained to me that eventually, I might be able to drink first, even before any actual reconstructive surgery. Was there light at the end of this long tunnel, or more aptly, water at the end of this dreadful desert? On the more depressing side, TPN was also straining my liver, and its long-term effects were detrimental. When lipids were added to the daily IV blend, my liver enzymes would skyrocket. TPN was never supposed to be a permanent solution. We needed answers, and my dad went after them. He took me to the top doctor he could find—Stanley Dudrick, the inventor of TPN himself. Leave it to my superhero father to locate him, right in Waterbury, Connecticut, and score me an appointment.

Dudrick was a large, loud, jolly man, with a resemblance to Santa Claus. He reminded me of that loud uncle who comes to Christmas parties, as he pinched my cheeks and boasted amiably about his work. He is the man who coined the term, "surgical disaster," a phrase I fondly adapted as my medical "pet name." He said it with a chuckle, comforting my fearful apprehension. Miraculously, a "real doctor" was giving us the assurance that somehow I would be okay. In inventing TPN, Dr. Dudrick created more than just a portable bag of nutrients. He paved the way to saving countless people's lives.

After the usual shock as he looked over my medical history and confirmed jarring facts and numbers with my dad, he sat us down and was the first person (besides my mother, of course) who looked at us and said, "She *will* eat again."

When my parents described the emotional pain I was in, not being able to drink, how the orange drain refused to stay bone dry, and how we were hoping for a plan of care leading to an answer, he kept his casual gaze, and said simply, "just try it."

"What?"

"Just try it. Start drinking and see what happens. That drain is never going to dry up. If you wait for it to dry, you'll never drink."

This was the first time we were hearing anything like this, from someone we were meeting for the first time. Were we just supposed to ignore everything we had been told from the doctors who saved my life and risk it with this new doctor's radical advice? If my father had not kept searching for answers there would still be no solution to my "surgical disaster" without a roadmap for reconstruction.

The relentless thought of finally drinking made me intensely nervous. I had survived so far through rigid thinking; it was the only way I could program my mind not to think about food and water. I could either be human, which meant being miserable and terrified, or I could be a robot that didn't think or feel anything. On or off. What on earth did it mean to enter this gray area of "try it and see what happens?" I was also terrified that once I took that first sip, nothing could stop me from gulping down gallons of water, then stuffing my face with food, causing my stitches to burst loose, and then... I was still frightened of my body, I couldn't imagine the impact of even a thimble-full of water on my disconnected, strained, stomach-less anatomy.

Dr. Dudrick took a mechanical pencil from the pocket of his white lab coat and drew a diagram of my anatomy for my father. He explained how, technically, if my esophagus had healed enough, any fluid I drank should bypass my abdominal cavity and go directly into the bag on my neck. We were skeptical, but totally willing to believe. We left Waterbury with trepidation but even more hope and encouragement. Could it be we had finally met someone as optimistic and clearly insane as we were?

Knowing Dr. Dudrick was a bit eccentric (and the perfect counterpart to Dr. Stolar, aka Dr. Doom), my father and I exercised a bit more caution and waited a few weeks before we went to the hospital for a barium swallow. I had never been more excited to drink barium in my life. This earth metal with a radioactive-sounding name was now the magical potion that was going to tell me whether I could drink. The nurse brought me what looked like a milkshake in a Styrofoam cup, and that thick, sweet, chalky fluid in my throat tasted better than any milkshake I've ever had. I gulped it down quickly, then stood nervously on the x-ray platform as the radiology tech told me to breathe in and out, holding my breath, while he took a series of pictures. I sat down again, and after about ten minutes, it was clear I wasn't going to die. The doctors then took their time looking through everything, but as with everything else about me, there was no clear-cut answer. We just had to use our best judgment. I might as well start to drink "a little" and see what happens.

So where did my first sip of water since my stomach exploded and I went into a coma take place? Not in an elegant restaurant with white tablecloths and crystal stemware. After we left the hospital, I took my first sip from a bottle of Poland Spring in our car. I poured it into a shot glass we had brought for the occasion.

I was completely let down. The water didn't taste like anything, except the leftover phlegm that always lingered in my throat. I really wanted flavor. Had I really waited months, no years, for spit? Shouldn't I feel elated? Nope.

I didn't experience any kind of bliss. But at least I was drinking again, albeit in very small quantities. It was frightening to feel the liquid enter my mouth and allow myself to swallow. Maybe I had built this moment up so much in my head that anything would have been anticlimactic. Or maybe on some level I realized that while this was a huge milestone, a one ounce victory, and I had so many other battles to fight before I could be normal again. All I said to my parents as we drove home was, "Well, that's that."

Okay, I will admit that feeling that ice-cold rush of liquid down my parched throat—left dry as a desert for day after uncertain day—was exceptionally refreshing. But I still couldn't eat, and even the biggest Las Vegas-style buffet could not have appeased my insatiable hunger at that point.

I was relying on this one small sip to fill the months of anguish that I had spent in hospitals burdened with memories of unquenchable thirst. The times I was starving for some kind of oral stimulation, and the glycerin swabs the nurses would give me just didn't do the trick. The times I would force whoever came in to check on me to also tell me what they drank with breakfast that morning. The times that every straw I passed, pleasantly reclined in a cool shiny glass of Pepsi, made my lips tremble. And the times every plastic bottle of Poland Spring firmly clenched in a visitor's hands felt like a glamorous magazine ad of a model flaunting the finest diamond necklace. I saw every slurp from a hospital Styrofoam cup in glorified slow motion like a hair model tossing her hair in the wind with an extravagant symphony of strings playing in the background.

Most important though, Dr. Dudrick was right so far. Nothing terrible happened. So, with caution, I adhered to his rules and allowed myself two ounces a day for the first week. I would excitedly prepare my water the night before in a tiny cup and refrigerate it so it would be ice cold the next morning. I would then take the cup out and place the smallest coffee stirrer straw

I could find in it. I transported it with me and tried to make those two ounces last the entire day. So far, it worked! I was drinking...and safe! This was the most exciting game of trial and error I had ever played—and the most nerve-wracking as well.

The next week, after nothing happened, Dudrick suggested I try four ounces of water, and the next week, six ounces. This was enough to make me feel human—human enough to lose any sense of willpower, my biggest fear. I drank a bit more than six ounces, then a bit more than eight, until I had gradually finished an entire bottle of Poland Spring. I didn't care what happened. Drinking without limits felt marvelous. And nothing happened.

Miraculously, just as Dudrick had predicted, everything flowed into the bag on my neck. Soon I started experimenting with other clear liquids, like juice, Snapple, tea, soda. The fizziness of Pepsi felt like Disney World in my throat. I even got inventive and heated up soup broth. Finally, after a full year of not even an ice cube, I was allowed to drink. It was *HEAVEN!* Ever creative, I started to have a little fun with fluids. Since anything I drank went right through the opening and into a cute little bag, I started drinking juices of every color so my bag would match my outfit. For Halloween, I took the bag off, drank cherry red Kool-Aid, and told everyone I was a vampire. I'm pretty sure I was the only one who got a kick out of that.

Perhaps there is a reason why one of my favorite songs at that time was Billy Joel's "I Go to Extremes." Stop & Shop became a dreamy playground. I would look through every aisle trying to imagine what might fit through the bag on my neck. I could have soup, smoothies, hot chocolate, even ice cream! I excitedly took a friend to Dairy Queen and ordered this large chocolate caramel ice cream Coolatta smoothie concoction. Hey, if it could fit through the hole in my neck, it meant I could drink it! The feeling of normalcy that came with slurping milkshakes with a friend was the healthiest feeling in the world.

At one point I added whole milk to cheese powder and started making my own kinds of soups, soy milk gelato, whipped cream, anything else that I might be able to fit through my neck. It was a weird problem, and eventually, my mom stopped me, worried that the gunk might clog the esophagostomy that doctors had worked so hard for in order to save my vocal cords. Of course, now that I had liquid, I wanted food. I told myself to take it one day at a time, even if it meant exercising through each one. I was hungry, but at least with fluids, I had become half a person. Exercising or not, my main job right now was to just get from one day to the next. I could drink, but I still couldn't eat.

TPN was not a game. It was my literal lifeline and also a lethal weapon. As it went directly into my bloodstream, the line had to be kept sterile. Changing the tubing daily was not a task to be taken lightly. Early on, I didn't understand this and treated the PICC line in my arm pretty casually. I would end up hospitalized for blood and PICC line infections where I went septic, nearly killing me. Soon, it was decided that my father would be in charge of administering the TPN. By the end of *Oliver*, my doctors had cycled the TPN down to fourteen hours: a major accomplishment.

I had always acted from a deeply felt place, and even out of the hospital, I couldn't play Nancy completely numb. I braced myself as I sunk my teeth into the character I was playing—ironically, a woman who clung to a man who was physically and emotionally abusing her. I couldn't help but think about Blaine and the impact he'd had on me.

I remember being furious that Blaine had brought me backstage at a Broadway show so he could talk to his student, congratulating her in his deep professional voice, while everyone shook his hand and thought, "What an engaging man, how clever and nice and smart and wonderful he is." That star student making her Broadway debut could have been *me*, and here I was, slouched over by his side, unable to speak. Brooke Shields happened to be starring in the show, but even though we were meeting a famous actress in an actual Broadway theatre, I had dressed myself as a worthless victim, with my hardly brushed hair and old baggy sweatpants, almost as a call for help. I felt like a dumb, invisible, filthy scrap he was dragging along with his heels. I also felt a tremendous surge of fury so deep and frozen stuck to my insides, filling me with heated tension.

I felt stifled, silenced, frustrated, mad, ashamed, and so alone, knowing I was the only one that knew his dirty secrets. As with nearly all abusers, he displayed no trace of the evil villain he was to the outside world. I was looking like a dirty little tagalong for all of these New York actors to see; they gazed at my pale, unkempt appearance and must have been wondering, "Oh, poor girl, what's wrong with her?" Blaine would eloquently respond, "Yes, bless her heart, she's just been through so much, between her family and everything, but she's really an old soul, and we connect on a special level, and she's my godchild." To which the outside world would coo back, "Oh, Blaine, you are such a noble saint the way you care for people like that."

Blaine tricked everyone far too well for them to know we had an inverse relationship: the weaker I got, the stronger he became. That is what happens when you suck someone's soul juice and feed on their blood like a vampire. At *Wonderful Town*, we were introduced to the stage manager and other cast members, which would have filled me with euphoria in a pre-disillusioned life. Now I was upset with myself over how little I cared. Where had all my values gone?

All the values Blaine claimed to hold were clearly disproven by his actions, secret actions that only I knew about. And by the end of the night, I was still the one who had to sleep with him, entertain him, listen to him, *and* wipe away his tears. I was still the one who had to go home with him and watch him transform into a temperamental infant. My cries were frozen in fear.

Why couldn't I snap out of it? Not once did I even think to myself, "Hey I am a Broadway-aspiring actress. 'Hi, Ms. Shields! Hi, Mr. Manager! I want to be on Broadway! Gosh, it's exciting to meet you!'" Nope, that part felt dead in me. Blaine, manipulating his control over my new zombie life, knew that. He planned it that way, strategically sucking away my goals, hopes, and dreams one by one so he could have ultimate power over me and my life. The man who had helped me gain my voice had literally stolen it and now showed me off like a charity toy.

These buried memories now pierced through me in hot flashes of light, possessing me with an overwhelming fire of anger. The paralyzing rage confined me in my room, jogging and pounding each recollection into my keyboard, simultaneously numb and furious with myself. Why was it so hard to fight back? I should have just been my bubbly self *and* have said, "This Blaine guy acts all big and tough but really he's a wimpy liar!" How could I be so mute?

Besides the rollercoaster of emotional traumas throughout the rehearsal process, my body was also in a dangerous state of flux. Throughout rehearsals, I was in and out of hospitals for blood infections, wound leakages, and other nuisances of being a stomach-less medical mystery still on the mend. And every time I had a medical crisis, my emotional traumas and memories of Blaine went on the backburner, which in a way, was a relief. Despite all the challenges, I missed only one rehearsal.

Of course, the day before opening night, I came down with shingles. I was in unbearable (even for me) pain while also trying to rehearse my lines. On opening night, I was still in the hospital but managed to be discharged just one hour before I had to perform. I went on stage like a champ. Apparently, the male lead had called in that day and said he "wasn't feeling so well," to which the director replied, "Unless you're leaking from all the orifices in your body like Amy, you better show up tonight." We both did a great show.

In, "Nancy," I had a safe container in which to think about the guilt that tormented me my senior year. But what continued to baffle me was my previous silence about my abuser.

Performing *Oliver* also reminded me I had loved musical theatre long before I met Blaine. That rush I felt seeing William Finn, how I adored his musicals, it was always in me. Blaine didn't create it. Which meant he couldn't take it away. He only pulled it out of me temporarily.

In spite of envying the other actors—their complete physical freedom, their chugging water bottles between scenes—doing *Oliver* was the saving grace I needed. I could channel my emotions through Nancy, the abusive Bill Sikes's lover, with a heart of gold. A selfless heroine who is murdered for trying to protect Oliver, Nancy became another hero I could embody on my hero's journey. Rehearsals were also a tremendous period of physical growth for me. Although walking up three steps was enough to leave me winded, by the end of the production I was jumping and dancing on tables, albeit with a limp (still excruciatingly painful) left over from my neuropathy.

I had proven to myself what I was still capable of, what I could hope for more of in the future. I remembered how it felt to take my final bows on stage as a high schooler, thrilled to be in a community theatre production, or the wonderfully innocent stress of memorizing lines, the day-of-opening-night jitters, or trying to go on vocal rest during an entire day of high school.

The stage manager kept trying to pull up my neckline so my bag wouldn't pop up on top with that little white circle of adhesive that didn't look very period with the dress I had to wear, and before I went on stage every night I would pull it back down a bit because I wanted to wear it like a warrior badge. I proudly had earned it.

CHAPTER 12

Hello Numbness, My Old Friend

MY SHOW WAS OVER, THE CURTAINS had closed, my costume was cleaned...and that was it. I was also without a group of people to commune with every night. I was back to square one—or maybe square two, since I now carried the joy of returning to acting inside me—still hungry, still isolated, still living in crushing uncertainty. So, I went back to my reliable friend: numbness.

My job was to pass the helpless days as smoothly as possible, which meant staying in my room all day, dazing out, and exercising.

I was shocked and saddened that I could never get my old, unwounded body back. But what really startled me was realizing what had happened to my mind. When I wasn't distracting myself with exercise and mindless activities that often became compulsive, I was forced to think, to consider what was happening inside my head. I knew what "trauma" was, but I didn't know it could cause so much internal dis-ease and dis-order—illness that I couldn't see, illnesses that had initials, such as PTSD, or Post-Traumatic Stress Disorder. I had never heard those letters put together before. Now I began to realize I was living them.

And that was the biggest shock to me—waking up not just in a new body but also with a new mind, a mind troubled by nagging, intrusive, disturbing thoughts that wouldn't go away no matter how hard I chased them. But what was the cause? Just as my body was broken and not working properly, my mind was somehow fractured, and constantly frazzled, troubled with anxious thoughts, associations, and memories. Overwhelmed with confusion, I used the best resource I could think of—a search engine. I didn't realize I was suffering from Post-Traumatic Stress Disorder until the Internet defined it for me. Reading about the symptoms of PTSD, I was able to realize I wasn't crazy. There were reasons why I was experiencing so many strange sensations that made me feel alienated from the rest of the world.

According to NAMI, these are common symptoms that PTSD survivors experience.

Avoidance: It was too painful to remember every setback and struggle, too overwhelming to recall everything I had lost with every surgery—my innocence, my old body, my sense of self. When I started to feel these scary memories at any given time, I felt like I had to avoid any stimulant that might make me feel anything at all. When I was unable to eat, this was a survival mechanism. If I felt, I might actually feel the deadliest sensation of all—hunger.

Dissociation: When trauma left me emotionally and physically wounded, I froze to protect myself. I went numb so I didn't have to feel pain, and so I didn't have to re-experience what had happened to me and mourn my losses. Through dissociating, I could avoid really feeling what I need to feel—grief.

Hypervigilance: Staying out of my body and dissociating was how I coped with anxiety. Feeling tormented by my memories, which felt like present realities, I was anxious and irritable. If I couldn't constantly fidget or find another way to "numb out," I would start to panic and would be overwhelmed with even more intrusive memories and raw, forgotten emotions. My anger would end up being misdirected at others when really I just wanted to shout at my circumstances. My anxiety manifested in all the wrong places—I couldn't sit still in classes and couldn't function as a calm, responsible adult.

Uncontrollable Rage: This same angry, panicked and bottled energy manifested in me as I hurled myself at anyone who tried to get me to come out of my room. I could see life only in swift, blinding flashes, like an animal. It was how I withdrew. I then felt smeared in shame for long after, petrified of myself. This irrepressible, unhealthy energy was controlling my life.

What to do with this New Knowledge

Just when I thought the hardest part of life was staying in my room coping with my hunger, my medical circumstances would consume my life again, and I would land right back in the hospital. With disconnected intestines, I was susceptible to every infection in the book. We still had the goal of reconstruction, but no doctor would think of operating of me if I was constantly getting sick. After *Oliver*, I spent the stretch between Thanksgiving through New Year's in the hospital, most of it in tremendous pain from pancreatitis.

I had just gotten the hang of becoming a "person" after coming home from the ICU. I had a chocolate business, I could bench press half my weight, I had gotten the lead in a musical. Now, hospitalized again, I lost my sense of who I was and took on "patient mode" as new nurses mechanically stuck me, assessed me, and documented my every move. I brought my chocolate business pamphlets and photos from Oliver to prove, "Look, this is who I am, I'm a fighter, please don't judge me!" And I put up all my old pictures on the walls for them to see. With every week spent in that hospital room, I'd add more and more photographs, magazine cutouts, as if I was collaging my identity, anything to show who I was. I was fighting for my personhood and my life.

This time around, I had a few new coping skills to take with me to the hospital. Just as my parents had secretly snuck me out of the ICU to go shopping a year before, now they brought a double boiler so I could make chocolate *in the hospital*. Doing *Oliver* had also built up my confidence in a major healing resource: music. I had finally gotten back most of my voice, and to my dumbfounded-ness, when I put on a playlist in my hospital room, and I would start to sing along with it, using my voice actually brought me some kind of joy. I was reclaiming it. I had forgotten there were ways to feel bubbly inside and full of vitality, rather than full of fatigue or pain. Singing caused a sudden brain chemistry shift, and suddenly the hospital halls were alive with the sound of music!

Now music, theatre, and chocolate were my "islands of security." Like a kid playing the "hot lava game," by leaping onto each creative outlet, I was safe.

It felt good to feel again—through my voice. The holidays were the loneliest, most stark time to be in the hospital, but showtunes filled those days with light and sound.

I had this huge musical revelation back at Columbia hospital and delved into my first instincts of tears and feelings. With music, I could dip my toes into emotions without worrying that I'd drown. When the emotions got too much for me, I'd go back to my safety valve of becoming numb through exercise. Rather than think of this as suffering a relapse, I realized this was progress: I was dipping into "feeling" a bit at a time.

Music granted me the promise of becoming more human, balanced with dazing out for spurts of time in the hospital too. *Healing happens in the stages we're ready for.* That was the powerful lesson I learned when once again stuck in the hospital for months. It was okay to have setbacks. I could still find small ways to reclaim who I was. This time, it was through my voice. Finally, after Thanksgiving, Christmas, and the New Year we were discharged. This time, discharge was to a place that had finally become familiar, our beach house, and my home.

Discharged on a sunny Wednesday, I felt how stiff and powerless my legs had become, as immobile as when I was first learning to walk. I limped upstairs and shut the door to my room. Safely within the dark confines of my bedroom, I put on a CD, and gently moved my arms around to the music rather than exercising compulsively in counts of eight. I felt pulled into the swelling of the music, and my body sailed along the pulsing rhythm. Soon, I found myself leaping all over the place as if thrust up by life itself. Miraculously, the more I moved, the more my energy came back to me, and I became so emotional I started crying. I opened my door willingly (which I never did) and ran downstairs to my mother, screaming "Mom, I feel Grandma for the first time!" not even knowing what that meant. Alarmed by this foreign feeling of vitality (something I had taken for granted as a teenager), and suddenly nervous as to where it might go, I left Mom there crying, ran back to my room, shut off the music, and went back to compulsive exercise for the rest of the night. Despite the joy of my breakthrough, it was safer for me to just stick with what I knew.

The game I was playing, like a dog chasing its own tail, was fighting the obvious: to seal the gap with this cement, I had to learn to tolerate being with feelings that were being brought up through voice and dance, feelings that surfaced when I stopped exercising to keep them buried. I had every right and reason to want to take breaks from feeling present by numbing out through exercise and allowing healing to happen in small micro-stages.

In the hospital, I didn't have any other options. I had to face the pain, so I had to deal any way I could. The sun is shining out my window, and there are no surgeons running after me with scissors and sutures. The engineer will not be wheeling in his gigantic x-ray machine. It is actually calm. I am in my room typing on an ordinary Monday.

As I started to turn to the present moment, I started to sense that finding the magic in the world all around us is an effective way not just to cope with trauma but to begin to heal from it, just as the Hasidic story I had loved about finding the holy sparks in everything.

The new year brought a new thirst for spirituality in my life—a yearning for a higher dimension, stemming from an instinct that there was something more worth reaching and fighting for. Once we got home from the hospital again that New Year's Day, I started to feel the first pangs of spirituality within me through nature, through song, through every picture I took on my digital camera which I now took everywhere with me on my walks that I had traded for room time. I was starting to find the beauty in life again, and in spirituality, or what Blaine had called "the higher things." I was starting to think more in-depth about Blaine and feel the first tears of emotion well up inside me as I mourned his loss. For the first time, I asked myself the simplest of questions, "What matters to me most in life right now?"

I answered: "Nature, music, the promise of food."

Autumn's such a magically sensory season. The smell of Thanksgiving turkey in the oven, jumping in a pile of earthy leaves crisp as paper. Life has become a spectacle in the truest sense.

This new grounded positivity was interrupted by more medical setbacks when my PICC line became infected again, and I spent another few weeks at Bridgeport Hospital. I remember shivering in pain the entire night in the emergency room but then waking up the next day trying to see life with new, healthy eyes, even in a stretcher connected to the pole. Asking myself that same question, "What matters to me?" caused a slow, steady shift in my days.

What do you do when you are so used to living life one way that you're not even aware that it could be any other? I guess that's how someone feels when being kept captive. You are so used to the abuse that you don't realize life doesn't have to be like that and it's okay not to suffer. You have no idea what happiness is and that anyone can achieve it.

Things began to look brighter as my mindset improved. I was adjusting to the most gradual transition of all: health. This color spectrum was my only concrete measure of time. It was the only hope I had and fuel to want to keep going.

I woke up and said, "Good morning, Grandma," and thanked her for any blessing that could come my way today.

Grandma was my new "art song." Nature and spirituality were another island of creativity that helped me feel and discover my new identity, but in between, I had to keep swimming.

When I feel anxious, I touch the points of my Jewish star. To find a safe place inside, I imagine myself as the grain of rice, gracefully diving through the viscous oceans of myself, tumbling into the abyss of myself, keeping my wounded bird safe inside of myself.

I had battled for eight months before looking to other resources besides numbing out, exercising, and feeling sorry for myself. Instead of torturing myself with the Food Network all day, I needed to block myself from any kind of outside stimulation, or any reminder of the outside, living, breathing world. So, I went inward. I brought my laptop to my room and started to type, just to feel my fingers moving. My thoughts raced at a lightning pace as I breathlessly tried to document every anxiety shuffling through my brain.

I didn't realize how huge the pile of thoughts building up inside me was until my fingers first touched my chattering keys. As I typed, I realized just how much I was holding in. With the floodgates open, I locked myself in my room from seven in the morning until 8:35 p.m., I would lock my door, shut the blinds to keep out all external stimulation, and type, trying to unpack these thoughts I couldn't keep down.

Bubble, bubble, toil, and trouble; I cannot wait to write today, my fingers are getting the jitters! I love how the keys are rattling like skeleton teeth right now as I get excited.

I began writing everything down because, so afraid of feeling those emotions in my body, I transferred any physical sensations to the keyboard as a way to emotionally contain them. I didn't realize how numb my typing kept me, until turning the fan on caused me to burst into tears, just to feel the cool breeze spinning around the room stroking my body with a rush of air. Every bone in my body trembled, and now I could feel it.

Journaling became a compulsion, to document circumstances in my life that were unfamiliar, a way to process a life that I had been suddenly catapulted into. With the power of words, I could articulate my reaction to my life. Through words, I could start to create who I wanted to become.

Typing gave me a place to contain my thoughts. I quickly realized that by documenting all my thoughts, I didn't have to feel them. I could just expel them and be done. Even though I was out of the ICU, my survival as a human being was a minute-to-minute job. To stay on track, I had to create rules for myself.

I must keep moving. If I don't stop, then I won't think. If I don't think, I won't feel. If I don't feel, I can make it through another day.

Every morning I would start the same automatic routine. I imagined myself as a frog leaping from lily pad to lily pad, determined not to fall into the ocean of empty space. As soon as I woke up, I'd jump onto my first lily pad of safety—my yoga mat. Within its safe perimeter, I'd stretch for ninety minutes, limp downstairs in my bare feet, and pull open the freezer drawer to quickly snatch an ice cube, dreaming of the day I could open my fridge. From there, I'd run back upstairs, while rubbing that single ice cube over my cheeks, shut the door, and hop to my final lily pad of safety: the floormat with room for just my laptop, a standing desk, and my two feet.

Now, the job was to keep my mind on track. I would try to write about anything, free-associating just to stay alive. Whenever my mind wandered back to the tempting sound of the microwave, or the smell of the toaster, I'd panic and find something to type about. I could go on for twenty pages about the shade of green on my bedspread.

Soon I was hopping out of bed and jumping right to my laptop, anxious to record every feeling, emotion, and sensation. If I could document my life, it meant I existed. Unbeknownst to me, I was starting to create a narrative. It made me remember who I was and what exactly my uniqueness was. I was the only one who could document the insanity that my life was. If I didn't write about it, who would?

Since my leaving the ICU months before, my mother and I had regressed from being healing partners to the point where I would quarantine myself in my room and not talk to her, or anyone, all day. I hid myself in the two artificial worlds: the world of the ICU and the isolated world of my bedroom.

Every day I would type over sixty pages of thoughts, ramblings, questions, childhood memories, hopes, dreams (though I tried to resist letting myself dream too much), and stories I would make up in my head. By the end of the day, I'd have an entire packet that I would print out and slide under the door to my mother. She, in turn, would read my writing, circling things she liked, and commenting like a middle school teacher, then sliding it back under the door to me. We became pen pals in the same house, worlds away. The more I wrote, the more fantastical my writing became, and through words, I started to create a world of my own design within the four walls of my room. Fourteen hours glued to my laptop made each day pass. I was astonished there could be so many thoughts inside one little mind the way Max's room morphs into a jungle in *Where the Wild Things Are*.

Although it started as a way to kill time, the more I wrote, the more I realized I had a story to tell. I was remembering things from the hospital I had forgotten about for years. I realized that things I thought I had dealt with in a cinch had actually affected me emotionally on a deep level. I realized that the chaos of the past few years was now part of my story, like the Central Park Jogger, and that I had a worthy story to tell. By writing compulsively every day, I was telling myself that I was not the only one who had ever experienced pain, uncertainty or frustration. I was so alone, yet through my words, I felt more connected than ever.

As I wrote, I discovered ways to handle difficult situations successfully and to learn from my situation and grow. Strength is the ability to keep a positive attitude towards a situation that proves to be hard and manage it in a healthy way. Strength is the ability to overcome fear. The more definitions I was able to write, the more empowered I began to feel.

CHAPTER 13

A Book Starts with a Journey

I WAS WELL-ACCUSTOMED to my routine of pacing through Barnes & Noble. As long as there were aisles I could walk I was safe to venture out and move around in public realms as long as I kept my mechanical pace. But just as *The Courage to Heal* had stopped me years before, in another body and life, I was unprepared for one oversized coffee table book in the "Bargain Books" section.

It started with a ten-dollar mythology bargain book because I liked the pictures. In all the archetypal stories—folk tales, fables, mythology, children's books—an obstacle is an adventure, and it becomes the whole plot. Every obstacle or suspenseful twist is different, and memorably unique. A Greek god might have got trapped in the sun, or a chicken thought the sky was falling. Whatever the conflict, they were dealing with hurt, fear, pain, uncertainty, and so was I. And best of all, reading stories gave me something else to think about besides my own internal musings. I could turn my focus outward, yet still feel these stories related to what I was going through.

Mythology. A large picture book with ancient, romantic oil paintings. Figures reaching for one another, shields, armor, swords. Heroines and Goddesses. Flying horses, mountaintops and lightning bolts. Sweat, tears, determination, battles. Spring and rebirth. Darkness, graveyards of bones and tragedies—Greek tragedies—all of which I knew from the Disney Hercules cartoon, and that was about it. But what really struck me was the art—the Mayan murals of corn and rain Gods, the Norse gnomes and funny-shaped trolls.

I nervously stood with this heavy book weighing in my hands like cemented power. It was one of the few times I had the patience to tolerate the wait in the long (one person, but to me felt like ages) checkout line. Purchase finally in hand, I threw the book into a shopping bag and paced outside, waiting for my mother.

My mother tilted her sunglasses slightly over her nose as she stared at my bag. "You bought something?"

"Yeah." I tapped my toes on the seat as we drove the calculated eight minutes back home.

"What did you get?"

"I don't know. It's fine," I mumbled, my eyes focused on the road ahead, waiting to spot the front door, and planning the "complicated" trail out of the car, up the three steps to the front door, the staircase to my room, and that satisfying, safe relief the moment the door could slam and I could be alone.

But this time, I wouldn't be alone. I had a companion—a book of painted pictures, gods, and stories.

Me, My Laptop, and The Book in My Room

We pulled in. The car door slammed, then the front door, and finally the door to my room. At last my jogging feet, affectionately nicknamed "daggerfooting," could recommence their movement. As I dropped the book on my bed, the thud amidst the quiet, the rhythmic pitter-patter of my ASICS alarmed me as I stared at the cover.

MYTHOLOGY. How could one simple word contain all that lay within this volume? I couldn't help reading the caption under a Thor painting, and then the stories of Buddha, Prometheus, Quetzalcoatl.

I froze at a painting occupying an entire page. Jonah and the Whale. I read the margin note: *Jonah is swallowed in the belly of the whale. A hero's journey.*

Hero's journey? My feet kept moving, and the pages flipped faster. As I stared at the photographs, I was beginning to get the gist of these stories. Someone is going through a difficult time suddenly, after life was normal. A new dark world, like the belly of the whale!

In that world, this protagonist encounters multiple hurdles until he's literally spit out from darkness (or at least Jonah was!), then returns to the world changed by his experience. Simultaneously humbled and empowered. In the dark belly of the whale, Jonah was spit out and transformed.

That was why all these captions, paintings, and stories seemed happy and revelatory, even amidst death, darkness, tragedy, and unexpected changes. Within one big bargain book there were ghastly struggles with Gods and demons, whales and spiders, but every victim who was "preyed" upon ended up with some kind of treasure, lesson, or positive mission going forward.

The characters and places and specific events were different, but the stories all somehow felt the same. Even mine.

Flipping through, these were all stories of people taking actual trips—journeys that required persistence, faith, and resilience. A journey that wounded people, so they could by journey's end, be healed.

Discovering the Hero's Journey

Looking down at my body, I knew I had a lot healing to do but had no clue how my final "transformation" would take shape. Reading story after story, I got a feel for how a dark, unexpected journey could go.

That book initiated my shift from writing about my day locked in my room to writing made up stories. The words seemed to flow through me and never stop. By each night's end, I was exhausted and relieved as I spilled my entire soul onto my laptop screen. After I had drained myself of my own thoughts, I filled myself up with the stories of others. Every story had a hero. Learning about their heroic struggles, their failures and their triumphs, I began to form a roadmap for my own hero's journey.

Though it all felt new to me, I soon learned I wasn't the first person to discover this single thread that seemed to connect all of humanity, even me, to the world I peered at through my bedroom window.

All I had to do was jog my "daggerfeet" back to my laptop, Google "heroes mythology story," and there he was, Joseph Campbell. I clicked on a YouTube video: "Bill Moyers Joseph Campbell interview, 'Man and the Power of Myth, Part One.'"

In the documentary, Campbell described the hero's journey, and used the word "archetypal," a word I had never heard before, a word I later learned was another way to describe stories that felt universal. As with all things that helped me heal, I soon became obsessed with this foreign concept.

According to Campbell, "The Hero's Journey" is a recurring pattern of narrative that appears in drama, storytelling, myth, religious ritual, and human psychological development. It describes the typical adventure of the archetype known as "The Hero," the person who goes out and achieves great deeds on behalf of the group, tribe, or civilization.

If Luke Skywalker, Little Red Riding Hood, the Central Park Jogger, and any other famous protagonist could be heroes, why not me? I was a warrior on a journey battling to reclaim my identity.

Looking Back Gave Me Courage to Move Forward

As I pushed myself to move forward, I also allowed myself to think about my life before trauma. This was my pattern—yearn for the outside world, taste it just enough to be overcome with emotion, which would scare me too much to feel anything.

I was determined to keep pushing through the unnumbered days into the expansive void of future. I realized it was not the uncertainty I feared, but that things would never get better. Was I tough enough to stand that possibility? If I wasn't, I had to become someone who was. So, I created a brave warrior self and named her "Tiger Lilly." She gave me the courage to go forth believing things would, somehow, improve. With the hero's journey as the archetype for my struggle, I finally had a roadmap for surviving and overcoming trauma.

Becoming a Warrior: Tiger Lilly

A personality trait is a characteristic that is distinct to an individual. To create my new identity (since my old one had been stripped away), every day I gave myself a warrior trait.

I wasn't a patient, I wasn't a victim, and I wasn't a survivor. I was the protagonist of my own story who was being tried and tested: a warrior. Always fascinated by their ferocity, power, prowess, and beautiful black and orange stripes, I identified myself as a tiger, inspired by the fables I was reading about animals and myths I was reading involving animal gods and spirits.

If I was going to "do" the hero's journey, I was going to do it full out. After all, I was an actress.

Coming out of the hospital, I had felt like "Wounded Amy," a fragile, small, wounded bird with an injured wing. Now, I was "Tiger Lilly: A Professional Wounded Healer" (it even said so on my handmade business cards). And it was the job of Tiger Lilly, the thriving hero of the story, to rescue the wounded bird in a heroic act of bravery. Now, healing seemed thrilling, adventurous, and exciting. My room was a real live jungle. No trespassers allowed.

What traits define a real warrior? For each of my warrior traits, I assigned myself a different symbol, going through the day as a poet on the hunt for metaphors. Everything I spotted became a magic compass to guide me on the next step of my hero's journey. My warrior traits became my timeline, my roadmap, my game plan in a realm of no answers. Like a calendar, they marked my time until that magical day of reconstruction—the day everything would be normal. Each trait built up so much courage, that for the first time in months, it became a struggle to stay hidden in my room.

The Courage to Leave My Room

Finding the next warrior symbol became the purpose of each day. Once a symbol spoke to me, I'd devote the rest of the day writing poems about it, paying homage through art and stories. As I read more chapters of the mythology book, my own hero's journey began to take shape. I envisioned myself crossing further and further over the threshold into the unknown and emerging from the other side, somehow triumphant. This gave Tiger Lilly courage to start emerging into the scariest place of all: the world outside my room.

My expanding thoughts were becoming too large for the confines of my four walls. My mother had been asking me (in a handwritten comment on my printed-out journals, of course) if I wanted to accompany her on a small shopping trip. Saying no was automatic. It was dangerous and unthinkable to venture out of my room. But slowly the hero's journey was empowering me with the courage to leave and see the big wide-open world I had been reading about. I was keyed up for a thrilling, action-packed experience the day I finally left my room. After all, I was the hero reintegrating back into the outside world!

What I found instead was an ordinary life with me in it, not the old me, not the hero me, but the broken me I was still trying to get away from. A wounded bird that didn't belong in the big open outside world, where everyone else was healthy.

I was looking forward to going to the mall because I thought it would give me all of this life experience and I'd see all the objects come alive in my mind like the animatronics at Disney World, but I'm too hungry to live in the world now.

Tiger Lilly could provide me with all the strength in the world, but at the end of the day, it was like being asked to sit at that fancy Italian restaurant for my parents' 40th wedding anniversary, staring at a glass of water I wasn't allowed to drink. It wasn't fair, and there was little I could do to make it any easier.

I didn't let myself get too discouraged. I went to a china shop with my mother the next week with a different strategy: I pretended that every sight, smell, and action around me was a magical symbol, a good luck totem, or a mystical prize left for me by a genie of warriors who would help guide my way.

You have to believe in magic for it to appear. Without magic in our lives, we're lost. The more I forced myself out of my room, the more comfortable I became; and I soon became acquainted with an old friend: joy.

I made that trip to the china shop the most magical experience of my life. Like a genie, I decided to grant a wish, my own wish, and make it so. "Poof." How could Tiger Lilly turn this china shop into an enchanted far off land?

Now outings with my mother were scary in an exciting, bone-thrilling way—an epic adventure! The outside world no longer intimidated me, because I had turned the uncertain real world into an entertaining scavenger hunt. I wasn't lost. I was *exploring*. It was a warrior's shift in mindset, and I could handle this!

Finding the symbolism in everything made life burst hidden magic and wonder. I could escape through the fantasies in my own mind when hunger and life-pangs rang too deep—the hero's temptation.

Once I started leaving my room, even though my circumstances hadn't changed, I was happier. I finally felt connected to the world. I remembered what was important in life, and who I *really* was, even if only for a nanosecond. As difficult as it was or me to venture into the outside world, I didn't realize it was hard for my mother, wondering what people were thinking of me.

I was too invested in the bold task of self-discovery that came with every outing to care what others thought of me. Tiger Lilly's mission helped me take the calm pauses in my day I had been running from out of fear they would be filled with hunger cues. Connectedness was my holy grail, coating me in the security and protection I had been searching for so long.

A warrior keeping herself captive in a comfortable bedroom in a nice suburban may seem odd. Was I losing my mind, deliriously creating fantasy worlds every minute? Had years of being stuck in hospitals caused me to lose it? Maybe. But how else would you advise someone to go forth into the outside world, deal with drains, wires, IVs, while missing school, unable to work or maintain any normal routine, with liquid coming out of a bag on your neck, and unable to have a morsel of food for an indefinite amount of time? There was no course of travel for me. So, I mapped out my own. Thinking of my endless expanse of "healing" time as a journey rather than "limbo" was massively empowering. A hero is someone who goes through a trauma with a purpose—to reemerge with a gift that heals others. Becoming a warrior was my way of finding the beautiful adventures behind every painful transition. I wanted to live life as a seeker because, after all, life is what you seek from it. At last, my seemingly shapeless life had a shape, a structure. Thanks to Tiger Lilly, I had a purpose.

CHAPTER 14

Creating Frank

WITH TIGER LILLY'S HELP I could now call myself a "hero." But the body I was in, a body hooked up to tubes, a body that couldn't eat, it didn't feel like a hero's body. It couldn't be. If "Tiger Lilly" helped me see myself as a warrior, maybe I needed to create another "friend" who could help me process what had happened to my body and the person inside this now unrecognizable shell. So, I wrote about "Frank," a long-lost friend whose story was remarkably similar to mine.

For the "separation from the known" part of the journey, I sent Frank, my alter ego, on an African safari, where, although all signs clearly state that "Feeding the animals is forbidden," Frank ignores the warning and leaves the safety of the trolley after being captivated by an intriguing lion he spots, singing atop a passing hill. Frank walks forward into the vast savannah while the tour guide screams, "You're not supposed to leave the tour!" But Frank keeps walking until the trolley vanishes off in the distance. He's stranded but still curious, and he wanders over to the lion, a stand-in for Blaine.

Though the lion seems intimidating, he turns out to be friendly and takes Frank up to the sky, to his magical kingdom in the clouds (the lion can fly, of course), and transforms him into a songbird. They float together in the heavens with music and magical eggs and sunshine. The lion's mane grows as big as the rays of the sun, and Frank discovers that this lion is actually the ruler of a musical paradise where the winds turn into the staffs of sheet music which turn into little rafts they can float on using the music notes as oars to row through the air. As a bird, Frank is granted the ability to lay magical eggs with music notes inside of them. Lion Blaine, with his fiery mane of music, inspires Frank to unexpected heights and becomes his mentor.

Doodling this cartoon lion, I visualized his tail coiling slowly closer to Frank, the songbird, and was struck with one thought: *I know how this story will go.*

The lion's tail reached towards Frank, and Frank and the lion become close, connecting through musical staffs, and he takes me under a cloud. His tail grows longer and turns a sickly green until it morphs into a snake that seizes Frank, the songbird, and thrusts him inside of a cloud. Trauma strikes as Frank's tears turn the clouds to rain.

Through this image, I began to process Blaine's betrayal and surprising transformation. Just as the lion's tail had morphed into a vicious snake, Blaine had taken advantage of my trust and locked me in a paralyzing situation. I put myself in Frank, the wounded songbird's position.

In the thunderstorm, the snake bites my wing, and it starts to bleed so I cannot fly away, and instead, I fall into the forming ocean of my tears. The snake rips open the eggs of my soul, and all the music notes fall into the water. They turn into lightning bolts. I am now the wounded bird with a bleeding wing, and the blood pours into the ocean and spells out "This is your blood." As the snake sips the blood, it grows the monstrous tail of a serpent.

The snake follows me underwater as I drown and turns into a sea serpent who locks me in an underwater sea cave. My body freezes in the trauma while my soul bird flies away into the ocean, symbolizing the trauma forcing me to leave my body. My body then turns to bones, frozen in shock in the cave. The wounded bird hides in the ocean, desperate to collect her blood again, but I am stuck dead and lifeless as sardine bones, cut off from my soul, too frozen to feel anymore.

This was how I visualized the damage that Blaine had done. I knew he had touched my body, but I was not ready to fully acknowledge the harm he had done. By letting the cartoons guide me on a journey and allowing the story to unfold, I discovered that in his act of physical invasion, I had suffered emotional damage as well.

That's it! When Blaine started to abuse me, I felt paralyzed because his tail trapped me and then coiled around me in circles. I finally understand why the compulsive exercise started, and the mechanical "circles" my mind started racing in.

The damage those circles did went further than I thought. My visualization started to connect the dots; the serpent plants poisonous seeds on my bones and piles bricks into me. The seeds just weigh on me, heavy, like secrets. He is trying to get whatever soul juice I have left, but there is nothing. I am just a skinny, shriveling fish. As the lion flips me around, he tries to snuggle with me, but his skin is slimy, cold, and slithery.

The abuse had caused such a buildup of guilt and shame. Ugly feelings paralyzed me. The snake strangled my voice, filling me with secrets until something in me wanted to burst. Not being able to tell anyone about what was happening during my voice lessons was keeping my voice and anger inside, which was manifesting in all the wrong places.

As I visualized the angry, toxic seeds, I started to feel them in my core where my stomach once was. Pieces started to connect. The seeds in my stomach felt fiery, hot, sharp, and strangely similar to the severe stomach ache I'd felt when rushed to the emergency room on that fateful Passover night.

The medical trauma, my stomach exploding. The sexual trauma, the buildup of anger and secrets. Was it so far-fetched to connect these eerily similar physical sensations?

This visualization provided me with a healthy distance from which to view my trauma while still letting me confront what had happened to me and piece everything together.

In Frank's story, the volcanoes burn up all of the water, and the fire turns the ocean floor into a desert. The coiled lion's tail reminds me of another "wiry" invasion—medical IV wires. This unifying wire was now connecting the sexual abuse to the also paralyzing world of the surgical ICU. I understood how the surgical ICU made me freeze and numb out in the same way Blaine had. I knew Blaine's abuse had immediately caused compulsive exercise, and these snake-like medical wires had done the same.

Back in the waterless desert, those seeds within me cannot grow into plants and thrive, and instead, scorpions crawl into my skull and move me around, representing how I had no control over my body because the surgeons decided exactly what to do with it. As I drew the scorpions, I started to connect the dots, both figuratively and literally, as I felt the red tension crawl up and down my legs like ants and make a knot in my chest. The red ants have the same effect as the poisonous seeds, and they keep crawling all over me, the living embodiment of the nervous tension and anxiety that overwhelms me and my feelings of helplessness through my medical trauma.

That was it! Through my pen, and Frank's hero's journey, I was starting to figure out where these nervous red ants of tension were coming from. Things were making sense, and wires were starting to connect, just as my cartoons guided me from frame to frame. Running in place was keeping me frozen. And now my pen was starting to connect this frozen state to the heated, paralyzing pain I had felt the night I was sent to the emergency room.

I'm helpless to swat the ants off of myself, so they stay and lay millions of little eggs that lie dormant in me. Meanwhile the snake winds around me so tight that it gathers up the desert sands and creates a tornado. I try to use my daggerfeet to escape, but they only make everything spin faster, and the more numbers the snake pumps into me, the wider the current of the tornado.

"Daggerfeet" were my body's attempt to get free. But spinning around with these wires just created a tornado that was slowly sucking me into its eye.

That "eye" I was stuck in kept me further from the river I wanted to rejoin. But I couldn't. And cartooning the songbird, now a pile of bones in the desert, I started to remember my ways of coping when I was discharged from Bridgeport Hospital.

Locking myself in my room, I had stacks of empty notebooks I was anxious to fill, with pens and pencils crammed into tumbler glasses where water should be.

Keep the pen moving and don't look at your watch, I'd remind myself, as a warm glaze of numbness was every so often interrupted by the sound of a bird out the window or the phone ringing downstairs.

The pace of my scribbles accelerated with the exciting realizations I was making through these notebooks, literally tracing back what had happened to me as I tried to doodle my way back to a life of control. With my pen, I was unafraid. I could access the next difficult memory: How did I start losing weight? When did Blaine start abusing me? When did I "freeze?" I didn't know. *But the pen did.*

Once Blaine, the slimy sea serpent snake, bit Frank, the glorious songbird, his wing bled in the ocean. The snake sucked the wounded bird's blood up, and the bird turned into a skinny little wounded fish in the dark, wide, vast ocean. Then, the serpent locked the fish up in a cold underwater sea cave in Manhattan.

The skinny fish turned skeletal as it got colder in the cave, and as the cave got blocked off more and more, the snake didn't even have to try to prevent the fish from leaving the cave. The fish was frozen, just as I was frozen with the secret of abuse.

Creativity allows you to be fearless, reckless, unashamed, and gives you a kid-like will to think out of the box. Cartooning these stories was fantastical and childlike and so far from reality. I created symbols that helped me piece together my life, guided by the pen, the hero's journey, and the inner knowing that others had been on this path before me. Where did I want to go after all this? I thought of Grandma and wondered where I would find my liberation. My pen did the rest as it drew what became a temple. Frank gets stuck in the river just as he is about to approach the temple and finds himself sucked into this white-water rapid vortex that lies hidden beneath the river.

Swimming along the river means surrendering, and listening to your inner voice, following your true, wet and watery instincts to find your way back home, to your temple, in order to hear your deepest, darkest secrets, to Blaine and his abuse. Drawing Frank swimming to the temple himself, I felt like an athlete with a single-minded focus on that glorious finish line. I saw the "temple." I didn't know what was inside, or when I'd get there, but I knew that aiming for it would unwind me out of the terrible cyclone I was drowning me in. I had something to look forward to!

Through my cartoon, I realized why I didn't think about Blaine's betrayal when I was numb dealing with my medical circumstances.

When I was just bones in the desert, unable to eat or drink, how could I have noticed a spring? I couldn't.

I was ready to claim back my life. This warrior was all set to go, back to body, back to living! This is my blood! Maybe this darkness I was going through could become a warrior's adventure!

I started structuring my days like a hero's story—Frank's Journey. Now, the hours flew by in my room! But even Frank's Journey wasn't enough to stifle my frustrated angst, which I tried to drown out through movement.

As my health improved, and I felt physically stronger, I could no longer contain my frustration in my writing. Even though I couldn't eat, the TPN gave me an excessive amount of energy and stamina that at first, made me uncomfortable. Thankfully, I found a yoga class.

With as many looks as I received, I still bravely toted my IV bag to hot yoga until I was kindly asked to come without being connected to an IV line as that might make my classmates "uncomfortable." Ninety-six-degree yoga without a sip of water down my throat was torture, yet gaining calm, poised and centered physical strength gave me a new kind of peaceful confidence. Yoga re-introduced me to my body in a way I could feel strong, mindful, firm, yet relaxed at the same time. It was a healthy way to channel my energy, become centered in my body, and with each asana, I found a place of comfort within myself.

My manic energy would eventually be explained to me in a book, *Waking the Tiger*, by Peter Levine, which would become my warrior's manifesto. He explained that in the time of a very traumatic event, an individual uses such an abnormal amount of energy to persevere. In PTSD, the individual becomes stuck, frozen in that moment of terror, and that energy is never discharged. Therefore, when the traumatized individual is persisting on life after the trauma, they exist in this state of frozen, manic energy, which comes off like an unnatural state of hyperactivity. This is how I existed for years, and it surfaced as "jogging (daggerfooting) in place."

For a normal human, this might have seemed like an effort: jogging while writing philosophical essays about the hero's journey. But at the time, it was more anxiety provoking for me to stand still. I was looking for any way to stomp out any empty space in my day. Stillness meant quiet. Quiet meant time to think or feel. And that meant death.

For now, mastering the art of survival meant distraction—constant movement in any way possible. The feeling that I most needed to distract myself from, besides hunger, was unbearable sadness, which posed a constant threat of friending me with un-cried tears.

My numbness served as the greatest protection to the news that would prove to be more devastating than any news I had received so far: the deaths of my grandparents.

The day started like any other day, typing, numbing out in my room, with a half hour left before I would dart out, bypass the kitchen, and head straight for the car for a ballet class, hopping from activity to activity, passing another day, out of breath, exhausted enough to sleep. As I was mentally preparing myself to open the doorknob and race out nervously into the outside world for a brief hour, my mom knocked on the door so softly I could barely hear it.

"Amy," Mom said with trepidation in her voice. "I just want to tell you...that...Grandma died."

I couldn't say anything. I was so numb I didn't know how to absorb it. This could not be happening. I didn't even get to say goodbye.

This was the biggest reality check I had gotten so far. It was the harshest realization that, things are different post-coma. I'll never get back Grandma. But I couldn't grieve. I was so focused on getting through that the buildup of tears in my chest terrified me. Immediately, I tried to stomp out the despair with preoccupation about getting to ballet on time. When the class ended, I rushed back and locked my bedroom door, leaving the blinds down for extra darkness, exercising for the rest of the night until I was sure I had coated myself in numbness. I believe if, in that moment, I had made the space in my heart to cry, I would have never stopped. Just like losing my dog, Gabby, a piece of my childhood was forever gone, and I wasn't ready to leave my numbness and bear the massive weight of grief.

So, I did the only thing I knew how to—run.

Thinking of Grandma

GRANDMA WAS BECOMING MY ANGEL, giving Tiger Lilly a new, spiritual direction.

Lately, I feel her presence in a subtle way that sometimes stabs me in the heart when I least expect it. I think I am starting to feel a deeper presence with everything I do and trust God more and more. The invitation to do more than just "get through" life is on the table for me. I don't see anything else I can do but take it sooner or later.

Grandma became the new symbol of hope on my hero's journey. I elevated her to mythological status, and through this frame, I was able to grieve her.

What could Grandma, my personal spirit guide, do for my loneliness and despair now? She would always say she wanted to dance at my wedding. There's a wedding going on inside of me marrying all of my different selves together, and she's in my heart dancing, giving it a lively beat.

A Thanksgiving with no Food

I could only ascend so far without a stomach. My life was constantly about negotiating to not get too carried away and eat my feelings. Whether we wanted it to or not, time was zooming right in front of us. And we were stuck. Then we'd hope the same for next year, thinking we were much farther along than we actually were. However, it is that hope-bordering-on-insanity/denial that sustained us.

My mom and I would also mark time by the seasonal rotations in the mall. After Christmas, Hallmark would release their Valentine's Day cards, which would quickly transition to St. Patrick's Day, Passover, then graduation cards, Fourth of July, and then we would be back at the harvest-themed Halloween, followed by Thanksgiving, and back to Christmas cards. One year, two, three... With each passage, we were left flat-faced, scrambling to be a part of the real, forward-moving scope of time in society. The changing cards showed us that while we waited in limbo with a half-completed digestive tract, life would not wait, yet left us waiting, and window shopping with envy.

With nothing else to do, my dad took me for a walk down our street. That was all we knew how to do to distract. Walk. But this was the worst time to take a walk down our street because everywhere we looked, people were stuffing their faces, heartily enjoying their Thanksgiving dinners. Through the screen doors, we could hear the football games coming from the TV. I held Dad's large bear-like hand as tightly as I could and cried, "When will that ever happen for us?"

As hard as this was for me, I couldn't imagine how hard it was for a father to not be able to reassure his daughter when she would have Thanksgiving again. Not only were we the black sheep family on the street, but we were also this inhuman tribe of nomads displaced from the world of normalcy where people were able to pick out cans of pumpkin from the store, bake pies, and have a reason to have people in their life and at their dinner table. Life for me was as sterile and dark as that rainy day.

For someone who had always loved life, I felt guilty waking up each day just trying to kill time. Yet that was what I needed to do to survive. I wanted to scream, "What would you like from me, God? What would you do in my position?" How was I was supposed to feel human knowing food would kill my body?

Grandma was now my close-up, personal version of God, but I could no longer hear a message from her. As she watched from above, I questioned whether she was ashamed to see me like this. Grandma always loved life even after enduring her struggles. Here I was, alive, yet trying to kill every hour of the precious time I still existed on Earth. Could her angelic spirit bear to see me numbly exercise my way through every day?

Part of me yearned to hear her voice, so she could tell me how she would handle a trauma like mine. I needed to know that as dead as I tried to make myself feel inside, there was still something larger above and around me. I needed her guidance to assure me I was hanging in there for a reason.

One tall tree stands at the end in a clearing. And Grandma's arms come out of the tree, and I am running to her as fast as I can like a little child with the wind running through my hair. The tree turns into a soft figure, into Grandma in her flowery kitchen robe, who hugs me into nighttime and sings me a lullaby. When the sun comes back up, Grandma is not there anymore, but birds are peacefully chirping in the sky. I hug the tree and her spirit comes out and says, "I will always be with you."

Progress was slow, if at all, and TPN was causing my liver enzymes to elevate. TPN was never meant as a long-term solution, even though it was saving my life.

Leaving it to my dad to find some creative answers, he found a doctor in the radiology department at Mt. Sinai who came up with a radical procedure they weren't sure would work. Nobody wanted to open me surgically at this point; it would be too much of a risk. But if they could get a feeding tube into my intestines, they could give my liver some time to heal. Feeding my gut was much healthier for my body in the long term than feeding me through my veins. Miraculously, they were able to insert a feeding tube without surgery. Although I intellectually appreciated that this was somehow a step forward, I was frustrated because, at the end of the day, I still couldn't eat. Now, not only did I have to be hooked up to an IV pole for TPN every night but had to spend all day with a feeding tube in a backpack for twenty-four hours each day at home.

But soon, twenty-four hours became twenty-three. When you lose your freedom then get it back, you discover newfound gratitude. How could I forget the joy of me doing my first cartwheel a year later when the doctors finally allowed me to cycle my hours with the feeding tube? How amazing it felt to rip that feeding tube out of my hip for an hour and turn myself upside down like that! That cartwheel made me feel like a giant Ferris wheel, so boundless and glorious because that was my only hour of the day I didn't have to drag that backpack around. I had forgotten what it felt like to have the open summer breeze blowing on my bare skin.

CHAPTER 16

College Revisited

BY NOW, A YEAR HAD PASSED at home, and my friends had already finished their first year of college without me. With all the reading and writing consuming each day of my homeschooled "life education," I found my thoughts moving from Grandma and my past to college and my future. University of Michigan's musical theatre program had always been my first choice, and even with an IV pole and a bag on my neck, I was determined to make it happen.

I had been out of the hospital for a year, and now my family and I flew to Michigan again, this time with an esophagostomy bag on my neck and a PICC line on my arm. It was my first post-coma plane trip and a new ordeal in itself. The biggest fuss was passing security. I didn't realize that all of the medical bags attached to me filled with liquid would set off the sensors, and I was given my first official "pat down." I was an equal mix of nervous and excited as my parents followed behind me with three heavy bags of extra luggage, filled with medical supplies and IV bags. From that point on, we realized we'd have to allot several hours for passing through airline security.

I was still convinced I would be able to attend, even though I couldn't eat or drink and was sustained only by IV nutrition. But there were some things I hadn't factored in. For one, I didn't realize how exhausting getting around campus would be. I could no longer run up the stairs to the theatre building as I had when I first visited.

Michigan was a bittersweet reminder of the gap I felt widening between me and the rest of the world passing me by. The students were eager to meet me, and many were the same ones I was meant to enter with the previous year. Now they were "experienced" sophomores, and they kindly gave me a tour. Besides discounting my physical limitations, I hadn't thought about what would be most difficult for me in college until it was time for my tour guides to grab lunch at the cafeteria, or they wanted to take a study break at Starbucks where all I could do was eyeball their drinks and try to explain why I couldn't have a sip of anything without them thinking I had an eating disorder.

I was happy to see the chair of the program, Brent Wagner, for whom I had auditioned in what seemed to be another life. Although kind and gracious with his time, he could not hide his sadness. Throughout my visit, he and the entire department treated me with the utmost respect, and a month later I received a letter from the department. It politely informed me that, although my spirit was extraordinary, it would be implausible for me to keep up an intense conservatory program with my current medical situation and concluded that it was best I *not* attend. My theatre dreams were crushed.

Michigan's compassionate letter didn't stop my parents from believing I could go back to college that year. Before my coma, I had also been accepted at Northwestern University in Chicago. The NU theatre department willingly accommodated me and even arranged for a visiting nurse to come to campus. A few forms and countless duffel bags later, my freshman year of college began!

Recognizing that I hadn't even spent one night on my own since I was in the hospital, and because I was still dependent on potentially dangerous IVs, my devoted mother booked a hotel in Chicago and committed to staying for as long as I'd need her. She found a gym, cozy cafes, and made herself a home in the Windy City. I made it through orientation, albeit winded trying to keep up with my classmates. I was thrilled to be a college student yet couldn't shake off feeling like an alien. It wasn't long before I felt safer hiding in the bathroom. My fellow students were shocked to hear my story and admired my courageous spirit, but no one knew what to make of me. I had been so out of touch with the real world and people my age for so long that I didn't know what to talk about or how to act. All I had was my story.

On the first official day of my college career, walking around campus and managing my courses took much more strength than I had anticipated. Sure, I had jogged in place thousands of miles (while writing!) on a floor mat at home, but the energy to be present, engaged, alert, and connected took ten times more energy than the stamina it took to exercise myself numb. Unable to focus, I began dissociating, walking around in a fog, inundated by so much stimulation, while at the same time, protecting myself from it by tuning out. People waved as I robotically passed them, addressing me as though we'd had a previous conversation. I had no idea who they were. That time remains so blurry to me I can't even tell you what courses I signed up for.

It's one thing to be in a numb daze at home, coping in your room, but when you're on your own, a thousand miles from home and in charge of keeping your PICC line completely sterile circumstances become dangerous and one careless incident becomes life-threatening.

Mom: Matthew came to visit, and I suggested going to her dorm to see if she was okay. I had a bad feeling. We went up to her room and walked in to find her on the floor almost comatose. She was lightheaded and out of it.

We called a taxi and rushed her to the hospital. They told me we'd saved her life.

Barely breathing, I was ambulanced to Evanston Hospital. When labs were drawn in the ER, we learned that I had a serious PICC line infection. I remember telling the doctors that my professor was going to be so upset if I was late to his 5 p.m. lecture and asked if they could make sure I was discharged in time to get there.

Northwestern Hospital was a new and unfun reality check. A new doctor was introduced to my medical saga—Dr. Buch. Right away I didn't like him.

"Eating on your own is like pissing on air," Dr. Buch's said, laughing at the idea of me ever being able to get all my nutrition from food. So much for bedside manner. He put me on IV nutrition with four huge pumps attached to one pole, more IVs then I remember ever being chained to at once. I felt as if I was being put in jail, but this flood of nutrition did stabilize me after an infection that nearly ended my life. Great! I'd learned my lesson. *Now, I can go back, right?* Then the second reality check got cashed: the NU administration, alarmed at how I had been found, kindly told my mother over the phone that perhaps attending college was not the safest decision at this point. What?!

I was angry. Two college experiences had been yanked away. Would I ever be able to live a happy, healthy, independent, normal life, or would I be doomed to live in hospitals forever?

Despite these setbacks, my indefatigable dad was continuing to play the hero, trying to round up all the medical opinions he could because he was convinced that one day, I would be able to absorb food and eat on my own. My dad would not rest until he found someone who agreed with him. Besides being crushed by my second "expulsion," I resented the hospital for keeping me for so long, on constant TPN, away from my home, my family, and my college dreams. I wanted to stop caring. *Was I ever getting to college?*

I wanted to escape my situation so badly that I did some things that weren't so smart, like taking a break to go out when my mom and dad were visiting me in the hospital. I was feeling so angry, anxious, stir crazy, and frankly, just plain crazy that I snuck my IV pole downstairs to the lobby, out the door, and into an adjacent Walgreens. Imagine a seventy-pound girl pushing an IV pole twice her size across a city street and through drugstore aisles! As I cruised the store pulling that motherlode four-pump TPN pole behind me, the tubes shattered, and a lady freaked out because I got saline on her pants. I frantically tried hoisting the pole up so I could get the hell out of there. I didn't expect the pole to be taller than the entrance. The ensuing crash sent my IV pole hurtling to the ground and the contents of the tiny vials smashing onto a customer.

Like the antibiotic vials, I was busted. I was also shocked, terrified, and mortified. Worse, I was going to be in major trouble if or when everyone found out about this. So, I tried to hoist up my IV pole again and walked (I couldn't run) as fast as I could along the sidewalk. Soon I was being chased by staff on their walkie-talkies, hearing "she's heading upstairs!" and hiding behind an elevator as they darted past me. Somehow, I made it back to my room before my parents returned. To this day, I cannot remember how I explained my broken IV pole to my parents and doctors.

I do remember a statement Dr. Buch made to my parents, words that have always stuck with me. "I don't think she's bought into this 'life thing' yet."

He was right. When we were ready for round three, my parents and I envisioned Columbia University as a reality. I had been accepted there, and the administration was understanding of my condition. Most important, it was much closer to home and felt feasible given my medical needs.

I fell into a coma two days before I had to turn in a deposit to one of the colleges I was accepted to. I received a scholarship to Columbia University, and they have generously offered to take me every year. And every year, because I was right in the middle of a medical crisis, I had to defer. However, I just got another letter still offering the scholarship to me. Next fall, God willing, I AM GOING TO COLLEGE!!!

After agonizing consideration, my parents decided college would be too risky until after surgical reconstruction. Sadly, I had to defer Columbia once again.

I had gotten more than enough life education, and my mother and I had crafted our own college curriculum. We met daily, reading piles of self-help books, filling out writing prompts, and creating our own assignments. Our bookshelf was covered with everything from Buddhist philosophy to Julia Cameron, and every book from the "Healing" section at the bookstore, along with books on finding yourself, losing yourself, art tutorials, and everything in between. We had established our own self-serve treatment center in our Westport home.

Next year I'll be a Columbia student. But till then, who am I? Being a chocolatier for a few hours a day isn't going to cut it. I need a real job!

By now, I had been out of the hospital for two years, and life had begun to take on a normal pace, as normal as it could be without food. With IVs, feeding tubes, and daily nurse visits, I couldn't be a student, but perhaps I could be a teacher. After all, I was teaching myself lessons every day as "Tiger Lilly," the warrior on her hero's journey. After discussing with my parents, we decided that despite my medical condition, I was ready to have a real job (besides Professional Healer/Warrior).

What can you do in the real world without a stomach? What role in society could keep me connected but not taunt me with hunger?

Then I had an idea. On a shopping trip out with my mom, I spotted children running out of a school building. The euphoric sound of their laughter made me realize I had to work with kids.

I applied to be an aide in a local nursery school classroom, and they hired me! Three-year-olds reminded me what matters most in life. I learned how to be present, the value of play, what it means to have a friend, and the healing that comes from honest communication and cooperation. After only speaking with my family and medical professionals for years, I regained a sense of innocence by connecting with children and their wisdom.

One morning, an adorable three-year-old named Isabelle with dark brown hair and piercing blue eyes was sitting tucked inside her cubby, staring down at the floor with her ankles sadly crossed.

"I'm very sad today."

"Why is that?" I asked.

"I can't think of any *Star Wars* adventures to dream about, so I don't know what I am going to make-believe today!"

I was touched by how Isabelle depended on the safe haven of her fantasies to pass the time, the adventures in her mind as the highlight of her day, and if she couldn't find those dreams in her that day, then the day was lost. I envied how she clung to that importance, and it made me wish my imagination was vivid enough to be my world, a world I could play in, rather than fret over medical circumstances beyond my control. I realized I needed to find my *Star Wars* adventures dreams like Isabelle.

Teaching nursery school, I learned to re-trust my own buried-away fantasies and allow them to send me soaring for the day, not caring where they ended up landing. Sometimes, all it takes is a daydream to make us feel the joy of our aliveness. Other times, we just need to tuck ourselves inside a cubby with Isabelle and wish for more dreams to replenish our souls. For the first time after my coma, I realized I didn't "lose" my sense of purpose in the operating room but, rather, that my purpose had taken a new direction, a beautiful, child-like detour. Isabelle would have said I was going on a treasure hunt for health, a heroic journey, an epic *Star Wars* adventure daydream.

My students also taught me that it's okay to be out in the world and just have fun spinning around in circles until you are so dizzy that you fall down and get grass stains on the back of your pants. It's not about what we accomplish, but what we dream because those dreams are seeds of a soul we can only know through unashamed play. On another day, I set up a big bucket of dried rice with plastic spoons in it. This bucket of rice offered infinite possibilities, which they eagerly explored. The children had to trust that whatever decision they made would be the best decision possible, all because they chose it.

In the classroom, I learned that creativity happens in unplanned circumstances when children help each other discover things that enlighten them in a way no teacher or lesson plan can. Watching my nursery school children make rice-scooping decisions, build playful relationships, make creative discoveries, and laugh at beautiful mistakes, I gained confidence in my life circumstances. I learned that happiness is not such a lofty ambition. It was as available to me as the nearest package of dried rice at the grocery store.

When asked to serve Lorna Doone cookies to the kids, unable to have one myself while the kids requested seconds and thirds, I would still gladly comply, even to the point where the other teacher told me they'd had enough.

But I couldn't help it; snack time was my favorite time of the day, and I found the greatest joy in giving those kids cookie after cookie. I loved watching the joy on their face as they casually munched away. Seeing the crumbs around their lips, how they could eye it with admiration for a long meditative pause, and then devour one in two bites, how if they were hungry, they would wave their hand in the air and ask for more. I ate vicariously through them, longing for the feeling of cookies just tasting sweet, crumbly, and good.

Fortunately, we were now talking seriously about "reconstruction," creating a new, functioning digestive system for me out of what I had left. It would be a complex and unpredictable process of trial and error, not unlike the board game Operation. My dad had started to call doctors and figure out what a plan might look like, to which the doctors responded: "We can't plan much of anything until we open her up and see what's in there."

Still overwhelmed by hunger, I dove into every available distraction. By the time I saw that a local theater was having auditions for *CATS*, I was already weightlifting, tap dancing, and power yoga-ing with enough energy to burst through the ceiling. A year before, I could barely limp up the steps to my *Oliver* audition. Now I was thrilled to put my new stamina on stage, prancing and howling around as a singing, leaping cat. I was confident at the open dance call, twirling like everyone else. Other than knowing I would have to be hooked up to my IV pole within the next hour, life felt good. I was cast as Jellylorum, and the only tricky part was the fact that we all had to wear skin-tight bodysuits, which weren't exactly compatible with the IVs all over my body. I could even drink, although since everything went out my bag on my neck as I drank it, I had to be careful not to drink during the performance so my neck bag full of orange soda wouldn't splatter all over my cat-striped leotard.

As I went back and forth to doctors between rehearsals, preparing for my reconstruction surgery, I wondered if this would be the picture of my future life: being back in theatres; drinking, eating, dancing, and having nothing sticking out of my body. I was getting so close, and I had already come so far.

Theatre gave me hope. These were the small islands of creativity that got me through, and finally, I was seeing the shore!

It had been almost three years out of the hospital now, and my father was starting to "shop me around" to other doctors, hoping enough time had passed that we could start planning my reconstruction. To capture the excitement, a local news station, Channel 12, decided to chronicle the few months before my life would be magically reassembled. They followed me through a day of yoga, weight training, dance, karate, and finally back to the house to make chocolate.

The morning started as usual, in the dark, blinds closed, kicking in place, watching the Food Network. "Amy! Can I come in?" my mother said through the door.

I figured today was an "out-of-the-ordinary" day. I would be letting people into my world and talking to them face to face. I could tell my mother was nervous.

"Can you dress up nice? What are you going to wear?" She gently cracked the door open and held a Macy's dress on a hanger, one of our many "retail therapy" ventures. She had been hoarding dresses like Christmas presents, waiting for a day I'd need them. The camera crew was coming over at 11:30 a.m.—a welcome deviation from my mechanical routine that typically lasted until at least 3 p.m. each day. The anxiety suddenly melted to pure excitement once my mother let them in. A blonde reporter, a stubby man with a camera, and a third woman trailing behind with a notepad became guests in my world. Instantly, it felt like home.

I milked every second of that interview—I forgot how exquisite it felt talking to people! As I proudly displayed my chocolate creations, suddenly, I wanted my world to expand beyond home and into the light.

The crew stayed into the night. My mother beamed as she watched my eyes become aglow with animation, heard bits of my laughter, and witnessed actual spontaneous conversation that felt normal. The march upstairs to my room, after the stubby man had packed up his camera, had never felt more weighted. I slammed my door, trying to block out the warm, open feeling that had overtaken my heart with the opening of my door. Luckily, I was fully immersed in my numb routine when I woke up the next day. And now everyone was going to get a glimpse into my world! (Or at least houses that had Local News 12.)

This was supposed to be the "before" segment of that magical thirteenth reconstructive surgery. After this procedure, life would be normal. I would eat! I would drink! I'd be done with this medical saga! As it turned out, not quite....

My dad reflected on the theme of Passover as it related to my exile from eating.

Dad: Passover had always been a big holiday for us. We usually had big crowds at our house, and it seemed ironic that this all happened at the Seder. Not eating was hard to say the least, and it consumed the whole family. With Passover 3 months away, we held hope Amy would eat soon. Amy was always artistic, and she began working on a large diorama. It showed a family at the Seder table with all involved eating a big dinner. She labeled it "Passover 2006."

At the end of every Seder, we say, "Next Year in Jerusalem," to voice our hope of spending the next year in a land of freedom, whatever that means for each of us. Every year that I couldn't eat, I would tell myself, "Next Year in Jerusalem," which, for me, meant, "Next year I'll finally eat, we'll finally have our Seder again, all innocence will be restored, and everything will be just like I remember." But I soon learned everything can't go back to how it used to be.

CHAPTER 17

Holding out for Hope: Awaiting Reconstruction

LUCKILY, I HELD ON LONG ENOUGH for my father to find some creative answers. While I coped from day to day, he called more and more colleagues, seeking suggestions. Reconstruction was no longer just a pipe dream, but a goal we could actually aim for realistically, as tangible as "I'm going to apply to college" or "I'm going to get my driver's license."

But what did "reconstruction" actually mean? All we knew was that somehow, someday whatever bit of my intestines remained would be rearranged, rewired, and reconnected so I could digest food. I would leave the specific logistics to the professionals. And what would life be like after reconstruction? With an esophagostomy rerouting my digestive system, I felt like a kid in a candy store as I discovered more "liquids" I could drink. I could have soup, smoothies, hot chocolate, even ice cream! But, I wondered, would a surgery with unknown repercussions take away the one thing still working in my favor—the gift of taste?

As excited as I was, I couldn't help the nervous feeling that, due to the nature of surgery, things might not go as planned. Should I back out now while I still have a choice?

As reconstruction approached, I would go to Stop & Shop more frequently to load up on drinks by the gallon—our fridge was packed to maximum capacity—because deep inside, it felt like a last supper. There was a part of me that was relieved when the surgery date kept getting delayed, thinking, "Ooh, more time to buy apple banana Juicy Juice and ice cream and flan and gelato and popsicles and milkshakes and all that fun forbidden stuff." But the other part of me couldn't wait for it to happen. I had already waited so long.

> *Dear Amy,*
>
> *How can I be there for you in this time of crisis? I know you don't want to look like this, and I want to give you a voice. I want to let you through because your soul is so penetrating, I can feel it in the beautiful autumn sunlight. And I promise, I will not let you miss the fall. We'll go apple picking and to petting zoos and, most importantly, smell the air, and reap the harvest.*

I shook off my fear and stayed excited about what was ahead. I thought if the reconstruction surgery was successful, life would be perfect. But how could I know that being allowed to eat would open Pandora's box and let out a swarm of memories and feelings and fears? I was too preoccupied with medical concerns to think about the trauma I had experienced before my coma. I had no idea that memories of my abuse were lurking in the background.

As doctors started returning my dad's calls, they started to make a plan for me, and I couldn't help but think back to the years of numbness I forced myself through while I avoided food. What would it be like to not have to avoid anything?

Sometimes a coping strategy outlives its usefulness, but you don't want to lose it.

"You're a trouper," everyone would tell me as I put up with anything in the various hospitals. But I'm not a trouper. I'm a warrior. I fight through things. And I'll take whatever means I need to fight. When you ask your doctor day after day when you will be allowed to eat, and he simply replies, "I don't know," as he copies down the various data displayed on a screen just above your head, you must find a way for your soul to accept that it could take years.

To deal you have to fiercely ignore your inherent need to feed yourself, your need to moisten up your throat with some water in the ninety-degree heat. You fight with any means at any cost. If you have to exercise all day to keep your mind off your body's pleas for food and nourishment, so be it. Any move of desperation to block out hunger otherwise become your darkest enemy.

With Blaine, I was a trouper by meeting whatever his unhealthy needs were. Sometimes to survive you have to be compliant. But inside of me was a warrior who forced that compliant daze of numbness on me to get through and made sure I would resort to anything to keep that daze up. But can the trouper lower her guard?

I realized that my numbness had shielded me from my lost innocence all these years. The innocence I mourned was that of a happy family before a monster shattered it. Was it such a crime to be comfortable in the life I once lived?

The five stages of grieving are denial, anger, bargaining, depression, and acceptance. With denial comes shock. When I went out of body during my abuse, I was frozen in shock. And before I could move to anger, my stomach exploded. Since I didn't get the fiery anger out, a fiery volcanic eruption exploded in my belly instead. So, while I was trying to get the anger out from the Blaine trauma, I experienced the shock of my medical trauma. My soul was trying to combine two grieving stages into one. As a result, the anger from Blaine got distorted. I felt anger, but because I was out of my body, I took out the anger in all the wrong places, namely, on myself. I was in the whirlpool, stuck in every time frame except the present moment because I was still trying to deal with demons from two different pasts. No wonder I couldn't be present. No wonder I couldn't hear my soul bird singing to me and guiding me.

I knew if I stayed numb, I would just be a victim. I couldn't let Blaine win, so my anger motivated me to look forward to reconstruction as a warrior and heroically surrender my numbness for a greater prize—myself.

I have to accept that the old life is gone. I have to find a new spotlight now because old has to make way for new beginnings. The bus always comes around, but if we don't take these new opportunities out of fear for the rest of our lives, we stay frozen.

I was used to my life now, but the risk of reconstruction and possibly losing all my progress could also promise big rewards—the return of happy Thanksgivings, going freely to auditions, fun little sibling arguments—a world that was loud and bright.

I was torn. But I told myself if I pushed away reconstruction, I would remain stuck and push away my life. I thought of the archetypal wounded healer. Maybe this scary path of reconstruction would somehow give me the heroic wounds that would ultimately better myself and the world. Trusting this was the hero's journey I was meant to take. So, for guidance I followed the roadmap of one of my favorite childhood stories, *The Giver* by Lois Lowry,

In *The Giver*, everyone in the village was assigned a particular job, a certain role in society at an early age, and each child got a mentor to teach them that skill so they would be prepared when it was their turn to take over the task. The book's protagonist gets the job as the Receiver of Memory, but it is harder than everyone else's job because it involves transmitting the memories of feeling to the now unfeeling society. The boy has to feel all sorts of pain and undergo tests and trials, while all his friends are learning how to be teachers or store managers. But he is the only boy in the village capable of storing memories for society so he can deliver these gifts of feeling to his community and preserve them for posterity.

So maybe God is my Giver. Maybe I have been blessed with the task of carrying the weight of a giant healing message on my shoulders to share with the outside world. I'll fight hard, so I can give back too.

CHAPTER 18

Deconstructing Reconstruction

DOCTORS WERE NOT SURE WHAT I had left, or what was connected to what. Pre-surgery procedures, CAT scans, and MRIs could only show so much. We weren't sure what to expect, but I was hoping for a miracle.

In August 2006, I had just finished bouncing, crawling, and pirouetting across the stage in *CATS*. Once I had prowled off stage and made my final bow, I was sure ready to be rebuilt. My father had been researching surgeons all along who were up to the task.

Dr. Lobre, the GI doctor from Columbia who had saved my life, worried that if surgeons tried to reconnect everything at once, too much strain would be put on my body, and the wound would open right back up as I tried to ingest food once again. So, he recommended *two surgeries*. If I was hooked up from the "bottom" first, and then we waited a few months to reconnect my esophagus, my intestines would have time to heal and recover after surgery. It would be an overwhelming procedure for my body in the first place, and Dr. Lobre wanted this to be as safe as possible. Of course, I anticipated the agony of recovering from part one, then waiting in limbo for part two and another recovery. I wished they could connect me as easily as LEGO bricks. But one stage or two, I just wanted to get it done.

Dad: Dr. Wink at the NIH was helpful and said I need a "surgeon's surgeon." Someone who only takes the most difficult cases, someone who other doctors call when they need help. I set up an appointment with Dr. Slem at Yale who fit all of the criteria. After multiple scans, x-rays, and exams, he agreed to do the surgery. He said it would be complicated, but we didn't know what else lay ahead for us.

Meeting Dr. Slem, he was kind and soft-spoken with a lyrical South African accent, nothing like the gruff, blunt New Yorker Dr. Lobre. He was compassionately realistic, and like every other surgeon, he could make no guarantees. But flipping through my thick charts and dozens of diagrams, his confidence was comforting as he described what parts of me should be attached to what. My parents (and my disconnected intestines) were excited. Dr. Slem was exactly what we needed—someone to boldly think out of the box. His plan was to create a pouch from my intestines that would enable me to at least partially digest food.

We all knew reconstruction was a risk, but we all understood the greater risk was not knowing if I could ever live a normal life. Slem agreed to the surgery but wanted to wait until the TPN had built me up enough nutritionally so the stitches would actually keep everything closed once the procedure was over. His advice was to stay positive and hope for the best—something I had become quite good at.

Finally receiving a reconstruction date was more exciting than the day I got my bat mitzvah date. On September 19, 2007, my family and I waited eagerly for this portentous day of new beginnings. I finally started to look at food with new eyes (hopeful but not too idealistic), with the mindset of actually buying it, bringing it home, cooking it, and eating it. I allowed myself to imagine planning my day around meals the way everyone else did. For the first time, I gave myself the freedom to believe I would really eat again.

The night before my thirteenth surgery, I went to bed nervous about surrendering control of my body again, since surgery was always a crapshoot, but also ecstatic at the idea of waking up to a new, fully functional me. We spent that weekend packing pajamas, sneakers (my parents knew I'd be darting around the hospital as soon as I could), and enough distractions to last us months (since experience had taught us that wasn't such an unreasonable expectation). The next morning, my parents drove me in for lucky surgery number thirteen.

The morning was filled with standard pre-op procedures and hours of waiting that only served to make us all as nervous as possible. This was not like any of my other surgeries. I was not being rushed to the ER while in crisis. This was something I had deliberately scheduled and represented my decision to risk the functional life to which I had adjusted and surrender myself into a world of uncertainty.

As I once again assumed the role of the medical marionette, I couldn't help thinking, "What the hell am I doing?" I had built myself up with weight training and dance. My vocal cords felt vital, flexible, and unburdened by the strain of a tracheotomy or ventilator. I had just been leaping across the stage in CATS. I couldn't eat or drink, but I was still feeling strong healthy and energetic. I had no open wounds. I was just "anatomically disconnected." I dreaded the steps it would take to recover from surgery and knew it would be an arduous process.

After being wheeled into the operating room, my parents gave me a kiss as I was rolled away into the sterile white light. I wouldn't see them for another nineteen hours.

<u>Dad</u>: Once Amy went in, no one came and went until, finally, we got our first update: "All was going as planned." More than 7 hours later, at midnight, Mom and I fell asleep exhausted. At 2:30 a.m., Dr. Slem woke us up and told us Amy would be in recovery soon. He felt he had succeeded. We were incredibly relieved.

Waking up, I felt paralyzed. The worst part of recovery was always coming back into consciousness. I could hear things but couldn't move my lips. I remember hearing nurses saying there was bulimia in my chart from so much damage done to my esophagus. I was a singer! Why would I be bulimic?

After hours of lying in the recovery area, it turned out this surgery was way more "involved" than expected. It took nearly a whole day—nineteen hours and three shifts of nurses and doctors, nearly the entire hospital. Now, I was hooked up from the bottom up. As I was recovering, every other person came up to me and said, "I worked on you! I worked on you, too!" I was a celebrity, though not the kind I had hoped to be when dreaming about my career on Broadway. This surgery was meant to lay the groundwork. Now, I just had the second part to go, and with luck, Chinese food was right around the corner.

As boring and uncomfortable they were, the first few days after surgery were probably the easiest. I was too foggy to understand how the surgery had affected me. It was only when doctors suggested I try to get out of bed that I faced the immense physical pain and hopelessness of how far I had to go.

This recovery was beyond painful. It had never been so tiring to breathe. Once I was alert, the respiratory team insisted upon testing my breathing by giving me a handheld inhaler-like apparatus with three balls. To strengthen your lungs after surgery you're supposed to blow hard enough in it so all three balls lift up. It was hell. Waking up from surgery is usually a time when you'd rather not be bothered, but ironically, it's the time nobody will leave you alone. As soon as one doctor opens the curtain to leave, another one presses the Purell sprayer by the door and makes his grand entrance.

All that poking and prodding left me with no choice than to develop the Nietzschean mindset: What doesn't kill you makes you stronger. But then that took on the distorted form of: You are great and honorable the more pain you take. And that was what I based my worth on. Surgery number thirteen was a failure and I began to numb myself again. To top it off, I heard the same dreaded "I don't knows" that I heard back in the days of the Columbia ICU.

To deal with the fear, uncertainty, leaks, and limbo, my "dazed cyclone eyes" were used as a shield over my wide, blue, trusting eyes, once beaming with hope. The iron box was once again locked around my heart to numb me from the devastation, anger, anxiety, and hopeless grief which now overshadowed any looking forward to the future of food and normalcy. And my daggerfeet were once again strapped on because, in constant motion, life would stay a blur. I just had to keep moving so my heart could stand still. My trauma survival kit was all I had to shield me from the physical pain during a torturous recovery.

Reconstruction, much like after the Civil War in the American South, was turning out to be a disillusioning transition.

Being discharged from Yale, I was tired and sore, but underneath it all, I was hopeful. After surgery part one, the bottom half of me was connected. I was told it would only take a few months for the bottom to heal before I could get my "top half" reconnected. I was now back home, but after guzzling gallons of soda just weeks before, now I was not even allowed a drop of liquid.

I was truly back to nothing and life was stalled. I told myself, "It's just because I'm healing. Once I've healed, I can go back to drinking. That will make things a little bit better."

However, my wound didn't heal as I expected, and I suffered a series of serious setbacks. I remember lying flat in bed as my dad went to dress my wound, always something I dreaded after surgery. Twice a day, he'd unpack dozens of compressed gauze sponges and re-dress it. I would spend the rest of the day dreading the moment when he'd have to unpack it again, scared to look at the gaping wound, something I never could get used to.

With every dressing change, I would sneak a look at my wound, hoping it had gone down in size or was somehow looking healthier.

"Ame, the skin around the wound is looking much pinker," my dad said with a warm smile. Dr. Dad's encouragement was a big part of his nightly dressing change regimen. "You're healing and it's..." He stopped in mid-sentence and began to squint looking more closely at my wound.

"What is it Dad?"

He became very quiet.

"Nothing. Just looking."

I remember it as the first time I saw my father truly frightened of what was happening to me. How could my own father, a doctor, not have answers? This turned out to be my first fistula.

What I didn't know was that it was the first of many setbacks that would threaten to put my life on hold forever.

Fis·tu·la: *an abnormal or surgically made passage between a hollow or tubular organ and the body surface, or between two hollow or tubular organs.*

The day I saw my wound open, I felt as if I'd been cast in a dystopian horror film. This could not be my life. Was everything I feared before my surgery coming true? Had this surgery been a huge mistake?

For this fistula to heal, I would have to stop drinking indefinitely, and part two of my surgery was put on hold until we could arrive at a solution. With liquid taken back out of my life, trying to pass the time was torture. I had placed all my hopes on this surgery making life normal, and this felt like a monumental setback. I even tried to make a stick of gum last forty-five minutes. My days were filled with a variety of x-rays, procedures, radiology trips, and messy dressing changes—more leakages than answers. But the most agonizing part was knowing I was making no progress towards Part Two of reconstruction. When I wasn't in the hospital, I was going to Beardsley Zoo with my parents, visiting malls, and returning to my chocolate business. I tried my best to fill my days and not let myself think about how frozen I was in time.

The following months were filled with radiologists trying to insert tubes into my fistula—but my wounds were opening like volcanoes leaking into piles of gauze taped onto my body. My nightmares were literally leaking into my life. Every time I moved; I was playing with fire. I didn't trust my body and was constantly scared it would fail me. We had finally been clearing out our house of hospital supplies thinking we were getting over the hump, and now we were right back in the hell of medical anxiety and uncertainty.

The idea of a *regressive* surgery once life was approaching normal was unfathomable. I expected Part One to be long, rocky, and painful to recover from, but I figured if surgeons took nineteen hours to reconnect my insides, they wouldn't need to go back and disconnect anything. That wasn't supposed to happen. Now that I faced my first fistula, (I would have many more to follow) our fridge, which I had jammed with every possible juice and liquid that would fit through my neck, was once again emptied out refilled only with sterile, bulky, yellow bags of TPN. The kitchen? Deadly once again.

The neighbors must be able to hear us arguing, as my family and I cry together, searching for answers, angry at our situation, sometimes taking it out on each other. If only they could see us sometimes holding each other and shaking our fists at the sky, demanding that something will give and let us back into our former lives.

While I was pouring chocolate into Christmas molds for gifts, my parents had to tell me that my inside parts, which I thought were staying inside for good, would need to be cut up again. No one knew exactly what was causing liquids to leak out of me, or why my stubborn fistula wouldn't heal, so the doctors came up with a "solution" that seemed like a death sentence for all my hopes and dreams.

My dad came down to the kitchen with my mom. I knew something was up because they never bothered me when I made chocolates. They knew it was my coping time. "Amy, can you put that down for a second?"

"This chocolate mold has to set. Later."

"Things aren't working like Dr. Slem had thought. And...he wants to operate again."

Dr. Slem had reversed every bag on my stomach. Now, he needed to put them back on.

"I don't want a colostomy!" I cried as I slammed a chair and ran upstairs.

Since my coma, surprises had constantly been thrown at me. And I had fielded them all pretty well. But now, I was hearing that I would need another surgery before Part Two, which now wasn't even being discussed. This wasn't slipping a few feet while nearing the summit of the mountain. This was having my ropes cut and suffering a devastating fall back to base camp.

When my parents told me about the colostomy, I was so furious at a situation I was once again helpless to change. But instead of giving up and holing up in my room again, I turned to my creative work to heal what I could. I couldn't stuff my face with ice cream or drown my sorrows with a double martini. Instead, I had to be resourceful.

Molding chocolate was the best way I knew to come to grips with what I was feeling. I could find some kind of joy, lost in a process, embellishing each peanut butter cup with glossy chocolate coating.

So how did I survive the years without a spoonful of anything besides IV nutrition? I figured out how creativity could satiate me...for just one moment at a time. Creating ruthlessly, recklessly, shamelessly, and resourcefully working with whatever I was given.

As much as I protested, I had to accept that getting my colostomy back was the only way I could even think about planning for part two of reconstruction. So, with far less effort than it took to schedule, plot, strategize, and plan for the previous nineteen-hour procedure, number fourteen was quite "routine," and perhaps my most "normal" surgery yet. It was "only" a three-hour procedure, and I breezed through it, Amy-style. My body went back to how things were before the extensive reconstructive surgery, so I could find some solace in what was otherwise a devastating reversal.

After the colostomy, it took me less than an hour to recover. Once alert, I got off the operating table and went shopping. Now I could begin to think about Part Two of reconstruction at Mt. Sinai where they would hook me up "from the top." But months went by, and I think we exhausted every mall in the tri-state area. Time passed, but the fistulas never fully healed. Still, after much debating and much more time, we decided to go ahead with the second part of reconstruction and hope for the best possible outcome.

<u>Dad:</u> In 2007 or 2008, your GI system was stable—everything was diverted from your neck. We were soon directed to the only doctor who could do this—Dr. Woo.

Dr. Woo felt confident, after going through all of Dr. Slem's notes, Dr. Lobre's diagrams, and my ever-growing stack of medical records that he could complete the work that was started by seven hospitals so far. I breathed a sigh of relief as we marked a date on our calendars. Surgery number fifteen promised "normality," a year and a half later than we had originally planned.

Compared to everything else I had been through, surgery number fifteen was no big deal and only took a few hours—for me, a cinch. We were discharged within a few days and this was supposed to be the final "put my life together" moment, spitting me back into the outside world. When I "healed" from this surgery, I could eat. This would be a normal recovery, I was assured.

I realized with time that nothing for me is normal. Changes in my physical identity also affected how I perceived myself.

The wider I can stretch out my arms to latch onto more concrete things in the outside world, the more secure and substantial I'll feel. So much is missing. So much that I've had before.

For the first time since my coma, I didn't have a bag on my neck. Oddly, I sort of missed it. I had even begun to draw on it with sharpies, writing new designs with every bag change. This bag had become part of the new me.

I was beginning to find a comfort, even humor, in my condition. I had my muscles back. I could sing. I journaled, had a chocolate business, and a newfound interest in Billy Joel. I couldn't go through life hating my condition and myself. I liked the girl I had become, but I had decided to give her up and take the risk of surgeries thirteen, fourteen, and fifteen because I wanted—needed—to be able to eat and drink again. But the thought occurred to me: Would I have been better off settling for the "medically stable" life I had?

These were the questions that raced through my head as my dad drove us home from the Mt. Sinai unit on the Monday morning after my surgery. Part two was done. I was weak, bandaged, and sore, desperately thirsty, but forcing myself to be optimistic and patient. I had grown accustomed to having patience at this point, but it didn't make things any easier.

My neck had to remain bandaged, and I was forbidden to eat, drink, or even have gum this time around while the stitches healed. I counted down the days until my follow-up appointment, desperately dry and starving. I was so sick of my TPN bags and pole. I allowed myself to dream of the day, now approaching, I could nourish myself on my own. When I finally had my follow-up appointment with Dr. Woo at Mt. Sinai, CBS cameras followed me, as well as CT News 12. I had become a news story. The plan was to film me going food shopping at Fairway right next door after I got the go ahead. To my disappointment, the world watched as Dr. Woo said I could drink clear liquids but would have to wait a bit longer for food.

A total letdown, for sure, but for me, even just having water again was a blessing. "Better than nothing!" I told the news cameras.

A few weeks later we had another appointment—on my twenty-first birthday. I was given the green light to eat. I brought a mini frozen waffle with me to see if he would let me have a bite of food right then and there, and with Dr. Woo's nod, I had my first food in three years. There's no way to describe how chewing and swallowing felt after all that time. But now, with my frozen waffle, I was cautiously optimistic. I took a bite, self-conscious as the cameras followed me again. I wasn't sure if I was supposed to swallow, or if I would die if I swallowed it, and my parents looked at me eagerly and anxiously. After I didn't drop dead on the spot, Dr. Woo congratulated me and said I could eat. Done. Or so we thought.

CHAPTER 19

Building up an Appetite

I WAS HOME, AND FOOD WAS MINE! After three years, I couldn't believe I had taken my first bite of real food; on national television! I had told myself I would finally be happy, normal, and at last satisfy years of cravings. And I did. But not quite. That little frozen waffle I took with me to my doctor's appointment signified my return to the world of eating. It was exactly what I wanted.

It was a birthright that I was coming into all over again. I was finally growing up after going into a phase of infancy in the hospital. But after that bite, I realized I had to start with baby food. Chewing took work! After all, my body had gone years without one bite. On top of that, because I no longer had a stomach, I didn't have the muscle contractions the body uses to move food along through the digestive system. I quickly learned that food would stay stuck in me until *I* moved around to pass it along.

To be safe, I started on a puréed diet. So much for my frozen waffle leading to a whole buffet. Still, food was a thrilling rediscovery. And I was home, in my kitchen, entitled to every morsel anyone else was. I was finally human again. I rummaged through the groceries we had haphazardly thrown in our shopping cart at Fairway and delved excitedly into that once-forbidden trove of treasures.

Food had always felt innocent, joyful, and exciting to me growing up. All the way up to that fated "last supper" at Blaine's studio apartment, I was a well-fed teenager, partial to Chinese food and non-alcoholic Shirley Temples. Of course, as a Jewish girl with a (very) Jewish mother, I didn't expect hunger to ever be something I'd become intimately familiar with. But then again, I didn't expect my life, free of any medical problems whatsoever, to be blown apart and rerouted when my stomach exploded. Now, finally life would start for me. The countdown was over!

Food brings up emotions. That's a good thing and a bad thing. Food connected my mind, which was great! But it also connected my emotions, which was a double-edged sword. I had underrated food's potential, not only to satisfy my intense, years-long hunger, but also to awaken memories, both pleasant and painful.

> *I take a sip of burning hot chocolate, and happy memories of skiing in Vermont with my family flood my body. I bite into the warm flaky crust of a biscuit and see my grandmother's face. I didn't realize how much I missed her! I was too numb to even cry after I found out she had died.*

The first place food went? My mind. I had no idea it had taken so much effort to keep my focus before I had real nourishment soaking my brain cells. My world quadrupled in size, richness, and complexity. I was intellectually stimulated for the first time and suddenly wanted to learn about everything. My first time back at Barnes & Noble since I could eat, I was doing a literary supermarket sweep, running down the aisles and grabbing books from every delicious genre. When both arms could no longer contain my stock of eclectic reads, I plopped down on the floor with a pile of books twice as tall as me, everything from sign language to Spanish history to knitting to politics. When a passing bookseller gave me an odd look, I stammered, "I'm just really excited to be here!" I started feeling the wonder of the world again. I forgot that food could make you feel!

As excited as I had been about that first nibble of frozen waffle, I was still limited to a soft food diet, and since I didn't want baby food, my mother and I stewed over what else was considered "soft," and that is how I came to have the great pumpkin revelation. And my first home-cooked meal!

Around 8 p.m., I could smell it from upstairs in my room. Suddenly, my closed-off room felt dark and unfamiliar to me, a world I didn't want to be in any longer. Food was life, and it was downstairs!

Lured towards the most delicious smell, I reached for the doorknob. I knew my mom had seasoned that pumpkin with cinnamon and love and things in that spice drawer forbidden to me since we had moved here. It smelled warm, homey, and sweet. It smelled like how I want to feel inside. I was really excited to eat it for nothing but pure enjoyment. That really struck a chord with me. I realized what it felt like to really *want* something, to *know* what makes me happy. Even if it was just a silly scoop of pumpkin.

I had been through the struggles of someone three times my age, but I felt like one of my nursery school kids. Everything felt brand new and shrink-wrapped in wonder. Although scarred and weary, I was ready to start fresh, and with a hunger to heal.

I realized that for all of those years of not eating, my odd behaviors made perfect sense. I wasn't crazy! I was just coping with the unnatural task of starving myself!

I can freely enjoy what was a forbidden pleasure for so long. Pumpkin baking in the oven, makes the whole kitchen smell like Thanksgiving. I love scraping up the burnt edges with a spoon! Yum!

Now that I was eating, I was living again, and living meant feeling. With each visceral bite of food, I felt more involved in the process of life and less desire to write about it in an abstract, intellectual way. As I filled myself with food, I was filled by a vast array of emotions.

The trauma of not eating was finally over. But I had no idea of the tastes and flavors, some delightfully sweet, some horribly bitter, that eating again had in store for me.

My body is a treasure chest of hidden memories that I've clamped off by constantly shoving of any feeling I have back under water. But now I can't help it. I'll cry at the drop of a pin, and I don't know why.

Eating Becomes a Warrior's Challenge

Now Tiger Lilly the warrior was being tested. She had to be comfortable in her body, just being still in herself like a firm, sturdy, stable tree trunk rooted in the ground.

I thought once I could eat, I'd be done with TPN, right? Until Dr. Stolar explained to me that I couldn't just "get off" TPN. Yes, I was eating. But then I looked at my arm, still attached to a PICC line that had to be carefully dressed and cleaned daily. Being able to feed myself meant I had autonomy, that I was entirely my own person. But because it would take time for me to start eating comfortably again, I was still on a full cycle of TPN until I was able to eat a complete diet. But now that I had a digestive system, I wanted my power back, and my arm!

Pumpkin had been my aromatic introduction to the power of food to open up an entry to myself I had long forgot about—pleasure and warm, soft comfort. The next door that food would open was by an unexpected gooey gold mine—hot, cheesy pizza.

It took a really long time to work up to pizza, and I was terrified I would choke. How was I supposed to chew all that grainy cheesy goodness? What did those pieces do in your body once you bit them? How would anything be absorbed in my body that wasn't clear liquid intravenous fluid? My mom just ordered a standard cheese pizza from the neighborhood takeout place. This was so strange; this food that I had built up in my head was now here, in the proverbial "flesh," so close I could actually smell it. I stared at my flimsy white paper plate, already stained with grease, a *really* long time. Now that it was actually here, I was nervous. My mother's friend was at the house. She looked at me and said, "Well, why don't you just eat it already?"

So, I picked up the piece of pizza and quickly took a bite. And I seriously went crazy. In a good way, of course. This was my first social revelation.

Besides being the delicious cheese I had so fondly remembered, eating pizza was a lightbulb moment. Suddenly, I remembered every instant I had had pizza before—at parties, with friends, at a school function, ordering in delivery for a movie night with friends—food was social. I forgot about that!

The first thing I did was take a walk outside and call my brother. I was so giddy and flustered, rambling on, "Jeff, you wanna go out for pizza or something? I can go to a diner and be like, 'Hey I'd like to order pizza!' I can call some buddies and be like, 'Hey, let's have a game night, and we'll take in some pizza!' I can go on double dates to a pizza joint! I can have a pizza party! Heck, I can make my own! Once I can eat pizza, the world is an open door!"

Once the surgeons connected me, it was still my job as the "emotion surgeon" to piece back together the shattered pieces of food with food as my scalpel. Now that I was a social pizza butterfly...what next?

Real food was helping me regain physical health. Now that TPN was no longer my sole source of nutrition, there was finally color in my face, and even the energy in my body felt different. Food was a new life force. But I was unprepared for the emotional side effects of surgery—flashbacks and memories I thought I had repressed.

I had been making slow but steady progress as pizza had opened up a world of social discovery and every bite seemed to make my mind work in more dimensional ways. Now, my mom had picked up a small carton of French fries from McDonald's for me—a fantasy I had built up in my head over the years, daydreaming of casual activities that "normal people do" like go to the drive through at McDonald's and pick up a Happy Meal. After not feeding her daughter for years, Mom gave into comfort food in all its unhealthy glory.

Fries. They smelled so temptingly crispy, salty, oozing with all things indulgent and out of my reach for so long. The oil touched my lips, and I could taste a fleck of salt. What was that? Wow!

But one warm bite of a French fry jolted me into a flood of fiery red emotions. I panicked as a violent knot of anxiety engulfed my chest. Was I choking?

I learned that the French fry was my "trigger." (I hadn't even known what a trigger was, and now I was in an emotional war zone.) Up until this point, refeeding my body felt pleasant. Food had already made me start to feel. But now that I could "feel," the dam was unblocked. Now, I was feeling everything, including the pain I had tried to swallow for years of medical uncertainty, surgical interventions, and memories I thought my coma had permanently repressed.

As my trauma memories overtook me, it became clear that eating food meant not only reclaiming my life after my illness, but also reclaiming my life after Blaine. Just as I would strengthen my body, I would strengthen my voice once again, despite the man who tried to silence it. Eating would restore my nutritional and emotional independence. I had to prove to my doctors I could do this. I had to prove it to myself.

With every bite, I felt some emotion sink deeper into my soul. Food is soul medicine, I told myself, so my soul bird can finally run free. With every bite, I started recognizing my voice and allowing it space in my life. I started to see myself as a confident woman, holding a water bottle and sandwich— my warrior's bow and arrow.

Who knew that one fry would break down the entire wall I had worked so hard to build up through my numbness and exercise? Why did my heart panic when my body felt good, all because of a fry? The damage was done, and soon intrusive memories were unavoidable. I would be sitting in a car, buckled into a seatbelt, and all of a sudden, I would start to panic. I felt locked in, confined, and unsafe. Suddenly, I was remembering what it felt like to be chained to IV poles, unable to move, and constricted to a tiny space. My heart beat rapidly, and I panicked as my memories intruded on what appeared to be a perfectly calm moment.

Food was forcing me to feel that pain, betrayal, and deception *in my body*, and I started to resent eating for making me feel at all. I was used to numbness. I *liked* it. What was the point of feeling? It could only hurt me, as it had done every time before. Food was trying to trick me into feeling, and I couldn't let it!

I was far better off with my numb, dazed trauma survival kit, which shielded me from the hurtful emotions in my body. I knew I had looked forward to food as a cure-all to finally start my life again, but maybe it was easier to spend the rest of my life in my room. Faced with the other side, maybe numbness wasn't so bad. One French fry had conjured up enough anxiety, flashbacks, and overwhelming feelings of impending doom to scare me into reverting back to the coping mechanisms I had used to numb myself for all of these years.

With every bite of the fry, with every thought of Blaine conjured up by that fry, with the coupling of pleasure and pain, my body began to react as it did back in Blaine's apartment. I panicked and got anxious. Then I felt guilty for feeling this way, for eating the fry, which caused me to relive these emotions all over again. Physiological feelings of helplessness, shame, and guilt feel the same in your body; if you feel helpless in one situation, you'll subconsciously associate those same feelings with another situation because these wires are intertwined in ways we cannot imagine or anticipate.

Because I felt helpless with Blaine, I can't help but feel guilty about what happened even though I did nothing wrong. But the body doesn't know that because it thinks to itself, "I feel helpless," and it turns that into, "I feel ashamed." Eating that French fry connected my pleasure sensations to the sexual sensations because my wires are connected very differently than they were before the trauma.

Being able to eat transformed instantly to an intimidating terror because it granted me the unwieldy power of feeling but not the power to select which feelings I got to experience. Reaching my emotional threshold, it felt much better to block everything out, even the wonderful feeling of fleeting connection I had experienced with pumpkin and pizza. Running to my room, I immediately put on the daze I now wore so well. In my daze, I could freeze. I felt no hunger; no feelings. And not even the most aromatic French fry could interrupt my numbness.

Blaine was gone from the picture. How could the voice teacher still take away my voice?

Two Worlds

TWO WORLDS—A DRAMATIC STRUCTURE present in all stories—the clash between two worlds, the tension of opposites. A hero embarks on the gateway to the unknown, to the other side, to uncertainty, from the known to the unknown. Could one French fry transport me into an uncharted world? I desperately wanted and *needed* to keep eating. But I didn't want to go where the French fry was taking me. That fry had activated the scared "wounded bird," the subconscious part of me that was still in fight or flight mode, still unsure the coast was clear, that it was safe and beneficial to leave my room. I needed to tell myself, "It's safe to come outside and play, skip into life, and feel the hurt, pain, and *betrayal*."

How could food give me so much happiness and so much pain? I had never felt so out of control. I thought I had trauma all figured out! So why wasn't it going away? I could sense every fear in my brain, but it wasn't eliminating the fear. The problem was, my intellect wasn't able to outthink what my body was feeling. Even one surgical procedure, even one hospital stay, creates a separation from the body. Medical trauma causes numbness. When the body is injured, if it *explodes* (as mine did), or is cut open and repaired, *you become separate from it* as a survival and coping mechanism to avoid the pain.

But you can't appreciate the beauty of your body unless you're in it. It's a conundrum. To heal we have to get back into our broken bodies. We have to dive into our emotions, re-experiencing their *physical, felt sensations*, teaching our bodies how to have a different response. It turned out that food had a unique power over me. Food was able to bring me into my body like nothing else could, and my mind couldn't outthink it. This realization was major progress in my healing, but also a painful step on a scary journey.

Who am I? I am half a surviving victim who doesn't care about anything except keeping her mind occupied and her heart numb, and I am half someone desperately trying to learn what it is to live a full and happy life. Food has given me thinking skills, but now my brain hurts as it re-develops its feeling skills. I wrestle with the idea of what's eating at me. How do I swim out of this frightening whirlpool?

I soon acknowledged these triggers connected me to more than just the medical anguish. They went far deeper, unearthing a life I had forgotten about, even before my coma, which apparently no amount of surgery could alter or erase.

If I spent my life in a hole just staring at my writing, locked in my room, fifty years could pass and I'd never know it. My coping mechanisms of isolation and numbness blurred the reality of the present moment because my little wounded bird couldn't handle any more hurt. But she also wanted to fly.

Going back and forth between my two worlds was hurting me. I had to bridge them. I began journaling again and turned to nature, music, and stories as power sources to redefine my world as one in which I was not a survivor of trauma, but a fierce warrior on my hero's journey. This was Tiger Lilly's world, where fear was energy I could magically transform into myth.

Here I could move from unhealthy to healthy coping strategies. While I remained scared that food was bringing up feelings, I knew I had to work through it. I relied on Grandma's spirit and my warrior's journey to guide me. Trauma had programmed me to feel fear, but that didn't mean fear made sense. Maybe I could make sense of fear by turning it into something else.

When difficulties are overcome, they become blessings. Looking for miracles in nature helped me begin a healing dialogue with the fear that threatened to uproot me.

I gently informed my wounded bird that it was safe to come out by turning its attention to nature, which is always changing. What would happen if a tree just lingered down in its roots and never allowed itself to sprout up towards the sky? A tree responds instinctively to the sunlight, allowing its branches to be pulled up from the tippy top of its head. Yet it stays grounded by letting water deepen its roots into the soil. Each day, nature taught me how to never get stuck in the past.

Today's intention: Acceptance. It is gorgeous outside. I am going to ground myself outside in nature, connect with my gods and my angels, really feel Grandma today, and have single-minded concentration on each activity I am doing. Whatever is, just is. Relish the sourdough bread caressing scoops of peanut butter, how sweet it tastes smushed around in jelly.

Today's Intention: Breathing. I am run by breath, not fear. Just breathing in fills me with unshakable peace that settles me into exactly where I am. I will try to see something unexpected on what may seem like a routine walk. My breath is my safety ladder that connects me to the moment, my umbilical cord to the world.

Music was a container where I could safely experience any feeling without drowning in it. I created a playlist of songs for when I was outside to keep me present, aligned with my voice and breath. My playlists could become my guide, giving my body permission to root itself, and actually sing along. Feeling how the words vibrated and trembled on my lips, I'd feel the beginnings of a tear start to form in my chest.

> *Every time I fell into a moment, I felt the tears well up in my eyes, and I was thinking, "That's not going to happen. I don't feel anything." But before I even knew it, my throat was choking up, and I couldn't even get through the song! I didn't know what was hitting me. That's how the physical sensation of a memory feels.*

The more I sang and stayed within my "container" of playlisted songs, the more I was granted permission to be present in every note, every moment, and in the World of the Thriving.

I was at a crossroads. I could let myself be controlled by every thought racing through my head, or I could choose to let some go. I chose to not listen to fear, and when those intimidating thoughts passed, I felt set free. It took great courage to release the thoughts I had grown accustomed to running my life. But when I did, my thoughts changed. And through change there is power.

How Do You Know What Thoughts to Choose?

I decided to choose the thoughts that aligned with my mission: taking my power back against surgery and against Blaine. Food tested my bravery, and I was proving myself triumphantly!

I had to dump numbness for feeling...and healing. So, I came up with a multifaceted toolbox with healthy tools to replace the years of numbness. The most powerful tool? A universal story.

My mythology book was packed with universal stories. Myth is different from history. It's not inspiring stories of people who lived notable lives. Myth cannot be located, so it's ideal when we have no roadmap and need to find ourselves wherever we are. That is how my grandma became a mythological symbol of guiding light to guide me back towards food and myself.

This mythological wisdom energy lives in all of us. It's our own power, bound to a larger calling. Myths point beyond our field, to the transcendent; we look at the stars, wonder what's up there, and wish we could be a part of that, too. Allegory teaches us lessons, but myth is something we can embody and become.

I had always loved metaphors, and now I felt this whirlwind of anxiety as a very powerful metaphor—a whirlpool. I felt like I was drowning in a whirlpool of fear, a cyclone of emotions that I couldn't do anything about but swirl into its evil eye. Pre-trauma, life was a flowing river, unbothered by fear or triggers. How could I redirect the cyclonic current of the whirlpool and learn how to flow back into the river of life once again?

I can counteract this trauma vortex by planting my body in the present moment. Then, nothing can stop this warrior, armed with nature walks, iPod playlists, animal spirits everywhere, and Grandma guiding her at every turn.

Creating Wounded Amy and Thriving Amy

I was still grappling with the broken halves of me, desperate to rediscover wholeness and comfort in my own body. To keep working through my story,

I projected these halves onto other characters. Just as I made myself into Tiger Lilly, the warrior, to steel myself for the fight of my life, I now divided myself into two characters to reconcile the conflict raging inside me.

> *I get confused because I just had this strong and powerful thought of releasing into life, but that paranoid controlling part of me pops right back up like a kickboard under water. Which side should I listen to?*

Earlier on, I created "Frank" as an alter ego in a story to help give my own story a frame. Frank's story was my story, but I couldn't accept it as my story then. To feel like one whole person again, I had to write a dialogue between my conflicting inner voices—Wounded Amy (WA) and Thriving Amy (TA). As they talked it out with each other, they became the joint protagonist of my hero's journey, a complex, empowered female trying to put herself back together after being doubly blown apart. Besides the skits I'd force my brothers to perform with me as a kindergartener, this was the first "script" I had ever tried to write—for my eyes and heart only.

> *This is the raw truth of what I've been through, and this script will answer the open-ended question of what I am to become after all of this. A choose-your-own-adventure story, a tale that has no ending...yet*

In my play, the antagonist, the voice teacher and abuser, seems like a friendly, fatherly figure but uses those qualities to manipulate Thriving Amy. He is a lonely man who has access to all the words and music in the world but no one to share them with. He takes advantage of Thriving Amy's thirst for words, music, and a fatherly figure. Thriving Amy is a poetic, but lonely soul with deep instincts that there is more to life than what meets the eye.

Wounded Amy is in a sedated state in the ICU for most of the play, while at the same time she is reliving her sexual abuse. We never actually see her in the hospital bed to show that even though she is "there," her mind and soul are somewhere else, locked in a world of secrets she has never been able to disclose.

The thrust of the play is the two Amys "waking up," winning their life back. Thriving Amy "wakes up" to her abuser, causing Wounded Amy to wake from her coma, breaking free from both constraints at the same time. The final hero? Just one, full Amy. By Amy's own actions, she influences the play's outcome. By fighting her abuser, she wakes up and starts living again.

Meanwhile, this Amy felt like she could never reclaim her full self, still dependent on machines. I was determined to meet all my nutritional needs through real food. Doctors doubted this would ever be a reality, but I kept the hope alive. As much as I wanted my power back, I was terrified once again of leaving my room. Feeling was deadly. But I didn't want to stay chained to TPN, so I decided to force myself back out of my room in spurts, even if it hurt.

Still, everything I did had to be compulsively balanced. If I spent thirteen minutes out of my room, I'd force myself to "make up" those thirteen minutes in my room at the end of the night. I had created a game out of life with numbers to cover up any quest for meaning or worry about my future, or unpleasant emotions. Playing my "number games" were how I rigidly kept my attention away from anything serious, like pacifying a baby by dangling a golden chain before their eyes.

Once I did force myself to go outside, I was again overwhelmed by the sheer wonder of the world, what had always entranced me.

I see circles everywhere. In the footprints on the sand, in the scattered clouds, the circular dance of the seagulls atop the water. Empty circle in my heart, opening up to the world, trying the horizon on for size.

Even the most rigid of routines could not keep my heart frozen for long once nature got back into the picture. I realized that even with everything I had been through, I still had an ongoing love affair with the beauty of the natural world. My journey back to feeling, unlocked by food, was opening my heart, eyes, and soul in ways I could not control with numbers.

The smell of cloves, a tang of allspice
A burnt whiff of cinnamon
Just sit there and breathe it in
All the recipes I bookmarked on the net
All the cookbooks I bought but haven't opened yet

The hum of the stove, the scraping of a ladle
That familiar feeling of waiting at the table
All of the napkins I've waited to need
All the hunger I've waited to feed

Now it's mine to sink my teeth in
This will be my world, my reason
Now life can begin
So dig in.

Getting out was a welcome break from my rigid routine, but I soon turned my outside time into a rigid routine as well—another numbing coping skill that continued to plague me.

I was scared of making decisions, because I didn't know how to listen to my gut. So, to avoid making decisions, I had an all or nothing mentality. If I was going to go out of my room, *I was going to go out of my room*. No matter what. Making structure was my safety.

One cold wintry day, my mother and I had planned to go the dog park. We didn't expect the entire walking trail to be iced over when we arrived. My mother still remembers slipping on the ice, begging me to turn around, and seeing the look of firm resoluteness in my eyes as I kept walking ahead, more loyal to our scheduled agenda that day than to my mother's sudden fall.

With Great Freedom Comes Great Responsibility

I had three big questions: 1) How am I supposed to know what to eat, 2) How am I supposed to know what to feel, 3) With the door open to my room, how am I supposed to know where to go?

How do we know which direction to circle in? We can only judge by how we feel at every curve. Or we can just reverse directions and see what feels right.

Without knowing what I was physically feeling, I felt like I had lost all instincts and trust in myself altogether.

Horizontal ripples of the sea, like little commas in an everlasting sentence. Which side is life? The sky or the sandy shore? And where does the tide want to go? Where do I want to go? I belong with the tide, contently bobbing across the vast fluid waves, moving away from its heavenly source of light, floating to a world of life, a world of people.

As time progressed and I got used to eating again, my pull for life got stronger, but the fear of emotions was my constant undertow. Now not only did I feel like two separate people pre-trauma and post-trauma, but I also felt conflicted as to who I wanted to be now, and what I was supposed to do about it. In a way, it was easier when I didn't have any options. I had been told for so long to wait and not eat, completely dependent on doctors. Now that I was my own authority, the ability to make decisions was terrifying. There were just so many.

I see myself precariously balanced on a tiny horizontal wave, gripping its liquid edge to me like a warm winter blanket and riding it home. Homeward bound, whatever that means, as the wind pokes at my hair and carries me towards life, towards the soles and souls that wander along the shore. It's all waiting for me. But for now, I peer over it from my window like Rapunzel waiting for her prince to come.

Though I found the power to bridge my two worlds, happiness continued to elude me. I was eating sweet food again, but why had life suddenly gone sour? I felt so abandoned. The doctors' job was done. The news cameras had left. I could finally feed myself. But I felt like I needed more taking care of than ever.

The one emotion I hadn't allowed myself to feel was anger. What was the point of being angry about things I couldn't control? I was now at the point in my life where I began to understand everything Blaine had taken from me.

I'm drowning in this whirlpool, pushed by fears, but pulled by the joy of gratitude. What should I be feeling? I'm angry, and that's a righteous feeling! Maybe anger is the blast of energy coming from deep inside me that will break through my internal barriers and get me unstuck once and for all!

If only you had heard me scream.

Clinging to Trauma-Survivor Identity

I DIDN'T GET IT. The surgeries were over. I could eat. Life was good. Why was I making things miserable for myself? Why couldn't I let go of my suffering? Why not be at peace with the fact that things are always changing?

The doctors had done all of their work, so I was the one stalling progress. A tremendous sense of guilt washed over me. *I* was the one holding myself back, and I couldn't help thinking the outside world was thinking the same thing. Everyone had seen the news reports, right? All I could hear was: "Westport woman goes years without eating, finally miraculously reconstructed, and now has an eating disorder?" *How ungrateful! Why can't she just get her life started already?* At least, that's what I was thinking.

I had been able to eat for nine months, and while my body was physically better, I couldn't really say *I* was better in any way than I had been before reconstruction.

February 22, 2008—The snow is falling from my window so fast. I could stand by my computer all day and watch the snowflakes fall. You can only do so much when you are too afraid to leave your room. How many baby steps do you have to take before you take that leap of faith?

I had gained back food, but with it came bittersweet memories of loss. Oddly, or so it seemed until I understood trauma better, I missed the times I had with Blaine. I remembered lying next to Blaine in the dark, and I was very upset inside. I thought at least I could confide in him, just because *I had no one else.*

I didn't want to be faced with the guilt tormenting me for not fighting back or running away, even after I knew things had turned. Why had I gone back to lessons, still, regardless, week after week? Had I been I asking for it? But to my own abuser, I mourned my losses: "I really wish we could go back to being student and teacher. I don't know, I've just felt really not like myself since everything happened."

Blaine very "logically" responded. "Our connection was so deep that you know neither of us would have been satisfied had we just remained student and teacher. The pull was too intense. Neither of us could help it. It would have happened sooner or later. That's just the nature of soulmates."

And of my lost innocence, he unemotionally replied: "Well, I think it's time you grow up. Your house has this enchanted air of never-never land, like the boys who never grow up."

I didn't know what to say. I didn't know what to think. I bit my lip to not feel anything because there was no point. There was no one I could tell who would understand, so why bother. I turned off my feelers, my emotional radar, to save myself for the weekend. I felt like no one was there to watch me or help me, just like there was no one there to grieve with over my lost innocence.

I couldn't stand my abuser, but I felt like he was all I had at my lowest point. Plus, an ember in me kept hoping that one day Blaine the teacher would pop out of this monster's body and it would be like none of this ever had happened. I couldn't give up that hope because then my whole world would fall to pieces.

But I tried to tell who I could...however I could. That summer, I tried to tell my brother Jeff when I was visiting him in Washington while he was working on the John Kerry campaign. We were taking a long walk past all of the huge monuments, but all I felt was the panic in my heart and the shuffling of my feet.

"Jeff. "I don't think I'm very happy," I said while trying to catch my breath. "I've been spending a lot of time at lessons. With Blaine."

"Yeah, mom says you're over there a lot."

"Blaine said it was like...we were soulmates."

"What!?"

"No, I don't mean like seriously; it was a stupid joke, you know! Forget it, I was joking."

I scared him as soon as I even hinted, so I panicked and ended up covering up the terrible secret I was harboring. He walked ahead of me, with a jumble of feeling outraged, shocked and confused. I followed behind with my head hung in shame and regret.

So, I was left with an ugly secret half-exposed for the rest of the trip, and all I got out of it was an even tenser relationship with my brother, who has always been the smoke detector of the family. It's hard to have a relationship with a liar, he would always tell me, as he confronted me about compulsive exercise and all of my other destructive coping mechanisms. How could I be truthful to anyone if I couldn't even be honest with myself? I was desperately trying to not let myself realize that the "Blaine-Buddha-Teacher" I knew was forever gone. All of my destructive behaviors put me in a daze, which I used as a shield to turn my face from his demonic transformation.

My body was touched in ways it was not ready to be touched. I missed that body, but I also missed the innocence that went along with it. I lost the joy of the first time the man you love touches you. On *your* own body. In your skin. I gave that up for Blaine.

The first time I was touched was by a snake, and its venom poisoned my positive associations with romance. I lost my prom and the flirty girlishness to even score a date for the prom. My coma saved me from the last four months of that shameful senior year. I lost my pride with boys. I didn't even bother having crushes anymore, because I felt disgusting. I lost my confidence, the tough skin that protected my soul.

What could I do with all of these memories? I felt inundated, stuck in a whirlpool of long-forgotten emotion, sensations, and thoughts that were slowly spinning more and more anxieties for myself.

I wasn't ready for therapy when I couldn't eat or drink, but now that food was on the table, so to speak, I was more than ready for someone to help me. So, I called a trauma therapist, Rita.

Rita listened to my flustered ramblings, then calmly replied, "You have to tell your story. You have to say in words what happened to you."

I hung up and thought I would never talk to her again. She was oversimplifying things. I'm used to "thinking" myself out. I didn't know why I actually had to verbalize it. What could words do? I spent a few months pretending everything was okay, but it wasn't. Then I thought, *what the heck, I'll say it.*

I tried, but I couldn't speak. At that moment, I knew the therapist was right. Until I could use the power of words to express what happened to me, I would not heal.

To say that Blaine had molested me was…impossible. Speech is a powerful thing. I had to open my mouth and hear those words. It was terrifying because in speaking, it would be real, it would have happened, and that would be me, a girl who was molested by her trusted mentor. And it would make me cry and unlock feelings I did not wish to feel. So, I didn't speak it. I just kept writing. I hoarded journals of every shape and size with picturesque landscape covers and inspirational quotes, believing one day, these stacks of my written words would guide me right back to myself. But I still couldn't breathe, mouth, or speak what I was writing. Did I really have to talk about all this?

Rita, a psychotherapist specializing in EMDR (Eye Movement Desensitization Reprocessing) a friend had recommended, was the only real "therapist" I ever had. But our therapy wasn't traditional or scientific; it was all done through art and creative expression. We didn't talk. We spoke in hero's journey metaphors, body sculptures, drawing, and song.

The first day I met Rita, I was nervous. I knew anyone who had been through my situation should be in therapy, but I didn't know what to expect. I also wasn't used to speaking to other people. Rita seemed to understand that right away, and all she asked me to do was make a sculpture with my body of how I felt now. I curled up into a ball. Then a sculpture of how I wanted to feel. I stood straight up with my arms to the ceiling as I would for a closing number, belting on stage.

In our sessions, we spoke in metaphors—in literature, poetry, and art. We created fantasy stories, hero's journeys, signs and symbols everywhere. We did not mention the words "trauma" or "anxiety." She described trauma to me as a river that got stuck in a current and somehow the current can flow back into the river once you unleash the energy in a different way.

Rita: You develop certain symptoms as a result of the stuck trauma, and the Anxiety is due to this energy logjam. When you shut down and daze out, your logjam is stuck. When there is too much arousal going into the trauma, there isn't enough discharge of energy.

I lost trust in my body and became unfamiliar with how to take care of it. That is why pleasure frightened me. Now, I just had to report the sensations I felt like a "body weather report." If they were just sensations, they couldn't turn into a scary feeling—like anxiety.

This creative view of trauma actually gave me back control of my circumstances. It gave me confidence, and I was able to use the role I knew I could play as an artist and the tools that were natural to me to help create a way out of this mess. It became clear that art could really save my life.

Now it made sense why at the end of high school I had felt alone, unable to focus, and robotically leaving my classes. Or why I was numbing my mind by writing down calculations for my gigantic slime smoothies. At eighteen, I was scared of who I had become.

With each bite of food, I explored the high school memories that still paralyzed me with shame. Food finally brought clarity to the fog I'd been stuck in for so long. I could clearly see, for the first time, what a living hell life had been right before my coma. That, even before my coma, I had been running away from shame I didn't deserve.

Once Blaine started molesting me, I turned to exercise to not feel anything at all when I went back for lessons. Just as I used compulsive exercise to pass the years of hunger, I had used it to shield myself from my teacher's demonic transformation.

I remembered the inescapable torture I felt, confused at how each day had degraded into miserable stretches of hours to endure. I couldn't figure out how life became continuously fraught with panic. I couldn't contain the raging urge to pace around all day. I got desperately anxious if I didn't walk around nearby neighborhoods for hours or work out in the gym. I secretly wished and prayed for the gym to be locked every day and breathed a little sigh of relief when it was. Because it was like I *had* to, and if I didn't, I couldn't live with my guilt.

I couldn't believe, as I willed to go further and further into my memories, that I had actually blocked all of this out.

When you have a compulsion, you know you shouldn't do it, but you also know if you don't do it, you'll feel even more miserable and guilty. That's what exercise was for me at that time in my life. And no one knew my secret world of misery, and I didn't know how to call out for help. But I felt like I was running from a hitman, and I needed help desperately.

My heart would start to pound as I heard the voice inside my head: You better run out of this classroom, down the stairs, and into the car so you can exercise! And I would get scared if I took one extra second to tie my shoes or gather my books. If I wasn't ready to go by the time the bell rang, I would feel such guilt hanging on my shoulders.

And I would race to the car, and try to maintain a conversation with Mom, but I was so dazed I couldn't really focus. All I could hear was the voice in my ear about how hard the hitman was going to torture me once I hit the exercise room. I would have a panic attack in the car home from school every day. "How was your day?" my mom would casually ask. "Fine," I would mutter, wishing I could call out to her and express to her my pain and fear. I wanted to reach out for help so badly.

When my mom barged in on me in the exercise room and screamed in horror, "I don't even recognize you anymore! Your eyes are hollow!" it scared me more than anything because I realized I didn't know who I was anymore. I had no idea how I ended up with this imaginary hitman running after me with dumbbells. I didn't want to live like this anymore. I just didn't know yet how to escape.

When we went to Disney World that summer, it felt like for a week I was out of the death grip, free of the maniacal circles the exercise hitman was spinning me in.

I breathed a sigh of relief to myself and exclaimed to my mom, "look, Ma, a palm tree!" For me, it was a sign I was in a different universe, and maybe that horrible whirlpool had stayed in Fairfield so I could get a respite from the torture it caused me. Maybe for a week, life didn't have to be miserable. But my heart beat with such anxiety the moment I thought about how in just a week, I would have to return home and face it again.

I didn't have to wait even that long. The whirlpool penetrated the border of Florida and continued to drive me mad. I couldn't understand why I had to take the longer route walking around every street, and why I suddenly was unsure of how much to eat. I immediately didn't feel safe here either. Life was agony for me as I wrestled with myself over how to take care of myself, and it felt like everyone was out to get me. *Who could I trust?*

Why did it take so many years for such potent memories to surface, let alone cut me like a knife? Had I chosen to block all of this out? Had I lost myself long before the surgeries? Was I a hopeless case? Or was I a work in progress?

CHAPTER 22

Who was I After Trauma?

TO REGAIN MY IDENTITY, I had to confront who I was after Blaine. I had returned to school for senior year drained of all life force. I felt alone, in a black hole. The real world had no idea I was suffering in the whirlpool vortex, cut off from my normal river of life. No one could understand why I wasn't back to being myself.

"Where's my daughter? You've lost that spirit." Mom said.

Where could I find it? Even Jeff wrote to me in a melancholy tone saying that he missed "her." But I hadn't actually lost my bubbly effervescent energy, and I never could, according to the law of energy conservation. Now I was alleviating shame bite by bite. Each bite continued to bring back a pre-coma memory I had tucked away. Like the summer before my senior year, when Jeff stopped home for a visit. Fully aware he was watching my every move, I led Jeff out the front door on a humid August day and put on a smile.

"Jeff, wanna go outside?" Except I walked right past him and nearly shut the door in his face. I felt him judging me and forming his own conclusions.

"Amy, what's wrong? Sit," he said and sat on the curb.

"Not now." Panicked, I paced in front of him, anxiously.

"You can't just sit for a second?" He clearly wasn't getting up.

"I just said not now."

He was trying to connect with me, but I was stuffing down a trauma I had yet to fully understand, and all he saw was his sister as a pacing maniac, the result of the cyclone my river had become. I was confused about everything and felt helpless as Jeff became more aggravated with my back-and-forth steps. He thought I was doing it on purpose. *No one* does this on purpose. Looking back, I can see I was trying to create a misery that would outdo the real misery I was running from: Blaine.

I felt so alone in my huge room of undiscovered secrets, in this giant manic whirlpool, that I felt like no one could ever understand. I hardly did.

It's ironic, I prayed to God every night that Blaine and I could have a deeper, truer relationship, that we could be equals. Be careful what you wish for. Now it's all that and more. It's confusing. And disillusioning. I want my mentor and muse back.

I wish I had the power and knowledge back then to say: "It's HIM, HIM, HIM!" Whatever I tried to do to escape only sucked me in further.

One night that year, I wanted to be rescued so badly from my hell hole whirlpool that I crawled into my mom's bed before I "had" to work out. A furious panic attack came over me. All I could feel in my body was this red fire. My mom asked, "What's wrong Amy?"

In between heavy gasps and the intensifying anxiety about the next day, I stammered, "There's a secret! Se-cr- inside...I—gotta get...out! I can't do this—it's killing me!" I stared at her with wide, blank owl eyes, waiting for her to respond and urge it out of me.

"Amy, take a breath!" Mom tried to place her hand on my shoulder, with a mix of upset, confusion, and sheer fright.

I avoided looking at her but could sense she didn't know how to help me, and honestly, I didn't know how to help her help me. My helplessness turned into more frustration and deeper gasps as she tried pulling out a yoga chakra deck of cards. She took one more forced breath as though she was giving birth.

"Okay, sweetie. Should we try a grounding chakra card?" I couldn't concentrate. My body refused to be put into the here and now, and my voice was too frozen to scream, turning me into a stuttering, gasping mess for the rest of the night. Sitting cross-legged in her bed, trembling, we ended up watching an Adam Sandler movie together, *50 First Dates*. Unlike Drew Barrymore, who forgets everything that happened the previous day, I remember every moment of that film, not scenes specifically, but the encroaching feeling of fire coming from a deep place in my gut, impairing my ability to speak or breathe.

During that last year of high school, my parents kept sending me for lessons, unaware I was dreading each interaction with Blaine. I was convinced there was something wrong with me. Was I defective? Was it all my fault? Rita helped me see I had been a scared young girl having normal a reaction to being molested for months by a sixty-year-old sociopath. All that time I blamed myself for the mess my life had become. For the first time since starting to eat again, my brain was as clear as it had been with my first bite of pumpkin. My emotions were all on the table.

With Rita's help, I began to put the pieces together to see how I could finally break free. By remembering my trauma, getting all my secrets out, and disclosing my harbored feelings, I was able to state with a totally clear conscience: "None of what happened was my fault. Nothing." Speaking those words enabled me to take my power back.

The more I realized things weren't my fault, the more excited I was to dig up old memories, connect the pieces, and regain my sense of trust through alleviating my guilt.

As sad as it was for me to remember my pain, I felt relieved releasing it. With each secret, I uncovered a hidden feeling and formed another brick of the new wall I was building for my river. Rita also had the idea of thinking of it as a biological cell wall, with food as the nutrients that would repair the wall. She helped me see that by remembering my secrets and turning them into bricks I could rebuild my walls and redirect my river's energy towards the future, into both who I'd been and who God intended for me to be. Floating on the river of compassion allowed me to start moving on.

I had always loved biology in high school, mostly for the diagrams, which always looked like an action-packed superhero comic strip. So, Rita's suggestion of the cell wall worked wonders. Like a cell, the river could repair itself. I imagined myself a big cell, responsible for letting outside stimulation pass in and out of my numb, rigid membrane. I envisioned food as being the mechanism through which I could give the membrane the strength and nourishment it needed to rebuild myself, the strength to fight the strong, stubborn current of the trauma whirlpool.

As much as I had hungered for it all of these years, now that I was at the brink of life, or so it felt, I was scared. I had taken comfort hiding in my room all of those years. It was like asking a traumatized prisoner to come out of hiding or like how my parents and I felt when we had gotten a "day pass" to leave Bridgeport Hospital to go to the mall, and all we wanted was to go back into our safe hospital room nest.

While my work with Rita was beginning to bring me out of my shell, or at least helping me crack it open, I still wasn't quite ready. I needed to come out slowly and sometimes pull my head back into the safe refuge of numbness.

Taking a break from "Thriving Amy" to settle into my comfort of dazing out. Wish I could stay like this forever. Fun while it lasts.

I was terrified of what lay ahead, but I was more frightened of staying the same, of never escaping my cocoon where I didn't have to feel anything.

I was a stranger to myself, a stranger in a strange land. But not for much longer.

"Get Your Life Together, Amy!"

Now that I could eat, I felt the pressure to "get my life together." I tried various things to start "feeling normal," based on what I thought normal people do—go to school, get a job, do things with other people. I started sending out resumés for every kind of job I could think of. I registered for courses at a community college, but I still didn't feel normal. Although my mind was pressuring me to be "normal," my body was still swept away in the whirlpool of trauma. I was not ready to be in the real world yet, but I did try.

My first step toward reintegrating myself into the world was taking a class at a community college. Unfortunately, you can't go to school and run from trauma at the same time.

When you live life on the run, you don't have time to make any long-lasting worthwhile connections with others or investments in life. I couldn't get one thing out of my classes because I felt compelled to always keep busy during them. If I wasn't taking notes, I had to be doing other work. Sitting with extra energy having nothing to use it up for was like a death sentence. I needed to keep my pen moving to survive, and after class, I had to run away and start pacing up and down the stairs because getting rid of that energy was more important. I was still too scared to confront the energy of the past.

I spent most of my time in class cartooning in my journal. In my creative cartoon adventure, I, as detective, had ignited another question: Did Blaine make it that hard to breathe that night on my mother's bed? And... did Blaine cause my stomach to explode?

CHAPTER 23

Living in Metaphors

THE SURGEONS FINISHED THEIR JOB. Now it was up to me. My classes at the community college were a disaster and I didn't understand yet why things weren't working. So, I called Rita.

"I love my classes, but I can't concentrate! Will this trauma vortex thing ever go away?"

"No."

"I'm never going to get better? How is life going to change?"

"The answer lies in what the trauma vortex is made of: water," Rita calmly replied. "But just as water can race around in a vortex, water can also move in a variety of other ways. It can flow like a river, too."

I had had it with Rita's metaphors. I had been so excited to register for a full course load. But taking courses to get my mind off of my traumas couldn't push those same nagging anxieties out of my head. I cynically wondered what Rita's next brilliant remark might be. She continued, "If the trauma vortex is just water, it means you have the power to turn that water into anything. The trauma vortex doesn't go away. You just strengthen the healing vortex."

This was starting to make sense. Water can be a beautiful waterfall or a destructive cyclone—you have the power to change it—it's all just water, after all. I got out my notebook and pen and went back to Frank to really

AMY OESTREICHER

imagine this. How would I give Frank the power to change the raging waters into a healing vortex? I imagined Frank like Hercules or Zeus, seizing that river like a giant thunderbolt above his head.

With Rita's help, I began to understand how to use the healing vortex. I quickly held onto the mental cognition I was gaining. However, my body was still petrified to catch up to my brain power, speeding faster than even my anxious toes could carry me. I knew what I needed to do, but I couldn't.

It was much more comfortable to talk to Rita on the phone and intellectually "get" how to heal, but I chickened out of physicalizing this. The result: jogging around my room, having countless phone session "revelations" with Rita, but never having the guts to actually drive there, stand with her, myself, and stillness, and *truly* heal.

"How do I get rid of this awful whirlpool I'm drowning in?" I asked her as my feet jogged around my worn-down carpet.

"You heal from trauma by increasing the force of the healing vortex, like balancing a scale. One current overpowers the other."

How do you increase the strength of the healing vortex? By empowering it with every healthy coping skill and resource you can find, until your healing vortex has enough power to override the evil vortex of trauma. Rita explained that any small "everyday anxiety" I felt before my trauma became tremendously amplified in the whirlpool. The wonder of the river is that it can flow *around* normal obstacles like everyday anxiety. Water can break off around a rock, converge once again, and keep on flowing into the future.

I started to think of myself as a microcosm for nature. Physiologically, we are rigged up to heal, just like the earth. You have an earthquake or tornado, but the world can compose itself after that kind of trauma. Starfish grow back arms.

Armed with a visual metaphor of balance, I could begin to achieve a sense of control. When the power of the trauma was activated, I became panicked and terror-stricken. Now, I had to use that fear as healing energy that could counteract the trauma response. You can't stop an earthquake, but the earth will, over time, naturally heal itself. That is the natural process of life.

With my new understanding that achieving balance and allowing the healing vortex to do its work could heal my PTSD, I turned to my old favorite school subject: biology! Redirecting the current of a whirlpool of trauma into a calm river was how I could heal emotionally. And since I had the same cells that I had before my coma, the little micromolecules repairing my body within me were what I could call *home*.

The law of energy applies to me! I imagined every cell I had studied in my biology book now as a kind of home for myself.

I made myself think of the medical trauma and the pain I had first felt in my stomach. I imagined the cell walls inside me bursting. "Cytolysis!" I remembered from my bio textbook.

4:24 p.m. I had done it! Sat with that anxiety and stillness for (almost) two minutes!

Now, seeing that cell image replay before my eyes suddenly empowered a new motivation to eat. After the rupture, the cell loses its turgor pressure and becomes weak and flimsy. By eating, I could visualize those food molecules flowing in my body's bloodstream and repairing the cell walls to create a healthy working cell. I imagined me as a healthy cell trying to repair my wall with food to prevent evil invading bacteria from getting in. I was finally strengthening my healing vortex. But...understanding intellectually how to use the healing vortex was only the beginning. Visualizing could only take me so far. Now, I needed to feel healing happening in my body. To do that, I had to stop being so numb.

The more I worried and allowed any sensation to drive me to anxiety, the more I realized how afraid I was of emptiness.

Anxiety wants to trick you into thinking your life is meaningless and all you need is it. Because without you, it can't exist. Like viral DNA, anxiety has no life without a cell to feed on.

With the realization that dropping my courses didn't mean I had to stop learning, I felt warm heat fill my chest and flutter like a butterfly. This was not hot red anxiety, but a kinder inner glow. This feeling inspired Tiger Lilly the warrior to create a new god—enthusiasm, the god who rules over the healing vortex and who is vastly more powerful than trauma. The more my enthusiasm grew for life, the more my healing vortex grew stronger and, like a tree, more deeply rooted in my purpose. I began regain my *self* and ownership of my body and soul.

It became clear that without Blaine in the picture, I would have never felt the anxiety that raged through me during my senior year of high school. He had gained power over me as I lost my *inner goddess of enthusiasm*, and as he gained control over me, the viral DNA was replicating inside of my fragile system, into my vulnerability and innocence. Blaine was a virus: a force outside of me, not part of me.

I ran into the bathroom at the community college and paused in front of the mirror. The words, "Tell yourself I love you," rang in my ears. Doing so wasn't easy. I instantly felt a jolt in my chest.

I had to break past the wall of numbness to thrive. All I needed was a box of tools that could ground me in the present when the trauma swept me away in the past. Biology was a powerful tool for my healing current, and now I searched for more.

We think we are afraid of uncertainty, when, in fact, we are truly afraid of the certainty that we can't change, or that things will not get better. But a warrior possesses the courage to go into the uncertainty because they have the confidence they will be able to change things themselves, with the proper tools, of course. As a warrior on this journey, I needed to pack my warrior's backpack with all of the healing resources I could think of. It was going to take a fierce current to outweigh the cyclonic current of trauma.

No matter how hard I tried, I couldn't think or daydream or "write" my way out of being present. This final step connected all my thoughts to what I was feeling physically in my body, and this was the hardest part. Only when I was able to use my poetic metaphors and imagery along with feeling these images my body could I move forward. Body and mind had to heal together.

When I started feeling pleasure and it got linked to something painful or negative, I had options. I could feel my hands on the counter and tell myself I am here now, feel the temperature of the counter, notice how the food felt in my hand, and tell myself that it's with me now. Options gave me control.

Being in the moment was my secret tool. The key to being in my body without panicking was to experience awareness without judgment, to notice how my feet felt on the floor and how the floor felt on my feet. No emotions, just physical sensations. This exercise told my body it was not in the time of the trauma, but right here, right now.

No wonder why I loved exercising to the point of exhaustion; suffering and pain meant "safety." But it also kept me stuck and run by fear.

If I feel my feet on the floor, I can't fly back into the trauma that gets reactivated any time I do something that feels physically good! I have to notice the sensations in my body—I use to shrug that off as fluff. But now, I see that I haven't been living in the real world because my body has literally been somewhere else!

What did it mean to feel "out of body?" When you can't feel your body, the world is a scary place to be because you have no idea where you belong. I learned that being out of body had two dissociative subtypes: depersonalization (seeing your body from above, i.e. "This is not happening to me") and de-realization ("This isn't really real; this is just a dream").

Whenever I touch a part of me, I am always alarmed. It feels like I am touching a stranger or being touched by a stranger. I physically can't feel my body when I walk fast or numb out or stay in my mind. How weird is it that I am living in a shell that I don't even know? Home is your body that you can carry with you wherever you go. Otherwise, you feel unattached to anything.

With the five senses helping me feel my body, I wasn't alone, and I wasn't free-floating—two feelings that frightened me. When you feel your body, you are always home, you always feel like you are in a safe container. If you live in your mind, that is all you have, and anything can happen in your mind; fear can be a vicious demon who can kill you in your imagination because your imagination isn't anchored in your body, which should be a safe place to call home. But when you are in your body, you are grounded in reality.

Superhero senses continued to be my allies whenever my mind took over. Shame was in my mind, but power was in my body. My five superhero senses came along like imaginary friends, filling in the lines like an internal coloring book to make any moment beautiful, hence, my affirmation, "the present moment is all we have."

"I call the emergency line and say, "Is this the fab five senses? I need your help right away. There's a serpent on the loose! Can you help me be in the present moment save the wounded bird from drowning?" And those five little rock stars come flying through my window. With their hands on their hips and bright turquoise capes blowing in the wind, they declare in unison, "We hereby grant you the power of NOW!"

Once I let food into my life, it allowed in a sixth sense: nature. October came, and I started to feel the first pangs of spirituality within me through nature, through every picture I took on my digital camera, and through autumn blowing through my body. It was a gradual shift rather than a timeline, a gradual shift in colors, with things looking brighter and brighter every day. I realized that transitions did not have to be painful in a fearful way. To help myself understand the fluid nature of time, I looked outwards, to nature, to the seasons. I realized that a gradual transition can be a beautiful thing.

Autumn was the ultimate symbol of transition for me, and so I used this time as an opportunity to feel the gradual changes within me.

A fresh new day, a fresh new egg that tasted juicy with a warm mushy yolk that I swallowed down whole. It is in my body, my body is wrapped around it, there is no turning back now. A huge frying pan kept it warm for me, and I loved its fried crispy edges, forming a brown ring around the pure white blob. Determination is burning in my eyes. Since I feel myself more than ever, the Amy part is putting that energy towards making my blue eyes sparkle.

Eating had shaken my carefully controlled world like a snow globe, but now, the shaking allowed me to feel the snow of holiness shower me with inspiration, bringing me back to my *roots* (pun intended). Einstein said you can't solve a problem using the same thinking that originally created it. The change in environment from room to nature broke me out of my box of rigidity and returned me to my trees that had been my guides long before Blaine. Whenever I got out of control, nature grounded me.

I stretched out my hand to see what the universe had to offer me today, and God, like the stork, dropped into my palm a bundle of sky-blue light molecules from the clouds above. I do not like the feeling I get from just mechanically doing and not being, not being open to the spontaneity of the moment and just having my own agenda in mind. Where is the living in that?

When I surrendered control, I could enjoy myself. And it was okay! Now my family and I were moving along with the seasons, changing along with the world. So, we did as many festive autumn things as we could. We got pumpkins, and Mom wrapped leaf-studded ribbons around a glass jar of dried pasta sticks around the counter, and placed cider-scented Yankee candles everywhere.

Can you believe it? I went trick or treating on Halloween. In years past, I spent the night in my room, afraid of the world, exercising to get through the night, or in the hospital with shingles, or trapped in Blaine's apartment drinking Ensures. But this October, I put my foot down and said, "Dammit, I am living my life and I don't care what anyone has to say about it because I deserve it!"

With a Fresh Start Came Fresh Challenges

As I started "buying into life," the trauma vortex felt threatened and wouldn't let go without a fight. On paper, the question seemed like it had one clear, logical answer, but I remained torn between two worlds. I found that I had to hold onto all of my healing resources—my projects, writing, outside, shopping with Mom, to keep my mind off of exercise. That meant making a list of things I could do: walk a little, shop a little, do some cartooning. It was all about time and balance and keeping my day occupied.

When you embrace change, you look for the miracles within the changes, like little flowers that grow in between the cracks in the sidewalk. So, the question I asked myself every morning was: how is today an opportunity to learn, grow, and heal?

Trauma makes you feel kicked out of the human race in your own crazy vortex. You need to join a community again, even if it's not a community of people. (I joined a community of trees.) When you no longer feel shut out, you can open your heart and start to join the world of the living again.

I knew in healing from trauma, I was going to mess up. But if I kept moving through the messes, there was always a chance for a redo.

Yesterday at the dog park, the same one where my mom and I had that ugly freak out, I thought of a visualization that helped me. Every leaf that fell before me was a new experience, a new moment. That is my only job in life; to go through life moment to moment. The one leaf of now is the definition of happiness. It was a great day at the park.

CHAPTER 24

Letting Go to Take Control

IT WAS TIME TO START CONFRONTING high school memories. I boldly approached the colossal building, seeing it as though I were Marley's ghost, and could picture myself just a few years prior, holding my head in shame whenever I would see an old friend. In an instant, I was transported back to being a wide-eyed freshman, reconnecting with my old tree friends, hearing the symphonies swirling from their rough, rugged barks.

I can hear the crunch of the leaves walking to the entrance so clearly, and the exact lampposts with the clock on it, and the trees outside the glass doors, the same colors of the leaves, the clouds over the school, and I can even feel the exact temperature and textures of the breath I would inhale, the crispy scrumptious air that would invigorate my soul. I can remember the exact sparkle in my eyes!

I could remember a time when I loved myself and everything around me. I could feel tears welling up as I mourned that loss. Passing by empty classroom windows, I left the pre-coma Amy behind—the audacious, life-loving girl, and the dazed, trauma-stricken teen too. I walked away wondering, "Now who's left?"

I left my old high school grounds, unable to predict what was ahead, and that was okay. I now faced a healthy kind of uncertainty that everyone felt, not the uncertainty of not knowing if I would eat again. If everyone felt this uncertainty in life, then it couldn't be terrible. It meant that now I had normal people problems. How exciting!

The fall season that year taught me a powerful lesson: If I could change, I could grow. Moving from the trauma vortex to the healing vortex also helped me understand that change never diminishes us. I had "lost" my old self, but I had also gained so much in the process.

As I left more autumn memories, I was determined to give any change, loss, or challenge a magical energy rather than the "stuck energy" trauma had frozen me in. Now that this energy was thawing out, I had to use it in a healthy way. But which way was healthy?

Trauma had tangled the wires in my brain and now I had to rewire everything to make healthy choices. With school memories in one hand and a strong fist in other, I could use the rapidly unthawing energy to change the whirlpool's current, and that felt powerful.

Trauma was no longer an overwhelming diagnosis that threatened to overtake my life. In trauma, your energy can respond in three ways making you *fight, flee, or freeze.*

I could have immediately fought back against my abuser, yelling "no" or defying him in some way. I could have just run in the other direction as fast as I could. But I was so shocked by everything that happened that I froze. Like a deer in the headlights, I couldn't come to terms with the idea that a man that I trusted as my mentor could turn into a monster in the blink of an eye. I mentally left the situation, disassociated from my body, and became a passive bystander to a trauma that my body was directly involved in.

Understanding my compulsions didn't make them healthier, but the good part about knowing why you do something is that it gives you a point of attack when you're ready to start moving on from your unhealthy coping skills.

Now that I knew the traumas were not my fault, my body did not have to keep involuntarily punishing itself. Reading a section of *Waking the Tiger* by Peter Levine about "running movements" made me draw some parallels to my hyperactivity. He wrote about how when a gazelle is preyed upon in the wild, it plays dead, and when the threat is gone, the gazelle will gallop for miles, to discharge that frozen energy. Perhaps my "daggerfooting" was my own attempt to restore some kind of homeostasis. Understanding why something happened made me less ashamed to talk about it. Once I could talk about my compulsive exercise and bring it out in the open, I could finally start stopping it.

Nature was a comprehensive learning environment, and there was something to learn from everything. On my nature walks, I noticed that when squirrels saw a "threat," they would pause, notice what was happening, and then quickly move on with their day, rather than be frozen in fear.

The real work came from taking that nervous energy, which was formerly an essential trauma survival skill, and turning it into productive healing energy that once redirected, could color in a new world alive with melancholy blues, angry reds, uncertain grays, but also one of ecstatic oranges, bright yellows, and deep rich purples. Once I let myself feel the "bad," I made room for the "good."

Telling your story and disclosing secrets isn't an agonizing thing that your therapist forces you to do. Trying to think about old memories always paralyzed me. But when I described it as going into the dark dungeon of secrets, exorcising demons, finding a warrior's prize deep in the haunted house of buried, painful emotions, then it became a thrill-seeking adventure!

It felt courageous to keep writing heroes' journeys in the comfy cove of my mind. But speaking what I wrote was a physical act. To actually stand still and feel the silence around me so the words could echo deep in my gut, then say, "I was sexually abused" out loud and hear them resonate throughout my body was terrifying.

But terrifying equaled progress. I directed my unthawing energy into dancing, so I could start to creatively feel the joy that could come from reclaiming my body. With my turns and leaps, I shaped the words, "Healing is a physical act."

It I could get my body to start talking, it was only a matter of time before I could speak myself.

Can I challenge myself today and see how many moments I can stay "awake" for? How many times I can choose the right thought that my heart wants for me? Healing isn't so much about getting "better." It's about letting go of everything that isn't you.

Healing Through Creativity

TO BLEND THE WORLDS OF NATURE and creativity, two worlds I needed to physically reclaim myself in, I started creatively cartooning "Frank," my alter ego in nature. I kept a notebook with me at all times and created a graphic novel with Frank, who was really *me*. In my cartoons, Frank slowly came into the outside world, and I represented my struggles through his endearing little stick figure in a fantastical adventure story.

As I tried to take mindful nature walks, sketchbook in hand, Frank become my healthy coping companion. When I felt myself starting to "numb out," I asked myself: "Where is Frank today?"

One day, my mother convinced me to stop pacing and sit for a pedicure. I felt that anxiety creep up my legs as soon as I took a seat and the scented oil started warming my ankles. Thankfully, I was armed and ready with my journal in my lap, Frank waiting to guide me.

Frank got his toes wet! He built up the "POWER OF NOW" river a bit more, enough so the trickle turned into enough water to fill up a small tub for a pedicure chair!

As my pencil urged Frank to get closer to the trauma vortex, to dip his toes in it using the power of now, suddenly, the warm massage oil felt good!

Imagination 1, Anxiety 0

My imagination's powerful current flowed onto every page, washing anxiety away with every scribbled image.

Frank was holding my hand as we explored my "trauma vortex" together. In even simple activities, Frank encouraged me to stay present with the physical feeling of being touched. I drew him in the chair beside me saying, "This is how you'll get back into your body again." But the further I got into my body, the closer I came to the "core" of my trauma vortex: ANGER. Now, I needed a healthy way to get that anger out. *Frank, any ideas?*

I drew out "Frank" on one blank page. All I could doodle was a thin red swirling line wildly spurting off his shoulder. The panel needed a title: "Frank Feels 'Anger' for the First Time." Now, it was safe for me to "dip my toes" into the feeling of anger, too. It was frightening.

I love how my story keeps unfolding into new and dramatic counterparts, and the journey is always stretched out by one more challenge on the way to the temple. Like God is really testing me for the greatest warrior medal of all.

Releasing Anger Restores My Internal Balance

As scary as it was to finally get out that anger, for the first time I felt calm and balanced inside. By discharging all that "red swirling line" energy stuck in me, I was allowing myself to heal and move on. So, I drew Frank the next day with that red swirly line floating up into the sky, lightening his own load, and turning into a beautiful purple balloon soaring into the clouds.

My instincts were to waver, to dip back into that sizzling pool of crisis, panic, sharks, and snakes, to wade back into the danger zone. But Frank got that red angry doodle out of him and convinced me that I could, too.

Letting myself feel fear was petrifying. I felt like I was losing all sense of rigid control, that anything could happen. But my daily warrior traits were changing me from "wounded bird" to "fierce tiger." I resolved to push forward, to lean on my anchors: Frank, my five superhero senses, and my body.

Creativity as the Key to Healing

I sensed that healing required the courage to play, and cartooning was my first, creative attempt. And by playing, or playing things out through my cartoons, I was learning to make sense of how I coped. Once I shared my secret world through my drawings, I was no longer ashamed of it. As I doodled my compulsive exercise, I was able to understand the underlying reason why I "needed" to exercise, then forgive myself and move beyond it. Cartooning my secrets turned shame into adventure stories I couldn't put down!

Adopting Healthy Coping Skills

I was in my room looking out the window onto the street as Frank's journeys were becoming more exciting. In my cartoons, he was taking boat rides to uncharted territories, meeting new people, immersing himself in experiences he couldn't control. Frank was inspiring me, but how could I be as brave as he was?

Why was it still so scary leaving my room? How could I ever really feel like I belonged? I kept looking out my window, in front of which I had strategically placed my laptop. After a while, I started to make a plan. As I typed, my eyes wouldn't leave the window.

I created thirty "games," for myself that helped center me in my body. I kept all of these on slips of paper and would draw one out of a hat, especially whenever my mom was about to take me shopping. Some of my favorites?

- You are an astronaut on Mars, and everything is completely other-worldly.
- Go through the alphabet and name something around you for each letter.
- Pretend you are in a video game and all the objects around you are part of the game.

The more creative activities I did, the more I was transported back into the imagination-driven world of my childhood. My creative efforts also helped me confront less pleasant memories. My cartoon turned into Blaine's apartment. With Frank as my guide, I wasn't frightened to go there.

I have so many emotions knotted up from that era that still have to start un-folding like a curled-up yard of rainbow-streaked ribbon. The crayon won't let me run away. Frank, if you go first, I'll follow!

Flipping My Script—One Page at a Time

Sometimes you need to do something radically different and turn yourself upside down to gain a new perspective. I knew change was good, but was I better off with gradual micro-movements or totally flipping myself around? I found a happy medium: flipping myself around, but one cartooned page at a time.

If I had a mini book with me, I could just remind myself of something like "be in this moment" or "my purpose is to find the enthusiasm in everything." Then I would at least know what to do. I would take on the eyes of an artist and find the poetry, or notice how the light hits the ceiling, or find a miracle or something I'm grateful for.

I created a flip book for myself where each page was a floorboard in an intergalactic hallway, supporting the shaky steps I needed to take to that giant leap of faith. Another flipbook animated my Grandma visualization, where her glimmering spirit swirls out of trees lining a dark forest, illuminating my path I was getting better at loving myself and trusting myself, one step at a time.

Creating nature symbols as gods on clay beads, fabric blankets, and in mini flip books protected me whenever I "dared" to leave my room. When the outside world made me anxious, these gods centered me. They helped me realize that happiness was not some foreign, far off concept; it was in the present moment, a moment a could grab onto at any time.

I have my tree god (wisdom, perspective, balance), water-droplet god (spray-bottle, representing sitting in the sadness for a moment), passion god (Yankee candle flame), tiger god (stuffed animal to show fierceness and authority), stars in the night (light switch, to represent childlike wonder), Grandma (head of all the gods, guidance), moon (god of mystery and fear), wind (soul bird, god of breath, and body), and I think that's it! Oh, and my superhero five senses to remind me of the power of now.

My "gods" who now always surrounded me fueled a burgeoning motivation to understand why I coped in the past by hiding away. They propelled me forward, and their company overpowered the rising sense that I was losing something by moving on and being present.

Whatever I was losing, I committed to finding it again. I created spontaneous "exercises" to fill each moment with a new joy.

1. Notice 5 things you haven't noticed before as soon as you sit at the table.

2. Write about the feeling that is evoked when you open your fridge.

Now I'm excited when I feel the physical sensations of "fear." It means I'm onto something!

It became essential for me to have at least one thing that I was committed to doing every day, but also leave room for spontaneity and trying new things, and sometimes just *being*. I was closing the abyss between what I wanted and the choices I had to make by realizing I was the one who had control. I had tools to unleash the healing vortex and now, there was no way I could drown.

Stitching my Life Back Together

I was hooked on the idea of using creativity to heal. I looked to sewing as a way to create something whole out of threads. It got me out of my head, and I could concentrate on colors, textures and physical sensations My mom would take me to Joann's fabric store as our new mother-daughter bonding activity. Shopping together for fabric, sharing stories about my grandmother and her sewing, and going through her old buttons and thimbles brought us closer to my grandmother. We both needed her spirit to guide us on the journey ahead.

Going through old pictures was bittersweet; it helped me remember the happy times of my childhood but also reminded me of what I had lost. When remembering felt like "too much," I transformed my pain through creativity into figures on my new security blanket.

I sewed fabrics and ribbons together to recreate scenes from old family photos. These were tangible memories I could take with me, literally carrying my blanket into the big wide-open future. The more uncertain I became, the tighter I wrapped the blanket around myself.

Certain symbols kept popping up in my cartoon as Frank led me through my warrior's journey. I created a whole warrior tribe to protect myself.

- *TIGER—a warrior earning her stripes, fierce in the jungle with alert eyes and ears, ready to pounce, strong, powerful. Fiercer than a lion, firmly grounded in the earth, it lets out a powerful ROAR!*
- *BIRD—beautiful songbird flying in the clouds, graceful, spiritual, has an open throat to sing its song and brightly chirps all day long in the sunlight, free to fly anywhere, unburdened by worry.*
- *WHALE—a massive creature looming in the ocean, casting a huge shadow on the sandy ocean floor. It is big and mysterious, but it is the soul of the ocean, the heart of the sea, and the mammoth-sized river of beauty flowing inside of me that I have been afraid to tap into.*
- *LION—seems quite friendly. To the bird, the lion symbolizes God and a gateway to the clouds! But lions are clever and deceptive. Beware of the tail...*
- *CAMEL—has water in its humps. The support you need to help you cross the desert.*
- *RIVER—steady stream that a sailboat calmly sails along, pushed along by a gentle breeze, the warrior quality that symbolizes staying the path.*

Cartooning turned healing journey into a mega-size pop-up book, constantly surprising me with tucked-away memories. Every day, I would discover another flap to open or arrow to pull, leading me somewhere new.

Taking My Power Back

Cartooning was bringing my mind and body together, and the images were staying with me as empowering guiding symbols. I dared to leave the page, and nervously stepped foot in the "world beyond my locked room."

With my creative army, I was surrounded in safety. I trusted that my hero's journey would guide me, if I knew when to make choices, and when to surrender.

My surrender prayer:
Help me to flow like the river and let its cool, flowing, rippling water heal my thoughts and purify my heart. May the waters elevate my heart to the surface like a buoy in the ocean and make my heart sing to me so I learn how to embrace it and take it in fully. The world is a gift.

I asked myself, how could I pray more, and what did I really want prayer to feel like?

- *Like a sigh, or like God trapped in the glimmer of my sparkling blue eyes.*
- *Like an anchor of light to wake me up, a shock from an eel.*
- *Like angels singing a tune that carries me like a hammock.*

Prayer couldn't guarantee certainty, and that was okay. My own physical actions determined where the path led. I learned how to manifest optimism and trusted that if I stayed positive, it would come back to me. Now I could look outside and on a beautiful day choose to go out instead of staying in my room. It wasn't such a challenge to wrap my brain and body around God's gifts and feel completely safe in the sanctuary of nature.

Finding the Sacred in the Mundane

One day at Williams-Sonoma, where in the past I would have numbly paced around the kitchenware, my artist's eye immediately darted to the pots and pans set up on the shelves. They were so properly aligned, silvery and shiny, all their handles facing the same direction. It made me giggle as I imagined all the pots as a huge synchronized dancing chorus line, kicking their handles up in the air like fishnet-covered legs doing high kicks under the hot white lights of a Broadway stage. And I thought to myself, "How fun would this be to cartoon!"

I realized I could be talking to Grandma every time I saw an everyday object in a holy light. But whenever I saw Grandma, it moved me in another direction, a few millimeters toward mourning for her; something I was robbed of.

I stop and see the roses perched on top of the kitchen counter every morning, and by appreciating their wonder, I could visualize Grandma soaring out of it with her flame-like tail coming out to say, "Amala." How is your breakfast?" Then, maybe waking up wouldn't be so scary anymore.

Mourning My Grandmother

IT SCARED ME THAT I NEVER mourned my grandmother. I was tossed between numbness and a well of emotions, knowing I lost her in the midst of my own medical crises.

Maybe I couldn't deal with the loss of my grandmother, because I was processing so many other losses. Maybe Rita was right. Maybe I needed to fully go through all the stages of grieving to heal. I didn't want to get trapped in my past, but I didn't want to spend my life running away from it either.

I have to fully acknowledge it to accept it and move on. My heart misses Grandma more than I can verbalize.

I needed her more than ever now as a beacon of hope. So, I took the hardest first step to mourn her. I let myself feel again.

My mother and I often searched for Grandma's spirit in the many seagulls that flew around our tiny house by the water. We would pray to any seagull we saw, feeling my grandmother's presence in their glorious flight. The gulls helped us believe that my grandmother was still watching over us all in loving protection.

Lately, I feel her presence in a very subtle way. It sometimes just stabs me in the heart when I least expect it.

Grandma was everywhere now that I had opened myself up to feeling her loss.

Grandma swirls from only the trees that smell like chicken soup and are warm and wrinkly around their trunks. They'll hold me and I can hold on. I'm scared to let go, but I step into the center of a glorious field in my bare feet and she is everywhere! I just skip around like the giddiest child and think to myself, what was I waiting for? And that will be the day, that one day, I finally reach the world of the living.

When I couldn't access my feelings through creativity, I reminded myself that my best guide was being in the moment and allowing myself to feel the physical sensations of eating food. This made sense because I had lost food and lost Grandma at the same time. The more I ate pumpkin, the more I realized how food connected me to the earth, to myself, to things in the ground I couldn't even fathom.

I want to carve a pumpkin today and get my hands dirty. I want to toast pumpkin seeds and eat them because I want to eat something I've created myself that comes from the earth.

Of course, death was also part of the circle of life, and by indulging in nourishment and remembering how Grandma had nurtured me, I was connecting with her in yet another way.

Jews have a special connection with food, and eating is especially holy in the Hasidic tradition. Martin Buber claimed that "eating can be holier than fasting." Because by chewing the food and really enjoying it nourishing our bodies, we set free even more holy sparks. As soon as I was abused, chewing became uncomfortable. Feeling my mouth so physically triggered such dreaded emotional sensations that I would cram thousands of calories into a giant green smoothie to try and sip my life back up through a straw. Now, instead of focusing on the food molecules as evil Pac-Man monsters who unleashed painful, buried feelings in my body, I imagined chewing as the breaking down of God's gifts, the unwrapping of His presents, of His presence.

> *You can't destroy energy. It's always there, just in different forms. Just remember this, Amy. It's your safety net when you feel like you'll fall into the emptiness you fear.*

Eating actually made me *feel* holy because all of those sparks were floating through the river of *my own* bloodstream. Just as I was learning to balance the healing work I was doing in my mind versus in my body, I was balancing out the trauma vortex with the healing vortex.

Writing became an activity of choice instead of a compulsion. I was learning how to become more flexible and how to reap the benefits from doing so. I was discovering what happiness could be—little tastes of it here and there.

I had begun exploring my grief, but I hadn't cried as of yet for my grandmother's death.

> *I've tried to bargain with God a lot. But I need to accept that there are certain things I can't get back. To keep insisting on their retrieval is an insult to life, because life should be appreciated moment by moment. When you get hung up on one moment in particular, Mother Earth puts her hands on her hips and huffs, "What, you don't like all these other pretty things I'm making for you?"*

Being a victim is like the shadow side of the wounded healer. A "victim" wants to bask in a pity party about how miserable life is, feeling all alone in a gaping wound. But if you expand outwards to see the world around you, you discover little gems about yourself that otherwise would have been kept in the dark if you had not gone into that cave and claimed it as your own.

I thought of Grandma and felt that rush of grief.

Should I feel this? It's much easier to write about. But I am the healer, the patient, and the scribe. To fulfill all of these roles, I can't just stay at my computer and type. What kind of a healer would I be if I just sat at the computer writing out what might work with no way of knowing if I was really healing myself? It is my responsibility to get my own life experience so I can really play all of these parts. Am I going to own what I'm feeling right now?

I stepped away from my notes and did...nothing. From that place that a single tear could finally form.

CHAPTER 27

Using Stories to Heal

JUST AS WORDS CAN MAKE US FEEL sick, words can make us feel healthy. I couldn't physically control the way my body was healing, but by reframing my journey from a descent into mind-numbing trauma to an "adventure in healing," I was able to bring about changes in myself.

The more I read, the more I knew I needed to write—and tell. My alter ego became Tiger Lilly the warrior. My mission? There was a trauma vortex on the loose and my goal was to save the world by redirecting that vortex back into the normal river of life. Now, Tiger Lilly the warrior meant business.

Writing was essential to my healing, but I had spent so much time isolating myself, I knew I also needed to be out in the world living, proving to myself that my healing adventure was working. But how to balance those two competing drives?

As a healing storyteller I drew on symbols and animal guides to help me accept fear enough to face and move through it, fiercely and contemplatively, like a bull and a bear. A bear uses the inner energy of its soul to find answers, is strong and grounded, but is cautious and quiet, ducking into his cave for hibernation. A bull is strong and potent and has the stamina to reach his destination without burning out. A bull makes the earth more fertile, always having new ideas that need to be expressed, and can stand his ground in all life matters.

In all the stories I was reading and writing, obstacles were not the exception, but the norm. They were challenges for the hero to overcome, put in the hero's path for a purpose. Every situation could encourage me to build inner strength and integrity, if I was present with the world and its natural processes. Soon I was noticing miracles everywhere.

But no amount of miracles seemed to answer the unrelenting question: Would I ever know who I was?

Every adventure story has a heroic ending, and so would mine. In my cartoon, I decided to imagine Frank swimming around in the trauma vortex, searching for the break in the river, unwinding that deadly current by unleashing his powerful healing vortex, and ultimately flowing back into the river of life. Now healing was simple. All I had to do was draw him getting back to the river. The end.

Counteracting the trauma vortex took force. I had to take all of that restless energy out by using it for good, rather than taking it out on myself. The energy I was trying to "get rid of" through exercise and numbing out was the energy of anger I felt burning within me all along. But it had been too dangerous to let it out until now.

If I don't repress my emotions, they run me over and utterly consume me. Though compulsivity has its own set of problems and ultimately made me more of a mess, it's served to keep me from being a different sort of mess. But I've learned that life ought to be a beautiful, mad mess. That is why finger painting is fun.

It was all up to me. It always had been. The more anger I owned, the more I realized I did not deserve my guilt. Healthy anger was the key to the healing vortex. By integrating anger back into my life, I could make it less toxic and take away the power the trauma had over me.

It was time for Tiger Lilly to get serious about healing from trauma. Serious by getting angry.

The Battle for the Warrior's Soul

I was moving toward health, personal empowerment, and positive change. For the first time, as time was moving, so was I. But it felt more like walking stutter step through successes and setbacks, a push pull of progress and pain. Eventually, the pattern of the healing vortex emerged.

Normal people enjoy pleasure. The problem for me was feeling pleasure required separating the physical sensation of now from the painful emotions of the past. Was I addicted to pain?

"For you, pain and pleasure have been distorted because of what was done to you," Rita told me. "So, there is a crossed wire in your brain. You have to learn to switch back from pain to pleasure. Think of it as cycling."

Cycling was the superpower I needed.

We all have triggers. Just as a positive association triggers a happy memory, a negative one will trigger an unpleasant or unbearable association for a trauma survivor. The smell of pumpkin muffins might remind us of fall and a happy Thanksgiving memory. A car alarm might evoke the sound of an ambulance in the past and fill someone with fear.

When I asked Rita, how do I start healing emotionally, she had three answers. 1) Identify things in the "now" that trigger past memories, like that French fry, 2) notice when and how they come up for me, 3) Inform my body I'm living in a safer time now; past triggers don't need to paralyze me.

The trick was recognizing when I was being triggered and choosing a different response to shift the cycle. It was painful at first, but it helped to dive in and explore the bad feeling.

The more I examined my pain, the more I understood its cause: "re-lived trauma." I did not want to accept that I would never see my eighteen-year-old life again. I never even had a chance to say goodbye to it. All that was left now was me, food, and my chaotic medical journey. When all the sirens and beeping machines faded, and the discharge papers were signed, I was left with just me.

Trauma had left me empty. Now I had to rebuild my identity and learn to trust what I had inside. The literal, physical insides, my digestive system was "normal," but I was feeling more abnormal than ever. I knew I had the power to get through this. I just had to break through my triggers to do it.

Oh, hi smell of bread baking! You alarmed me because it reminded me of when I wasn't allowed to eat you. Let me take the time now to appreciate and honor this memory and know that now I can fully appreciate food.

I was able to see trauma as the trigger to my numbness response. I had needed numbness from all the surgeries. I was admired for rarely needing pain medication. I could go in one of those narrow MRI machines for over an hour stuck listening to Mom's cardio thumping music blasting through the headphones (she gave me the wrong music by accident), get CAT scans, even prick my own finger. In the real world, it is okay to feel pain. In the trauma world, you need to suppress pain to survive.

I did want to get better. I just hadn't known how. Now, I wanted the same respect and admiration I had received for being a medical miracle. I was a warrior in the process of healing her own battle scars. Jeff, loving but always one to look for "facts" and concrete progress, was the most impatient. He was always loyal to my parents and didn't understand why they were so patient with me.

"Amy, I think Jeff has a hard time emotionally accepting that you've been through all of this," Mom explained.

"He doesn't want to face the ugliness when I have to face it every day? If he wants to be a supportive brother then he has to love all of me, the good and the bad, even for the ugliest of times."

It's like the world has blinders on. They know I've gone through so much physically, but no one can accept that emotionally the work has just begun.

Trauma could be a gift; healing could be a thrilling adventure. The outside world just had no idea. And for that moment, I was able to have the empathy for my brother I hoped one day he would have for me.

We can't possibly avoid every trigger or negative experience. It's when we choose to embrace those triggers that we can actually move forward and heal. When I accepted this, I could move on and shatter the stereotypes surrounding trauma and healing; and the mounting fear of stillness motivated the warrior in me more than ever to take charge and win this hero's journey battle. Roar...

I was on the road, and my warrior's backpack was stocked. But I felt the pressure to be done with healing, to have a purpose, a profession already. I decided I was a writer and working on a book. Now I had a self-proclaimed career—*that's what people with laptops do*—but now, with a final product in mind. Amy's "real person" identity, found!

The more I wrote, the more I stepped into my truth. Secrets corroded. Holding secrets for so long is what made me sick in the first place. I had to write this book.

At first, writing a book had seemed like another coping mechanism to "keep busy" and another way to justify my endless healing to the outside world. Now I felt called on to share my hard-won wisdom with the countless other survivors who, like me, longed to break free of trauma's grip and start living their lives again.

I had to heal now, for the sake of anyone else who was suffering and feeling as ashamed, dirty, and helpless as I had been.

Everyone needed to know what an adventure healing could be. I thought about all the resources that had guided me so far and every tool I had gathered.

Now, when my friends asked what I was doing, instead of cringing inside as I said, "I'm still trying to heal from all this," I could say, "I'm on a warrior's journey!"

I want to show the world that healing isn't something you have to just get over so you can move onto your "life."

I wanted my family to celebrate my journey. I wanted them to witness Tiger Lilly fighting demons daily in my room rather than Amy jogging compulsively and never really getting better.

Every morning, I felt a manic burst of inspiration to work on my book. At first, my book felt like "the breakthrough" that would get me out of the loopy cycle of healing and put me on the mountaintop of "healed." But soon enough, I found myself numbly typing myself farther from that peak.

Everything turns into a coping mechanism, a numb way to protect myself, because underneath I am still scared of being hurt again.

This pattern of finding a healing strategy and pursuing it obsessively until it became an unhealthy coping mechanism, would follow me throughout my extended healing process. Only much later would I learn that eliminating fear was the key to stop vacillating in the vortex. For now, I had discovered yet another way to stay stuck without even being conscious of it.

Realizing that a part of me did want to stay stuck was the key to finally moving through it.

Jogging in my room left me more and more angry as I overheard Jeff and Mom fighting over what would finally "fix me." I took a breath as I heard Jeff say, "She'll never get better like this." *Oh yeah?* I thought about how much I loved my brother and how badly I wished I could come downstairs and sit with him. And then, I did it! Even though it was only for a *second.* No one could force me to stop numbing out or jogging. I had to do it myself. The pull for life had to become stronger.

Thinking of having old times with Jeff was a feeling of "pleasure," a pleasure strong enough to make me pause for a moment. Life with feeling was difficult but worth it. I knew that was the only way I would make a breakthrough into the next chapter, the next phase of the warrior's journey, which was stepping into that scary unknown to find the greatest treasure of all: identity.

But the more present I became, the sadder I felt as reality washed over me. While I had been busy staying numb, time had passed me by. Now I had to take yet another step and let go of the regret and self-blame over losing so much time. If I wanted a future, I had to stop letting the past define me.

My automatic pilot routine was a tidy container for the unwieldy mess I became once I had to be vulnerable to the moment. But the "tidiness" of staying on autopilot was an unhealthy risk.

I had to confront the emptiness I was running from.

So how do you go into the emptiness? You plan to "greet" the emptiness. Stick your toes into it. You must declare, "Okay, I'm brave. Let me see what the emptiness feels like. I'm up for a scare, I'm up for the challenge!"

I was ready to trade all of this crap in for something amazing. But was this the end of the "long bumpy road" that I had been forewarned about? The final destination—home, safety, myself? One road led to health. The other led to stuckness. The road forked before me and I had to choose.

I do wonder what God's plan is for me, how He has strategically shattered my world over and over again, like he wants me to excavate my soul from the rubble. He must be planning something extraordinary.

It was difficult to face all of this at once. Once I accepted the challenge, the true work began.

Often, when people heard my entire medical saga, their first instinctive reaction was to reach out with their condolences. They'd say things like, "I am so sorry you had to go through all of that." Immediately, I would want to fire back, "Don't be sorry. I'm happy this happened to me!"

Before I get led too far down that "Why me?" path, I stop myself. But slowly, I am learning to love the life I have. Why not.

"Why not" was the key to motion. Unlike the trauma vortex, the healing vortex was not a vicious cyclone. It had forward movement, shape, and purposeful direction. For the first time, I felt I was progressing into the future!

I guess life is about risking. You can't hold onto anything, just the trust that you can always create something to land on.

I suddenly recalled what the doctor had told my parents in that Chicago hospital: "I don't think she buys into this life thing yet." I laughed to myself. Because now, I was at the checkout counter.

Ironically, connecting my past and present selves made me more aware of how separate they were. As I felt Wounded Amy on my shoulder, born from traumatic events, I longed for Thriving Amy, my audaciously innocent seventeen-year-old self. How could they both make themselves at home in my soul? Being honest with myself meant listening to Wounded Amy, my wounded bird. Her answers, even if they hurt, gave me hope. She was filling in the blank spaces in my story that I had been too scared to face. Learning these secrets was scary but exciting. I was coming back from the dead with a chest of gold to share with the world that would illuminate secrets in the darkness.

I feel hope for the first time. I can't wait to write every day. Will Thriving Amy tell me her dreams, hopes, wishes, fears?

I realized the "final identity" would not be Thriving Amy or Wounded Amy after I healed. I needed to create a third persona to help negotiate them as I moved forward: Motherly Amy. Her job? To help the two parts of me work together as part of my new life by showing compassion for one another.

You are a part of nature, Amy. If you saw a tree struck by lightning, would you call it a freak? If you saw its limbs lying on the ground because a storm knocked it down, would you be angry at the tree? No. You'd feel compassion for the tree. When you do, you'll be hugging God.

"Your daze was just a freeze mode Blaine created," Rita explained. "You held onto it while you coped with your medical situation. Trust that now, you can make more compassionate choices for yourself."

"But how do I know I'm really choosing the right thing?" I asked.

She gave her trademark Rita response. "When you feel comfortable— with whatever decision you make."

CHAPTER 28

The Warrior Advances

AS 2009 APPROACHED, I decided this year would be the new beginning I was waiting for.

I don't want to live a librarian's life organizing documents and records of her existence. I want to thrive, and to thrive you can't be afraid of making messes.

Winter quickly turned to spring and with each month, I collected more "aliveness" by finding presence even if it was uncomfortable. Who I was, was uncertain. But I kept pushing forward, hoping I would find myself.

As Rita read through my hundreds of pages of journaling every week, she commented, "You write a lot about the story of what happened, but not the physical sensations. Uncover how this felt in your body, the pain and fear. That's your key that unlocks your healing." Just *being* in my body made me so anxious; all I wanted to do was exercise. Where was my payoff? I had to learn strategies from Rita to interrupt the "freeze" response and stay in the moment long enough to become "un-numb."

But feeling meant I had to strip all my coping mechanisms away.

Once I decided to be present again, regardless of pain, I reframed my circumstances and found greater meaning in the tests life had given me. That gave me the strength to carry on.

After a while, I realized the beauty that was waiting for me when I was ready to take a breath, regroup, and keep traveling.

Healing doesn't happen overnight, and it doesn't happen "for good." Healing is a process.

I felt alienated in my body after all of the surgeries. My body had changed so much over time that I could barely recognize it. Helpless and reluctant, but on the edge of something huge.

When I finally found the courage to look at myself, my old self, with compassion instead of revulsion, I stopped blaming myself for my trauma.

"Your body wasn't weak; it was just being normal," Rita said with a sigh. "It was just being used and abused by someone. You've reached the wrong conclusion."

I didn't stop Blaine because it was so confusing for him to be my godfather, my coach, my teacher, my mentor, *and* my abuser. It was like a shock. That's why I went along with it. Then I had to immediately dissociate from it to cope. Suddenly, I understood that the little wounded bird inside me was not the one to blame. She was just trying to survive.

I finally learned self-compassion. Now I was proud of my wounded bird for surviving. If we don't survive, we die. And if I hadn't dissociated with Blaine, I would have gone crazy and never come back.

I reassured myself: "I know that once you get through this, God is going to give you the biggest gift. You've just got to hold on and fight against it."

Rita read through my journals about how I moved into Westport unable to eat. "You had to turn off your hunger for years to be able to cope with no food or drink. So of course, it's going to be so hard to turn it back on."

I reminded myself to let that nervous energy from fear turn into excitement. Letting fear excite me meant I was tapping into a deeper memory that could move me forward. Now, Thriving Amy *and* Wounded Amy were sitting at the kitchen table together, ready for anything. As I moved forward, I had to constantly resource my healing vortex tools. Otherwise, my life would be run by triggers. So, I created a new story that would put me in charge—*Back into Life*, written by Motherly Amy.

My physical sensations were so scary for me because they brought up conflicting thoughts and memories about Blaine as both mentor and abuser. To fully move on, I had to integrate both sides of Blaine into my story.

How do I pick up the pieces? How do I collect all these scattered, random, broken shards of clues of who I once was, these scraps of hope and promise and dreams, and make a mosaic from it?

I remember having a checkup after I was discharged from the hospital. On the way, I convinced my dad to drive down Blaine's block. And by some chance, I saw him. Blaine was strolling down the street with his fanny pack. I wanted to chase after him, but—what would I do? Or say.

I know that if I do want him to see me again, I want to feel like I powerfully own myself and my blood again and I am fighting back. But a small sliver of me still just wants to keep tapping him on the shoulder saying, "Look Blaine, look what happened to me. Isn't that terrible? Can we just pretend like this never happened and make up so we can have a real voice lesson again?"

"Mark! Turn around—you don't know what he could do!"

"No dad—stop the car, let me get out," I pleaded.

My father heeded my mother's warning and we headed home. Later, we learned that Blaine's block was recent familiar territory.

My Father's Secrets

My father was waiting for his own confrontation with Blaine. Every time my father drove us to a doctor's appointment at my hospital in New York, he drove right back to Blaine's street, just pacing up and down the sidewalk, waiting for what we all were looking for: some kind of closure.

My father could never hurt a fly and has never been one to look for a confrontation. But that's not what he was looking for. We knew why he kept driving back. We knew he could never find what he was looking for and finding the resolution to our emotional aches would not be as simple as catching Blaine on his street.

Unthawing

Did I really want a last word with Blaine? I could vividly remember the last time I heard his voice—four years earlier. It was on a phone call, which at the time I couldn't even find the voice to respond to. I had already told my mother about Blaine's abuse, and we were waiting for him to call me after his vacation to Ireland. We sat on her bed, waiting for my phone to ring, just as his plane was landing. I gave the phone to my mother.

"Blaine! Amy, can't see you anymore."

"Marilyn! Is everything okay?"

"We know what you did."

"Marilyn, let's talk about this," Blaine shouted back in desperation.

But she hung up. They never did speak.

Surprisingly, the more I listened to Wounded Amy voicing her needs, the more power I could give back to Thriving Amy. Now with both voices equally strong, I needed Motherly Amy to help facilitate this dialogue.

Self-soothing meant lovingly understanding that my wounded bird was hurt. If I could love myself, I could trust myself. And if I could trust myself, I could listen to myself. For the healing vortex to work, the current of the river must grow stronger than the whirlpool current. For me, the upward yank towards God finally became more forceful than the pull down. The growing power within me signified that the trauma vortex was decreasing in potency. When you don't have a proper hold on your sadness, the vortex tries to draw you down and control you to stay rigid, numb out, and avoid feeling life. You stay frozen. I was ready to move forward.

The pain never dies, but the love for life gets stronger.

CHAPTER 29

Food Transforms Relationships

Today, Amy has truly recognized the value of the people she loves!

FOOD ALLOWED A NEW CLOSENESS with my father as we hit a birdie back and forth on the beach. Food highlighted subtle discoveries, like a yellow apple core on the sand, or scooping up the birdie and finding the unexpected treasure of a seashell. As I spotted little boys in their beach trunks innocently eating ice cream cones, I felt a spark-filled moment pulsing through me.

It hit me that healing was impossible in a vacuum...or in my room, and if I wanted to get better, I had to keep getting out.

Stepping out into daylight was the antidote to my anxiety. The physical work I had done with Rita made it possible for me to enjoy life instead of avoiding it.

Beliefs are thoughts we repeat to ourselves. "When you have energy, you have to walk fast." This thought-turned-belief became a compulsion, which now, I had the power to change. I could repeat, "I stand still to spot the miracles I've never seen before." I could use creativity to cancel my compulsions and change my beliefs. I could test how it felt to stay with anxiety long enough to feel the sadness behind it. I challenged myself to keep leaning in and trust that, like the hero on her journey, I could coach myself through each uncertain step.

Purposeful "Play"

When you're just surviving, life is getting through the next minute, hour, or day. When you're thriving, it's exciting to look ahead. Constant exercise had been my survival tactic, and it took a long time to disassociate meaning, order, and purpose from compulsive movement. I created a schedule of "fun" to find the purpose in just "having fun."

12:40pm: Focus on the bright color of the orange ball Jelly paws at. Turn on radio, so music becomes my safe container for playing with my dog.

Once I allowed myself to sit with anxiety, the fear disappeared, and I could find happiness. With a mature wisdom, I stepped back into my childhood self, and watched my trees fill with life again.

As a teen, I'd walk by through the snow full of wonderment, talking to the trees, my friends. I want to challenge myself today to stand still before a tree, to find that awe. I tried doing it yesterday, but I felt that red anxiety right away. I could sit with it for about ten seconds—an improvement. The more I do it, maybe I can increase it by a second every time.

I was starting to veer away from, "When I do ___, I'll be happy; when I get reconstruction, I'll be happy." I realized that happiness was a power I had inside me, not something dependent outward.

Isolation had helped me stay sane, but only connection could make me happy. The pull for life—and people—was stronger than the trauma vortex. I couldn't numb out to those I loved.

I relaxed on the couch with Dad, and I didn't even feel like I needed to write or flip through a magazine as I finished eating. I could actually concentrate on the movie and enjoy it, which I never am able to do—huge whopping deal! And as I ate my scrambled eggs and crackers and shake on the couch, I talked to Dad and found the movie engaging and relished the feeling of relaxing! The idea of feeling this wild rollercoaster of pain and pleasure in the living world around me is what entices me about nourishing my body now. It's like a pet you can't wait to feed because you don't know what tricks it will do next.

As I was journaling these discoveries on my laptop in the dark, Mom knocked. I looked at my watch, alarmed. This wasn't a designated time out of my room. My shoulders rose as I typed faster. "Matt's coming to the house. He said he'll take you for a walk on the beach."

A few minutes later, Matt opened the door without knocking. "You coming?" he asked. I felt exposed, like I was in one of those dreams where you show up in a school classroom with no clothes on. I ran downstairs.

"Okay. I'm ready." I took the plunge and went outside...

It was amazing! The minute I got outside; it was like the brain switch I had when I ate breakfast for the first time. I didn't realize how good the air feels on your skin.

After suffering for so long, it was hard to believe life could be...simple. Walking outside with Matt was so...easy. I didn't understand. I had based the "order" of my life on the idea that life was either suffering or numbing out to pain. On my beach walk, I even had to ask, *"Is this okay, God? It's okay to live like this?"*

Through food and people, I was drawn back into life. I am woman—hear Tiger Lilly roar!

As I reconnected with Mom, I learned that being feminine and womanly could be fun and relaxing...and that was okay.

"Amy, I'm taking you for a manicure."

Out? Now? I could feel myself shriveling in terror. But then I thought about the idea of nail polish—paint—creating art. Creativity was my bait. The manicurist didn't understand that I wanted tiger stripes on my nails, so my warrior self took charge and painted them on in the middle of the salon all by myself. I earned those stripes.

Not long after our nail salon outing Mom planned to take me for reflexology. As the time drew nearer, I was nervous about having my feet rubbed and a little skittish getting in the chair. But then I saw a bunch of other women doing the same thing and enjoying it, and I figured I've been through so much more than they have that it's okay for me to enjoy it. As soon as I sat down, I felt utter ecstasy.

Reflexology was safe while it lasted, but as I put my sneakers back on, my breathing quickened, and I suddenly felt tense in a place that had felt fine just a moment before. I was scared to go back home and face the snake.

My first try at reflexology was now an ecstatic experience for me; a spiritual high where negative feelings didn't run me. Reflexology had healed more than just me; it was healing Mom and me as two grown women at the manicure place. Arriving home, Mom sat on the steps of the front porch, leaning against the screen door, her legs outstretched as she laid the paper plate of turkey parts, mustard, and pickles on her lap. It felt like a lazy warm summer evening, the kind where you rock on your porch swing sipping lemonade and watching fireworks. Slowly, I trusted there was nothing to be so scared of. I was safe. *The world was coming alive.*

I had also been run by the compulsion to write for sixteen hours a day, frantically documenting everything because if I didn't write it, it wouldn't exist. Now I realized that there was another way to exist rather than writing—actually living it! I could just...be.

The feeling was so overwhelming that I bit my lip so hard, but it was of little use—the tears just flowed out of me so heavily, and Matt immediately saw how I felt. It was the first time I had cried in public. My mother had always reassured me that the world was, and has always been, waiting for me. I had forgotten what the world was like and that it could be mine and that I deserved it. Now, I was starting to remember and believe it.

Pleasure...Without Pain?

Has one of your relationships ever forced you to change your view or perception on something? Going to the beach with Matt, I had forgotten that there existed a type of ecstasy in nature of just feeling life soak into you and doing nothing more but being in the moment. I had forgotten that beautiful things happen when you don't plan; you don't always need to plan to live a purposeful life.

Beach walks with Matt embodied the lesson Rita had been trying to teach me all along—how trauma survivors put "pleasure" in the context of "pain," referring to the "pleasure" my body experienced with Blaine. This wasn't real pleasure. My body was feeling good, but the entire situation was painful. That was the dynamic of staying in my room versus going to the beach. The whole time I had been asking Matt about our relationship and when it got hard to connect to him and how we could make it better. But then all those worries lifted as we got closer on our walks on the beach.

Now that my healing vortex was finally strong enough, I understood and appreciated real pleasure.

There was more to life than just survival. Maybe that is why the fries felt so good in my mouth and on my tongue and all the way down to my belly.

I had fries today! They felt like real people food—a crispy outside, and a flaky top layer. But their inside was fluffy marshmallow mush! I felt so normal!

Reclaiming My Life

There is an Indian belief that everyone is in a house of four rooms: a physical, a mental, an emotional, and a spiritual. Most of us tend to live in one room most of the time, but unless we go into every room every day, even if only to keep it aired, we are not complete.

It was in the airing of those rooms that I made my heart feel whole again. My flowing tears could drown that snake drop by drop. As I reclaimed the rooms of my house, I could see the proof—at last—that I was home. Home in my body, I was no longer a stranger in myself. I was Amy again.

I have proof that I can be Amy in mind—look at all the writing I do now! I have proof that I am Amy in spirit—look at how beautiful I felt yesterday watching the thunder, lightning, and rain! I have proof that I am Amy in heart—I am fostering a relationship with Matt every night at the beach. I have proof that I am Amy in soul—certain songs still make me want to take off and soar. And finally, I have proof that I can be Amy in full body if I make the pledge to get there! Safe from the cyclonic whirlpool and free to float down the river any time I am ready...

Because being present had always come so naturally to me growing up, I hadn't appreciated that presence was key to connecting with people. After my coma, I had to rediscover what was second nature to everyone else.

I once had the door—the actual door to my house and the metaphorical one to my life—absolutely slammed shut, but now at least the front door was open, and I could see my mom, my new puppy Jelly, and the beaming potential of family. I saw myself relaxing into life through a screen door on the front porch, which I hoped to leap through soon.

Pleasure is just sitting in the car fiddling with my iPod, not caring that I'm not accomplishing anything. Today could have been any normal day, like when my mom and I used to drive to the city for auditions. Fuss-free, non-medical, mother-daughter conversation felt so good.

When my mother first started taking me for shopping trips, I felt anxious energy shoot up my legs, and trying to find something more "pleasurable" to focus on was an impossibility. I still felt like I was running from negative energy and trying to pretend like it wasn't there. But, sitting in the massage chair during reflexology had been effortless—as it was for most people. To me, this concept was mind-blowing. I felt like I was floating on an ocean the whole time, lifted up on the waves of pleasure and sinking down into the waves of pain, bobbing gently up and down in the open water in the warm sunlight. I was "cycling" successfully (thanks, Rita!) at last.

Now, when my mother took me shopping, she had *me* making all the decisions about where we were supposed to go. *Are you kidding, I can't be trusted with these kinds of decisions! What am I, a person?* We were like two women shopping together, it was crazy, we weren't in crisis mode or anything. There was no fire we had to run from or put out. Now what was *that* about?

Was I really capable of making healthy decisions now? I didn't know until I took a risk and tried. Now, like a puppy waiting for treats, I waited for "permission" to be let out of my room, no longer with anxiety but with eagerness.

Plugged into life you view everything differently—sometimes it even changes the funky rewiring job that the trauma did. Now, with family by my side showing me the way, everything that I once loved (that had scared me for years) was becoming a thrilling adventure again. I was reclaiming my appetite for food, for connection, for life. Healing from trauma means giving *yourself* permission.

Once I pushed through the undeserved guilt that came with eating, I was actually able to enjoy it. Just in time for my first holiday—Thanksgiving.

The final missing puzzle piece? Friends to celebrate with! I remembered the other Thanksgivings that I couldn't eat, walking down a dark sidewalk with my dad while we glanced into screen doors of celebratory dinners. Now, we all appreciated our feast with a new kind of thanks—like pilgrims setting forth into uncharted territory and claiming it as our own. The Oestreichers rejoining into the universe. Then it hit me: I was the one who had the power to heal us, empowering me with my superhero responsibility to get better and open back up the world so I could help my family heal.

We had gotten our holidays back. This year, Thanksgiving, next year, who knows...could it be...*Passover?*

The first Thanksgiving we could celebrate we were sure to have as much food, family, friends and chaos as possible—the good Oestreicher kind of chaos. We crammed thirty guests into our downsized beach house in Westport, and for the first time in years, I was able to invite my old high school friends over to celebrate. I was so overwhelmed that I wrote them all a letter, waiting for them at their meticulously set dinner places.

I don't know what my friends made of my long-winded "trauma-is-an-adventure!" letter, which just reminded me how different I was from them. Yet, with food at the table, everyone and every*thing* still came together.

I feel like all six of us being at the kitchen table together, even just for a moment, was like all the electrical sockets being put into place that makes the whole Christmas tree light up and cast a holiday glow around the whole

living room. There's no reason why we can't laugh now, love now, live now.
Just as the ICU had changed all of us, we could still change and heal together.

One particular meal we ate on the front porch, and I felt so safe finishing off my plate, that I didn't go back upstairs. Even my puppy Jelly joined us. F-E-A-R was just four big block cutouts of letters that my scared wounded bird used to hide behind. Now I was using each letter as a utensil to twirl up spaghetti strands!

Sewing Myself Back Together

Just as my grandmother had told her story through her sewing, I was now using a sewing machine and feeling more connected to her than ever. The physical act of feeling the machine bind cloth together was stitching me back up too. I began work on a fabric quilt as the threads of my story were coming together. Each cartoon panel would now be a fabric collaged square—a truly tactile way to physically bring my story to light.

Creating my fabric quilt was a concrete way to boost my tolerance for handling emotions. It was the prep work I needed when I had to dive into the next meal.

Jeff: The Hardest Relationship to Heal

Perhaps because Jeff was so close to the actual trauma—staying in the ICU and keeping a journal of the first seventy-two days—it was excruciating for him to see me struggle. As I grew closer with my family, Jeff and I were pulling apart. He didn't understand why I couldn't move on already, feed myself, or be less anxious every time I left my room, and his misunderstanding hurt. Was Jeff having as much trouble facing the wounded part of me I was?

My family was slowly gaining understanding—with the help of Rita's translation skills. She would explain to my parents why I needed to keep moving and why emerging from my room was so difficult. Then, I would tell her about my day with its triumphs and struggles, its anxieties and moments of presence, and she would help me experience the wide spectrum of emotions in a healthy way. I anxiously recounted to Rita how earlier that day, I immediately panicked when I tried to set foot outside my room.

"What did you physically feel?" she asked, making sure to emphasize the word "physical."

"Just...hot."

"Warmth is a sign of the parasympathetic energy being activated, so you're in a good place," she reassured me. "When the negative energy is activated, that's where the anxiety comes from. Sunlight is healing. By looking at the sun, you take in light energy, which is healing psychologically and physically, especially the eyes."

Now, warmth didn't feel scary—it was just a physical sensation—not anxiety, but aliveness. It warmed my heart feeling sunlight on my back in the wide hills. "Light is healing," I repeated Rita's words. "It brings all truths deep inside me to light, and I know that scares me."

The most painful part is when all that self-help starts to work and you actually start feeling of a healthier mindset, and so you start to feel like a giant stuck inside of a tiny dollhouse so out of place, and there is nothing you can do about it except eat your way out of the artificial world you've locked yourself in and widen up your eyes to what's out there.

Eating completely on my own, off of TPN, I couldn't believe how many people doubted me, including myself! I was capable of making my own decisions, trusting myself, and living fully—and I deserved to! My body became a safe space.

CHAPTER 30

Would Surgery Solve My Identity Crisis?

FINALLY, I WAS HUMAN! Free of TPN and independent of machines. I was no longer in limbo, wondering when or if I would ever eat again. Food had re-introduced nourishment, stimulation, feeling, and relationships, and I was no longer starving for connection. But I still wasn't what you would call happy. I kept asking myself, "What now?" If I couldn't find the old me, I had to find my new "normal." But I wasn't sure what normal really was anymore. I still had one more excuse to believe that things would feel "normal" when one more miracle was accomplished.

I decided, "Life will really feel normal, and I'll be happy when I reverse my colostomy." That became my goal.

I am the kind of person who can get excited about surgery. I'm not the one who has to do the work anyway. I just have to focus on the excitement of having a normal, working body.

Surgery number sixteen would be a life-changer—not only would I be eating like a real person, I'd have a real body, too. I hoped number sixteen would be as easy as number thirteen. Perhaps this time, I'd jump off the table, go to the mall, and be able to eat at the food court!

As I prepared for what I thought would be my final procedure, I grew solemn as the reality of the situation sunk in. I wondered if a surgical procedure could really make that happen. Then the exhilarating and frightening thought hit me: *If the surgery was a success, I would have to stop looking ahead to the next procedure.* What would I be able to say when there was nothing else to pin that hope of being normal on? Would all my coping mechanisms disappear when there was no more medical trauma to cope with? And when all the surgeries were finished, who would I actually be?

I didn't expect my anxiety to shoot up in the last days before my surgery. There is a burning lump of coal right where my heart is, and I am trying to let it go. I am nervous about having stitches, wounds and unexpected calamities again.

Despite my fear, I told myself to look forward, and even if I didn't know what to expect, I still deserved to expect the best.

However, I knew that while recovering from surgery, I wouldn't be able to eat or drink anything again. I told myself, that this time would really be temporary.

If things *did* go smoothly and "as expected," I would be the only one responsible for figuring out the next steps on my journey. That was terrifying too.

I knew my mother was just as nervous, so the night before surgery, I recorded myself singing some old standards that now had "new" meaning:

Mom, hopefully the surgery will be shorter than these two CDs, so you don't have to listen to all 34 songs. But here are my favorites:
God Bless The Child: May God bless this child for surgery, 'cause this child needs all the prayers she can get.

Chim Chim Cheree: Just imagine all those scalpels as chimney sweeps sweeping all the dirty crap out of me.
I Got It Bad And That Ain't Good....self-explanatory.

I went in for surgery number sixteen and it went as planned medically, though I wasn't exactly ready to run to the mall. There was one unexpected surprise. After recovering, I felt I had a powerful new tool, a lethal weapon in my hands—my body—*and it scared me.* Now, instead of a source of weakness, my body had become a source of strength. This was the first time I had nothing on me since before my life changed overnight. No IVs. No tubes. No bags! Just gauze, bandages, and stitches that would soon disappear. Could this really be true?

I didn't know whether to pinch myself to see if I was dreaming or hold my breath and wait for something to burst loose.

I felt...amazing. But I also felt so fragile, like a rag doll that could rip open at the seams with the slightest twist. I was terrified a single swallow might rip all my stitches. I missed the feeling of recklessly rolling down a hill like a log, not worrying about where my stomach was hitting or if anything on my skin was open.

My body had changed dramatically again. What was I supposed to do with a normal body now? Just be in it? Just live? I wasn't sure I knew how to do that anymore.

After a week of my stitches healing, I was told to "slowly" start eating and drinking again. When I asked the doctors to clarify, they said, "Take your time and don't go overboard." I wasn't sure what "little by little" meant.

Two weeks later, I flew to California to learn how to eat again. For most people, eating is not something you forget how to do. But I had been without a functioning digestive system and forced to suppress my appetite for so long that I actually needed to re-learn eating. It had been so long since I had hunger cues that it was impossible for me to tell when I was hungry or not. After much deliberation, my parents and I decided I should attend a program in California where they taught "intuitive eating." The idea of moving away intrigued me. "Eating school" might be the college I never had. We were all nervous boarding a plane with a freshly bonded belly, an arm free of intravenous feeding, and a mouth ready for the real stuff. What could plane pressure do to my new tummy?!

My parents helped me off the plane and into a car. We drove several hours past rolling hills and arrived at what looked like a horse ranch. My mom helped wheel my suitcases in, filled with brand new (two-piece!) clothing I now could wear with a real stomach—like pants! My dad followed with twice as many suitcases of medical supplies for post-surgical maintenance and "in case of emergency." Before I could process this new change of environment—girls swinging their legs on a porch with sunglasses, seemingly comfortable in "normal" life; I looked behind me and my parents had driven off.

At eating school, I lived with six girls in a small house, and I felt alien from the start. This was the first time in years I was interacting with girls my age, and I wasn't sure how to talk to people anymore. On top of that, I was trying to get adjusted to my new body, still fresh with stitches, and I was frightened of what would happen once food was reintroduced. But the meals were a dream for me! I had fantasized about freshly prepared plates of meats, fruits, grains, and snacks. I looked at my meal plan like I was holding my college degree! I drooled anticipating every bite, which I assumed I was now entitled to enjoy as a living, breathing normal human being. The trauma was over. Tiger Lilly was safe. She could finally put down her bow and arrow and savor her victory feast.

Unfortunately, I wasn't reacting to food like everyone else, and these grandiose meals didn't feel as satisfying as I had dreamed. Instead, they twisted each day into a distortedly painful nightmare. This was a "Farm Fresh" philosophy place, where they were feeding me tons of fruits and vegetables that that my new system wasn't able to process. With every meal, I started becoming physically pained. The staff didn't know what to do with me. Every day, I noticed my belly swelling a little bit more, but I affirmed to myself, "I am safe in the present moment. I deserve to eat fresh food and live a normal life again."

But my body was not quite ready to hop into the present moment with me because my worst fears did come true.

There I was, in my California paradise, reliving Passover of 2005. As I moaned in pain on the house front porch, the staff members were up all night with me until they finally rushed me to the emergency room. This was the first time I was ever in a hospital, let alone an emergency room, without my family and my father to always advocate for me. On top of that, the doctors wouldn't call my dad until they felt like it was "serious enough." Doctors who had never seen me before looked perplexed at my medical papers trying to figure out my situation. I feared what would happen without my father there to explain my unique medical history or to call his colleagues. Who would know what to do or what attention my case required?

I waited on a stretcher in the emergency room in unbearable pain for what felt like hours. Finally, an attendant came to ask me some questions and remove my gauze dressing, which had just been standard aftercare of my wound proceeding the surgery. I kept my eyes shut, afraid to look. As I felt the gauze being removed, I squinted and peered at what I had hoped I would never ever view again on my own body.

An opening. Another fistula. My wound had actually opened again. This was surreal and unfathomable. My body had failed me again, betrayed me. I had just learned to trust my body again, and now this? This was a disaster. Why had I even tried in the first place?

My situation was deteriorating, and after a few hours of blood transfusions, my father made arrangements to have me air-vacced back to Yale. I felt a flood of relief wash over me when I knew he would be meeting me in California to fly back across the country with me the next day.

I had never been in such a tiny plane before. I was claustrophobic, hooked up to IVs, and lying on my back as we flew east, stopping in Kansas so they could refuel and getting to Yale in the middle of the night with my parents by my side.

Once I'm at Yale, they'll take care of me and sort all of this out, I reassured myself. What I didn't expect would be the three months that followed of being a guinea pig prodded with every possible medical procedure and test in an effort to piece this all back together. I had gotten another fistula, and I knew this frustration all too well.

Yale was a confusing time because nobody knew what had caused this disaster or how to fix it. I felt guilty, believing I had messed up what Dr. Slem had so carefully reconstructed.

There was no "Amy" manual, yet I felt like, somehow, I had broken every rule. Did I have a body capable of being in the real live world?

Once again, I received the news that I'd have to stop eating and drinking until this was resolved, or at least until doctors could figure out what had happened. I didn't know how long I would be in the hospital, or what was going to be done. In my mind, this was just going to be solved, and I could fly back to California the following week. But nothing could have prepared me for the long summer months spent at Yale with my old friend—terrifying uncertainty. Reason for admission: Surgery gone wrong. Prognosis: Who knows? Doctors did everything they could to figure out the situation, subjecting me to arbitrary daily tests and procedures that re-traumatized me and made hope scarce as I saw them desperately seek answers. The lack of concrete proposals terrified me.

Another surgery was not an option, so an endless stream of non-surgical interventions was tried. They threaded things through me, scanned me, plugged things into me, poked me, X-rayed me, stitched me, and even glued me to try to close my wound. Most of my "field trips" were down to the radiology department where they would try to stick various wires into my fistula and have them come out a bag to bypass leaking all over my wound. Their hope was that getting all of the leaking into one centralized place would allow the wound to heal and dry. In theory, these procedures caused no harm because they were "minimally invasive." But the doctors overlooked the emotional scars that each broken wire, pulled stitch, or leaking tube would have on my tested patience and withering spirit.

It was hard to imagine that only months before I had been unbound by anything and freely able to feed myself. I was back to IV nutrition around the clock with a drain taped to my leg and various bags and tubes coming out of my belly that made it impossible to move or twist comfortably. The more stir crazy I got, the more I would push my pole for hundreds of laps around the unit just to make the day go by. Every day was a guarantee of futile experiments, another day on the assembly line being put back together and falling apart just in time for bed.

The best prognosis the doctors could come up with was, "Eat and it won't heal. Don't eat and it *might* heal. The choice is up to you."

Weekends in the unit were always the hardest. As much as I hated being bothered, I hated the silence and stillness even more. With all the major players in my case at home living their normal lives, it was just a matter of killing time until 6 a.m. Monday morning, complete with the diminishing hope we could find answers again. On Sundays, my dad was off from work, so he would stay the day and play card games with me so my mother could go home and have a break in the normal world, of which I was quite envious.

I built up an intense hatred for what my body had become. I felt trapped by it. Surgery was once again on the table. Just as Yale was confining my body, my body was confining my soul and my life's potential. The only life I had now was in my dreams.

Ultimately, the doctors decided against surgery. My old friend Dr. Slem felt that nutrition would eventually heal me. But I would have to spend more time in the hospital getting my strength back. Mom tried reading me self-help books to inspire me, and even the nurses looked forward to Mom's daily readings.

During the day, my mother and I had our quiet routine, gossiping with the nurses, trying to stall any huge medical decisions until my father arrived, greeting him in tears with the latest bomb dropped by the medical team. My father would often get the panicked call at work when the team would come in and demand to take me to some X-ray. We got used to Scattergories and had gone through all of the cards so many times that I had to make up hundreds of new categories. Magazines, games, talk shows—anything to get my mind off of hunger, once again, but more importantly, my situation.

Mom and I circled around the healing garden three times. I have so many tubes and bags on me that, at this point, I just want them out.

My patience, hope, and personhood were being tested. Could I make it through and preserve my humanity once everything I had worked for had once again been taken away?

Mom and I went to the healing garden and the raindrops looked so reflective in the pond. I made a wish for the drains to dry up. If all I can do is focus on getting through, then how can I live?

Between my ravenous hunger and restlessness, I convinced my mom that it would be good for me to get outside and walk at lunchtime by the food trucks lined up outside the hospital. After a week or so of sneaking out, the nurses gave me an official pass, and Mom was carefully allowed to take me on a short stroll. It was the same mix of torture/can't look away and starving/can't ignore food conflict that had dominated the earlier years when I couldn't eat. As difficult as it was, there was something refreshingly human about feeling the air hit my face and walking on pavement, even in my hospital slippers, and yes, even smelling hot food.

I came back from my walk, and I am leaking out of my wound! The doctors came in and said they wouldn't be too concerned because they just want the drainage to dry up, and they don't care how. I am NOT going home like this!

As time passed, I grew desperate for any kind of answer—even surgery. One day, as my mom and I walked past the food trucks, we talked about the agony of living with uncertainty and wondering how this was ever going to heal. All of a sudden, I started bawling. I began to think I might never have a real body ever again. I held Mom's hand and felt my heart break in two. I just wanted my body back. Was that really too much to ask?

I got called ROCKY again by the janitor. "I've been watching you—you're a fighter!"

My dad also took me on walks, past the classrooms, biology labs, big doors with an X-ray sign that said, "Do Not Enter," big nitrogen tanks, conference rooms with expansive open ceilings, and forgotten wings of the hospital. We were always back in my room in my time for the nightly dress-ing change. We even joked about coming out with a Zagat book one day on the best hospitals for walks, the wards with the most scenic passages, the ones that were the easiest to sneak out of. We knew them all well by now, from coast to coast.

Still, every day brought more tests but not progress. With every leak, doc-tors rushed my back to my room as they attempted to untangle the threads of my hopelessly bungled case, like amateur hitmen trying to figure out what to do with the body.

With every obstacle, I discovered a new opportunity. Stuck in that hospi-tal room for months, my mom bought me a set of cheap art supplies from the lobby. The day I picked up a paintbrush for the very first time, my world changed forever.

CHAPTER 31

Discovering Art in Yale

ART SAVED *ME*. Passing the morning hours at Yale was always the hardest as I agonizingly waited for the day to start, the sun to rise, the rush of doctors to come in like a stampede of chaos, and then to be left with time monotonously ticking away until the night shift of nurses arrived. I was used to waking up and feeling overpowering sadness. That's why as soon as the nurses could rearrange my wires at the break of dawn, I'd hop out of bed with my tubes dangling and leaking and fling myself onto the yoga mat I tucked beside the hospital overbed table. The sooner I could start moving, the less I'd have to think about—or feel.

One morning, my sadness was paralyzing. I didn't want to move at all. But if I couldn't exercise my way to numbness, what was I supposed to do? Just *be* with my feelings? I longed for the safety to actually feel, but Yale was a hotbed of too much uncertainty to even try. But if I ignored these feelings I would only hurt more.

I needed a Plan B before this despair threatened to swallow me whole. Some strategy to cope with emotions that were too big to run from.

I remember the exact moment I painted for the first time. My mom had brought in some cheap art supplies—canvases, a few brushes, and a set of kid craft acrylics with lids to screw off—along with various gadgets, games, and anything else she could find in the lobby gift shop to help us pass the time. For a while, the canvases and paints just sat there, crowded in a corner with the rest of the cluttered distractions. That morning, a solemn feeling of stillness washed over me like pale tint of blue paint. For the first time, even my racing, anxious heartbeat could not drown out my despair. I needed something to hold onto. So I went for the paintbrush, still wrapped in plastic, in the dark of the morning.

> I don't know what I'm doing. but I'm feeling something really strongly, and I can't run from it right now. I am just going to hold this paintbrush and whatever this feeling is, I'm just going to put it into this.

I remember holding that paintbrush so strongly that my IV was trembling as I pressed down hard on that canvas to drag one smooth wavy line. I don't remember letting go, as the brush dipped from brown to red to blue. What I created was "Singing Tree."

Nurses who had written me off as the restless manic patient now saw that I had a heart. A quick glance at my medical history should have been enough, but, as I made art, they found compassion for the pain I was going through. And, they really liked my paintings.

Suddenly, creating art became a way to express emotions that were too overwhelming for words. I found my voice again. The Amy I could recognize, who no medical intervention could surgically remove. I used everything in my art—even toilet paper from the hospital bathroom. I painted my trees that I missed; I crafted my inside and outside worlds, bursting with joy and pain, tears and hearts, lightning bolts and flowers.

Each morning before the medical team came in for rounds, I would take out a plastic palette tray and stare at yet another blank canvas, like the answers the doctors were coming up with. I would dip a small paintbrush into that kids' set of paints and paint a brown wavy line—always a call out to my trees to ground me. As the lines thickened, so did their trunks, and my sense of confidence. I could know where to go from here, even if doctors could not.

When I was done, I would put each canvas outside my hospital room. Soon the unit began to catch on. Nurses started walking their patients by my room to see what I had created each day. Having an impact on others through my improvised brushstrokes filled me with unanticipated satisfaction—a meaning. Art was sustaining my aliveness. My life had changed, but my *self* was still vital as ever in whatever colors I dipped my brush in.

Even though each onset of sadness would prompt me to paint, finding my heart in every canvas was the sweet reward.

The pieces I had the most fun creating were the ones that I had no expectations for. This started with random shredding and gluing of newspapers, magazines, coupons, plastic wrap, gum wrappers, and whatever else I was about to throw out. Then I spent hours painting layers upon layers of paint, trying to obscure some of the printed text. Eventually, a face emerged. It represented the process of finding myself—hard to find at first but becoming gradually visible with each layer applied carefully, tediously, and determinedly. With no idea of what was coming next from the doctor's daily visits, making art was the healthiest mindset I could have.

I woke up at 4:30 a.m. Dr. Slem said, "It is up to you whether you want to pull the drain out. You get the concept? It's to dry up the wound and divert it in that direction instead of out of the wound."

It was frightening to know the doctors were guessing as much as I was. To deal with the frustration of having no answers, I painted. My paintings were happy, whimsical, and expressive, but there were always teardrops in the background, broken hearts, and lightning bolts.

To this day, leaving a painting without a tear is like having an itch I can't scratch.

At first, I worried about how I'd pass each leaking, food-devoid moment. Now, one painting could take hours.

Now that I had art, I was emboldened with the courage to *know* what I was feeling, *accept* what I was feeling, and honestly *express* it through my brush strokes, rather than in my frenetic pacing around the unit. With my paintbrush in hand, I could feel myself materialize underneath all of the frustration.

My medical situation was getting worse but art was beginning to connect me emotionally with people, both my family and the hospital staff, and I could begin to hope that someday I would be back out in the world, exhibiting my work somewhere.

Once I started expressing myself creatively, I became more of a friend for Mom, who stayed with me every day and night at Yale. I realized she needed support, too, and now I could be there for her, and we could finally connect. I forgot how good it felt to have companionship; authentic human connection. Being numb keeps you safe, but it doesn't give you connection, which is what gets you through the good and the bad.

Mom said something poignant. She said that this time together has been like two girlfriends spending time in a hotel.

There were many times in Yale when I felt I was going insane. But the psychiatrist they sent me was anything but helpful. And I really didn't want his help either. I was beginning to heal myself.

I had been air-vacced to Yale at the end of June, and now it was almost October! We ended up spending Yom Kippur in the hospital.

This time, although my traditional prayers of healing my fistula were yet to be answered, I simply prayed through my art for something I could use to communicate with a force larger than myself. And for that moment, it seemed to work.

As I started to paint, I realized how sad I was without food. I drew the big blue teardrop I envisioned yesterday on a big tree inside of a heart. I covered it with toilet paper and matte medium, my go-to for added texture. I wasn't proud of it, but it will probably look cool when it dries.

Without art, I doubt I would have made it out alive. Now that painting started off each morning, my days had a different—even enjoyable—flow. I would get up and jump right into my art. It felt incredible to have something to do. Mom did her beadwork while I painted, and we sat together quietly, each focusing on our own projects. I even made my dad get into art when he came to visit, and our art sessions slowly replaced many of our sneaky after-hours walks in the medical school.

I was consumed by creativity and often the transport team would have to wait patiently while I finished glue-gunning the last scraps of felt and fabric onto my canvas.

We get back upstairs, and the nurse was admiring my artwork, especially how I had used the toilet paper! Everyone here says I should sell my artwork. To do that, I would have to get out of here, which means people have to believe that is possible.

But reality was still difficult. As painting began to stir up my emotions, I began to feel my old friend, hunger. My mother would always leave for her "lunch break" while I was swept away in my art. When she came back, she would try to finish her turkey wrap without me seeing, hiding her leftovers as best as she could.

Until my stay at Yale, I had never picked up a paintbrush in my life, and now, art was healing a part of me which doctors couldn't.

Soon, I didn't want to leave my hospital room. My antsy feet had found a way to express the energy of emotion, through art.

I added a snake—I guess today is a tortured day—and pasted words right out of a magazine with a lost little girl in the corner, upset. The snake is chasing the girl, who is holding a flower and running to the tree for a true anchor. I like how it turned out.

Every day I tried to face a memory a bit more. Dipping a paintbrush in my paint set, and "dipping my toes" in my trauma. Whether watercolored, collaged, painted, or sketched, every canvas was finished off with a blue tear. After nearly four weeks of tear-covered art, I drew a speech bubble for one, especially large, acrylic-outlined tear, simply with the words, "I am hurting."

After all this time, nothing was healing the fistula, so the doctors decided to try letting me eat. They didn't know what else to do. As relieved as I was, it was hard not to feel hope diminish altogether when the surgeons decided to allow me to just start eating again, "a little," and just "see what happened."

For the last week of our three-month stay at Yale, I was able to have a piece of bread and a slice of turkey once a day, as long as the fistula didn't seem to get any worse. Anything I ate that didn't make my fistula bigger was fine. But the real purpose of food was to make me feel human with some kind of semblance of a normal life, and that was enough for me.

It felt like my body's fragile state of being patched and stitched together was a trial and error game I was supposed to play. But this time, I had art on my side. My life somehow felt richer and more expansive than ever before.

I was discharged with bags and dressings attempting to hold my constantly leaking wound in place, a drain taped to my leg that unsuccessfully tried to divert the leaking to a bag (most of it just leaked around the drain, causing me to change my clothes frequently), and my IV nutrition.

Now that I was finally going home, Mom and I were forced to examine the feelings we had conveniently avoided. Instead of being able to make a limited number of decisions in the hospital, we were faced with the question of how we were supposed to go on living meaningful lives, even when things hadn't worked out the way we wanted them to. What do you do when you don't like your story's ending?

What did I come out of Yale with? A messy fistula that I tried to manage with gauze and a vacuum pack. A big green drain running up my leg. We also left with loads of art supplies. This was the first time I was coming home from a hospital as an artist, with something purposeful to pass the time. The biggest question was where to put all these new supplies since my mother had brought more and more to Yale every week. Art was now a way of life.

CHAPTER 32

Finding Safety in Art

ONCE AGAIN, I WAS HOME from the hospital with no answers, left to find my own way through the maze that had become my life. But this time, art was my guide. With a wound I didn't have answers to yet, art gave me the comfort to be with those feelings of uncertainty.

As my passion for painting grew, our kitchen table got stacked higher and higher with paint sets, fabrics, puff paints, and pencils. Soon enough, clearing the table became a lengthy ordeal, and I knew I needed a space for myself where painting could be my sanctuary.

"I have a surprise for you..." Mom took me downstairs where I could've sworn a furnace used to be. Now, the bare shelves were painted white. There were tall cabinets with empty pull-out drawers. As I opened one, the empty space seemed to transform and flood me with an infinite outflow of ideas. What could I fill each drawer with? It could be as simple as ripped out magazine ads, scraps of plastic wrap, and crumpled up notebook paper. When thrown on a canvas, who knows what it could become?

We got new lighting, a sink, and soon enough, our supplies easily fell into place. I chose to accent the room with anything red I could get my hands on. Red has always been my lucky color, reminding me of life, passion, and creating from the heart. I put up pictures framed of my family, both from before and after my coma. I did this to remember the innocent child in me who always created with joy and carefreeness, and also to honor the woman I had become from all of this, who still miraculously had a creative innocence, but also a deeper knowing and wisdom. To honor my grandparents, I placed my grandmother's old laces in my fabric drawer and hung my grandfather's big plastic bag of assorted buttons on a hook.

My mother and I sat together, reading biographies of artists every day, learning about artists who had also had "detours" in their own lives. Then, we'd sit beside each other, me painting in my studio, she making her jewelry, a hobby she had picked up at Yale. Together, we were healing through creativity. In my new "self-help" reads—artist biographies—I learned how many artists had healed themselves finding transformation and liberation through color and shape. Each struggle—Matisse, Kahlo, Van Gogh—was unique, yet somehow similar to mine.

Since I was developing a "holy" reverence for art and how it had saved my soul, I felt it was important to learn about those who came before me. When I wasn't painting, I was Googling art history or scavenging for the latest art books at Barnes & Noble.

What is it about creating in a time of crises that brings out the best in us? There becomes an obsessive need to produce, to document, because bringing a piece to fruition means we are alive.

I hadn't been able to go to college, but I had never lost my quest for knowledge, and learning everything I could about the history of art and all the artists I loved was my way of resuming my education.

Suddenly, I wasn't just killing time with my mom in malls in my "interim" phase of healing. I was actually a person, an artist, with a job, buying art supplies. Rather than pace through stores, insecure in who I was, I proudly had a role to fill in society.

Yesterday felt different, like I actually owned my personhood! I felt so proud when an employee at the store asked me if he could help me with anything, and I said, "Yes, you can!"

It felt good to be honest with myself and my intentions and my story. It felt good to come out to the world. It felt good to be vulnerable—a healthier and wiser vulnerability than the kind I had felt with Blaine.

My mother and I had created our own whole art therapy studio in our Westport home. Soon, I couldn't stop creating. Now, I was turning compulsion to my advantage.

I was a secret agent with an artist's mission: to get back into her body and into the world. Today's warrior mission: I will spend allotted amount of time sketching people at Starbucks. Mission—*expect the unexpected and YOU WILL FIND IT.*

1. Observe people's interactions. We have to find what gives people pleasure.
2. Find at least three different ways people are enjoying themselves.
3. Eavesdrop on someone's story and come back with one interesting fact.

The arts were always how I had connected to society, and now was no different. Spending months in the Yale vacuum had driven me almost to the point of insanity, and now I used my job as an "artist" to study the art of living and figure out how I once again was supposed to dive into that world.

Being an artist integrates the tools you need to recover from trauma into your day-to-day existence. It enabled me to create a roadmap for myself when there was no road at all to follow. I could anchor myself in my canvas, my sheet music, my notebook, my dancing, and then feel empowered, as if I had some control over my uncertain life. I actually started to daydream about the future.

Art was making all of these difficult concepts much easier. It was a way to take uncertain concepts and make them tangible. I learned I could be aware of my feelings but choose not to act on them.

Painting was the one area of my life in which I could move freely, non-judgmentally, with no exact game plan in mind or reason to have one. Art was really just for art's sake, and I still got to walk away with a product. Art let me be okay with imperfection, and okay with blurring every squiggly line.

The more I painted, the more certain themes started to emerge, which I realized were my values no matter what, where, when, or how I was. I realized I was deserving of being still and being in myself. Slowly, words formed, which I used as titles.

A new theme began to find its way into my art—my physical body. After every surgery, I would wake up with a new anatomy—a bag here, no belly button here, this missing, that added. I could explore how I felt about myself by putting on canvas what I looked like—to me.

I became fascinated with the figure as it relates to the world, nature, and the flesh. Seeing my figures look more and more body-like reassured me I was starting to feel human, accepting my body for what it had been through and calling it my own.

Everything I saw became material for my paintings. It was an exhilarating learning experience watching the subtlest of things—how people sipped their coffee, or what they did with their feet as they sat.

Art was breaking open my world and, at the same time, making me realize how broken my world was. I was overwhelmed with anger about Blaine. When I wasn't making art, I was obsessively writing in my journal. I convinced myself I was writing my book to help others, but the truth was I still had to focus on helping myself, on healing my inner wounds that, like my stubborn fistula, still refused to close up.

"Amy deserves to thrive." That's what Rita said. "Amy wants to feel." I just wish it wasn't too hard and painful.

I went so far with my book idea—a self-help book in adventure novel form on finding the adventure in healing through your own warrior's journey—that I even wrote a letter to a local editor. She never wrote back. I guess what I didn't realize was that I couldn't write a book to help others if I was still learning how to help myself.

Anger is an old survival mechanism. It helps get the body ready for the fight of its life to survive. I knew there was anger trapped inside me, but where it coming from?

I was angry that I had no clue how my medical situation would resolve. I was angry at what Blaine had done to me. Now I had a safe space where I could use my anger the right way: in streaks of red paint.

Art gave me the right amount of distance where I could engage with that anger through expressive metaphor. Healing became a creative dialogue rather than an angry confrontation with my past.

I let my feelings about Blaine unravel—feelings I didn't realize I had worked so hard to stifle.

Feeling invincible with my paintbrush in my hand, I boldly wrote in deep rich purples, dark thick blacks, and lots of blue swirling tears on the page something that I wouldn't have had the courage to do with a pencil, typing on my computer, or speaking aloud, even to myself.

R—the paintbrush seemed to curve on its own.

My thoughts told me otherwise, but for the moment, I pretended I was fearless. I continued my strikes until the color turned into the sound of sharp crackles: RAPED.

"Just go for it," I whispered to myself.

I filled up the rest of the canvas sheet with the green words: I WAS and messily streaked the rest of the page with those bold red letters. RAPED.

And then left the page wide open to dry.

Reclaiming Myself and My Power from Blaine

As my paintings became more vivid, I realized Blaine had been a parasite, not a mentor; an unanchored mask, a chameleon conforming to whatever he felt others needed. But he had nothing of himself to give. That is why he felt so empty. And why he tried to use me to fill his void.

I was no longer a hospital patient. I was no longer Blaine's victim. But I was far from feeling whole again. Art was helping me pick up the pieces. But what to do with them...

CHAPTER 33

Art Turns Me Inside-Out

NOW THAT I HAD BEGUN to wrestle with the inner world of trauma my abuse created, I started to feel safe delving into my real feelings of anger and fear.

I remembered the fire in my chest, which for years, had run me around in circles. I remembered the anger that consumed me and throwing a chair when I discovered I would be getting a colostomy that had just taken nineteen hours to reverse. I remembered the unexpressed anger I felt at Blaine that he had changed, anger I could only express with my running feet.

But through my art, I was moving past these feelings, doing the work to resolve them and turning myself outwards towards the world. I wasn't alone. I was connected, protected. With art and nature, I belonged. It's one thing to dream, imagine, and visualize. It's another to find an occupation that makes your dreams real. Art made recovering myself seem real and therefore possible.

My stays in the hospital had turned time on its head and forced me to create tools and strategies to get through each day or even each hour. Time had been my enemy. But through art, I was relearning the orderly passing of time through the changes in seasons. I was finally keeping up with and becoming part of the world around me.

Taking My World Back

Hand in hand with developing a clearer sense of who I was and how I fit into the world, I started focusing on what I really wanted—independence, travel, respect, love, honesty (from self), employment, to give more than I took.

Painting through obstacles reaffirmed compassion for myself and the world around me.

There was so much I didn't understand, and it was so liberating to let go of the not knowing and trust that I would eventually get to where I needed to be.

I would rather live in a world where my life is surrounded by mystery than live in a world so small that my mind could comprehend it.

Besides giving me purpose and a productive activity, art connected me to Grandma. I still hadn't accepted that I'd never see my grandmother again. Going through photographs didn't bring her back, and I needed her more than ever.

I snipped into a patch of purple felt to create Grandma's warm, tiny shape, and suddenly I could see and feel her by my side.

I held her old fabrics tenderly in my hand as I glued and cut them together to create a fabric quilt. I decided she would be a purple swirling figure that could come out of a tree like a friendly ghost. This symbol was another art motif added to my portfolio. Just as my teardrops and broken hearts popped up in every painting, now my grandma symbol would swirl out of every painting and immediately I'd feel protected. I created hope through my art, losing myself in the process, yet reliably finding myself in every moment.

I am carving new pathways for my nerves, so the next time I feel emptiness,
I have another image to relieve me; the image of Grandma holding me.

Uncertainty is not a safe feeling. Nor are anger and fear. Art gave me a safe space in which to let my feelings out, to explore and experience them, and to begin to make sense of my chaotic jumble of emotions. I would learn later how critical finding a safe space is for abuse survivors.

Trauma exists in a snow globe, inside of this glass. It cannot hurt me any-
more. Now, it is merely a scene. I can always find a place in my body where
I am feeling good, always finding a corner of my mind where there is safety
and happiness.

Whether walking through tree-lined neighborhoods or snipping pieces of felt fabric under bright lights in my makeshift art studio, I now felt Grandma with me constantly. And I could feel my sadness over losing her without the emotion completely overtaking me.

The fistula was just a small scribble on my canvas I could paint over. And when it got me too anxious, I hid away in my "safe room inside myself." This was not a way of denying my pain or sticking my head in the sand. It was instead a happy visualization—me swinging on a felt hammock surrounded by the comfy cottony clouds, looking out the window at the chaotic and anxious snowflakes, while I am all safe and warm inside of this bliss—sitting in the bliss and watching the anxiety from afar. I realized I was reclaiming my life for nobody else but ME.

When I was making my colorful sketch of my safe place hanging from my
tree branch, I felt a strange sensation: BEING in the moment. For a second I

went, "Hmm, I'm lonely." Still, it was a relief to feel! If I feel empty, I'll just fill it up with counting my blessings.

The new year was approaching and I began to experience life as a series of gifts. And I learned that it's not receiving gifts that enables us to be grateful. It's feeling grateful that enables us to appreciate the gifts we've been given.

Art was the only way I could explore the depths of myself and to find that perhaps there was really nothing to be afraid of deep down inside of me. That maybe the stillness and the quiet of my soul was really the key to all I had been searching for—getting my *self* back. I think we all are afraid at times of the stillness inside of ourselves.

Is that really the central lesson of life; to learn to be alone?

As much as I had learned to love myself, it was still painful to be alone, and feel the discomforting sadness that surfaced when I couldn't numb myself with distractions. When I was left with just myself, the truth of who I was...hurt.

I feel a tiny rubber band snapping inside of my heart. It hurts to have a conscience. It hurts to care. It hurts to be me, but I'm all I've got. I am enough.

CHAPTER 34

Ready to Put My Heart on Display

"I HAVE TO DO SOMETHING with this," I said to my mom while scanning the room full of completed canvases stacked against the walls. There were even more strewn about the rest of the house.

"What, Amy? The art? We're not done hanging it on the walls."

"People who paint; how do they show this stuff?"

"Like at Yale?" Mom looked truly befuddled at my question.

No. An art show. That's what artists had—something to show for what they created. I had spent all this time jumping from canvas to canvas, cementing my thoughts in paint and ripped out magazines. I wanted to do something with it. Something to get me out of my house. Something that would make an impact.

My Art Would be My Journey into Daylight

I called my first art show—*Journey into Daylight*. The show was a collection of sixty mixed media and acrylic paintings, thirty of which I had done at Yale. My mom had wanted to wait until I was "healthy," but what for? I had already spent so much time waiting. My father had a patient, Leona, whom he recalled was an artist. She came over one afternoon, looked at my whole portfolio sprawled out on the basement floor and didn't see why not. She remarked that my art was certainly busy and interesting, and more important, she had unwavering faith in me. So, to my mother's trepidation, we rented out the Westport Women's Club and made *Journey into Daylight* happen.

I hadn't done anything in the outside world since *Oliver* and *CATS*. And I had never presented myself as an "artist" with something to say. But I did have something to say...and that was what frightened me. My show would share my soul with the world—the feelings that remained unresolved.

Pushing my fear aside, I started preparing my first "art show." First, I had to write an artist's bio. I had never written a "bio" before. It forced me to summarize my long history of hospitalizations in a few short words and communicate what my "show" was about.

Next, explained Leona, I had to title my pieces and give a brief description of each. Wasn't the point of art to show what you couldn't put into words?

"Just give it a try," Leona pushed me. The first time I tried to put an image into words felt dangerously vulnerable.

But once I started, the words wouldn't stop. Soon enough, all seventy painting had titles, like "Broken Open," "My World Has Split," "My Trauma," "Can't Distract," and "Vulnerable."

I am Artist Hear Me...Paint

My show was up! And now *Westport News* was covering it. I didn't want those three gallery hours to end. I was so overwhelmed by having people back in my life. In my very first art show, people were discovering a huge, vulnerable part of me for the first time.

People I hadn't seen for years were looking right at me, saying things like, "I resonated with your experience, but I haven't been through anything like what you've been through."

It was over before it had even begun. We drove home once the last person had trickled out. I could tell I was feeling something that was growing more and more fervently. I still had not gotten used to these sensations of "feeling" brought on first by food and now by art. Now, how was I supposed to process actual *responses* from *normal* people in the *real* world?

My mother's words, "Amy, you deserve to be happy," rushed all over my body. That idea still felt odd to me. Was this what the floods of joy felt like?

Maybe art was my path to joy. This *Journey into Daylight* illuminated every lesson art had taught me so far.

My art show filled me like a blank canvas with a glowing wash of happiness. But I couldn't shake off the feeling that nothing lasts. For all I knew, even these people emerging into my life who had just walked by my paintings could be completely ephemeral. I had lived years in isolation. What would make this any different? Would I ever be "out enough" in the real world to stay there as a permanent fixture of society? Or was I to spend the bulk of my time in my art studio painting my life away while wounds kept opening, occasionally popping out for an art show and then retreating back to my trauma cave? I felt doomed as our car approached the driveway. My biggest fear was that once I came back home, I would never be able to rejoin the world. What was that tickle scraping my throat? Tears belonged on canvases, not rolling down my face. I covered my eyes with my fingers, still splotched with paint.

Dad parked and took out his keys. Here it was. Home. I jumped out of the car, feeling like my heart was going to burst out of my mouth. Still unsure of what was going on under my prickling skin, I ran up to my room, slammed my door, and bawled my eyes out. It was so overwhelming having all of these people in my life, and my biggest fear was that once I left, I would lose it all forever. The world opened up for just three hours, welcomed me with open arms, treated me like one of its own, and then spit me back out, forever doomed to be an alien wandering on the outskirts of the living, breathing, world. *Journey into Daylight* had made me an artist. Now, I just wanted to be a person.

CHAPTER 35

From Surviving to Thriving

YALE HAD OPENED UP THE WORLD of art as a gateway to new discoveries, new connections, a potential new Amy. Becoming an artist seemed to answer the question, "Who was I?" But my life and body had changed so radically that I needed to redefine the identity that was forming. I began by asking myself some essential questions.

I was finally regaining my health, and now that I was out of my room more and more, we were all getting too close for comfort in our little cottage on the beach. The members of my "close-knit" family needed their own space. My parents decided to sell our quaint beach house for a larger space in Westport, complete with an actual *dinner* table. My father even called it "our new Fairfield." So why was I still feeling lost, abandoned by life, without a place in the world I could truly call my own? Where did this new, reconstructed but still leaking Amy belong?

I had gotten used to our crowded, cluttered quarters in the beach house. The new house was empty, and so big that I felt overwhelmed, especially for someone who was so anxious about leaving her room in the first place. Packing up our Compo Beach house, a home that I could finally call "safe," was bittersweet.

I had lost both my childhood house and the comfort zone that our beach house had become. What was to come in the future? Trauma survivors thrive on routine to feel "safe." Suddenly, all my old routines were gone. My dad hoped the new house would be our new beginning, far, far away from the medical setbacks and leaking wounds—starting fresh as healthy, real humans. But was I ready?

I marveled at the newfound freedom I had, with no nurses or IVs attached to me every second. But I still wavered between being secure in myself and losing my sense of self-worth. With no tubes, wires, and machines holding me hostage, I now had to be someone in the world. I had to make a new commitment, not just to heal myself but to also make a contribution. But how could I give, when I had lost so much?

It dawned on me that I had to let go of my past and move on, both my pre-coma past and the years after in which I had fought and won so many battles, to step into my future.

Not only was my family moving houses, but we were all moving on in our own journeys. Trauma changed the course of everyone's life in my family. Matt ended up playing in the house band for Amateur Night at the Apollo in Harlem. Because Jeff had been devotedly by my side all through the hospital, he was inspired to go to medical school.

My mother and I threw ourselves into redecorating the new house during our daily shopping trips to HomeGoods, packing our trunk with decor to brighten our home. Our goal was simply to fill it with life. Tiger Lilly was setting off on the greatest adventure of her life: reintegrating herself back into the human world. Every vase I passed in each aisle could potentially be my newest warrior trinket to fill our new home with life.

As my family made our own personal transitions and settled into to a new house, we closed out a chapter of our life: we finally sold our Fairfield house.

We spent two months digging out dusty photographs, moving around furniture, and throwing away old papers I was still struggling to let go of. Fairfield was put on the market and eventually sold to a young family with children—just as we had been when we had bought it. I felt like my old life had been sold to the highest bidder. Just as I had tortured myself by cooking and melting chocolate to deal with hunger when I couldn't eat, I insisted on going back to the Fairfield house, even after the new owners had taken possession. I needed something from the house, but I didn't know what.

The house had already been lived in for a few weeks. Our plan was just to drive by and pass it, so I could take one good and final look. But I noticed that the owners' car was not in the driveway. So, I snuck behind the house, to the same path I would venture down when I got home from school and opened the gate to the back yard. There they were—my trees, as they had always been, standing there before me, hovering above my large pool, and the open sky stretched over my head. I took out my phone to record a video of myself stepping on the crinkly autumn leaves. I flipped the camera around to show the tears in my eyes as I stared into the lens and whispered, "This was my home." Tears could explode at any given moment, and I knew I was getting too close for comfort. Still, I wanted that closeness.

I ventured farther into the backyard of my old house and saw what I hoped I wouldn't see: a sign of new human life. I spotted a pair of baby shoes in the window of the basement—the room where I used to blast music to choreograph my dances, which was now converted into a children's playroom. Flooded with memories of having a physical house to call my own, and a body to house my soul that hadn't yet betrayed me, I burst into tears. I was a trespasser stomping on crumpled autumn leaves, like a child stomping on her youth. As I made my way back to the gate, wiping away tears, I saw my reflection in the kitchen window and thought about our round kitchen table with the underside covered in markers and crayons. I focused through the pane, with vacant eyes staring straight through and into someone else's life. I stood there for what felt like an eternity, until I could accept that my new life would not be found through this window, but somewhere else. I walked back to the car. And then Fairfield was gone—forever.

As we drove away, I knew I had gotten what I came for—a kind of closure. A wound must close before it can fully heal. It helped to try to make peace with the past, but now I had to heal in the present, and art showed the way there.

I was having an artistic renaissance after being the "resident artist" at Yale and mounting an art show for old and new faces in our new hometown. But my body was a different story. I was burdened with unsettled medical realities—a fistula that seemed determined to never heal and a big green drain taped up my leg. The darker the circumstances became, the more joyous my paintings became. Although the teardrops and lightning bolts were always streaked across the bold backgrounds, every tree seemed to be singing and dancing. To know I could *feel* at a time when every surgery made me feel like a robot, well, that just made me happy.

With my fistula a constant uncertainty, my mother and I tried even harder to remake and transform our lives. It was both a process of reclaiming the past and grabbing hold of the future. Now that being in touch with spirituality was a survival skill, I tried to embody this through the spirit of the home. We'd buy accessories that reminded us of Grandma and tie red ribbons around bed posts for good luck. I immersed myself once again reading mythology books, swept away by a world of symbols, creativity, and stories. I needed to know where my hero's journey was going to take me next.

But as long as food threatened to keep my fistula open, my hero's journey wasn't going anywhere. I went back to Tikkun Olam, the idea of repairing the world by finding sacred in the everyday and created symbols around me to make eating a holy experience.

We would bring lunch to our daily shopping trip to HomeGoods, where all of the employees now knew us. As I nibbled away at each slice of turkey I had excitedly packed along with me (along with emergency medical supplies), fearful of what might leak out the rapidly filling bag taped below my dress, I focused on the beautiful objects all around me, praying to each china plate and vase that with each bite I took, somehow, my fistula would heal magically or "with time and nutrition," as the doctors had promised. Nibble, wish, hope and pray.

When life felt stagnant and unmoving, at least I could count on the display in HomeGoods changing seasonally—from jack-o'-lanterns to Christmas ornaments to candy valentines. Symbols were everywhere.

With each tchotchke I bought at HomeGoods, I created another "god" as if I was creating my own, mythical, multi-god religion. I loved Mayan mythology and their nature gods, so I took the idea and ran with it: water, Earth, soul, Grandma (she was a force of nature!), moon, and child-like wonder.

Every warrior has a sacred space. For me, it was my new room. I had a large window that opened towards our backyard. As I looked out to see nature surrounding me, I could almost believe that, just maybe, God was on my side.

If you Build it, Anything Can Come

Using whatever I could find meaning from, I transformed my room into a shrine. These trinkets I collected created my visualization for a "safe room inside of myself." Once I brought them all together, this safe space material-ized and became sanctified.

I posted affirmations all over my new room to strengthen my ever-chang-ing healing vortex. Slowly but surely, I was gaining resilience with each transition.

AFFIRMATION: WE ONLY HAVE THIS MOMENT. THIS IS YOUR
FIRST MOMENT AND YOUR LAST. CHILDLIKE WONDER IS
NEVERENDING.

Still, I wondered, was God really with me? What was the point of praying and believing if life still seemed to have no answers? I created affirmations every day to help me on my journey.

My trip to California had been a well-intentioned disaster. I had come home from Yale with a million unanswered—and possibly unanswerable—questions. It was through asking and doing my best to answer the questions I could that I created the god guides that helped make my new home not only a safe space, but also a temple of faith and renewal, a place that would keep me safe and strong on my journey into daylight. My body remained a leaky, untrustworthy mess. Despite it all, my *self* was as vital as ever. I realized that all the questions I had been asking boiled down to one: What is *my self*?

CHAPTER 36

Inner-Conflict Continued

THE LUXURY OF SPIRITUAL "self-discovery" was only possible after creativity helped me face the practical issues of recovery: feeling comfortable with food in this unrecognizable body. But even the fantasy world I tried to create with my affirmations, gods, fabric quilts, and decorative vases could not stomp out the feeling that I was constantly running away from something.

> *My brain hurts as I feel like I am standing at the edge of the world. I am torn, conflicted, down, and it's all the whirlpool where that big knot of tension accumulates in my chest. I forget what makes me happy.*
>
> *I am sick of healing and just want fun with friends. All you need is deep within you waiting to unfold and reveal itself. All you have to do is be still and you will surely find it. I'll just pretend I am on a treasure hunt—a mysterious detective case where each spontaneous thing that happens today a message that God is trying to send me. I'll never hear it if I don't start exploring.*

When my anxiety sucked me into the trauma vortex, I grounded myself in my go-to warrior tool: gratitude.

What am I grateful for? Lavender sea glass, which would look beautiful in this glass vase that is just begging to be filled up. I honestly have no idea how I got so into home decorating.

Staying numb was a guarantee for permanent stuckness. I needed to view numbness as a hindrance, not a help. As a teen, I'd enthusiastically scribble out lyrics in the margins of my notebooks. Now, I couldn't think lyrically within a compulsive movement's panicky tempo. I wanted my poetry back, and that was enough reason reclaim stillness.

All this running in place has landed me just where I am. I haven't gotten very far, have I? I have to remember that being numb to life is only fine if I want to continue to live the rest of my life like this. Yes, I have the fistula, but that's no excuse for waiting for life to happen!

To trust these "risks," I created my "symbols" over and over again in any kind of craft I could put together, like a fabric blanket. I needed to create something comforting that could directly addressed the hurt I was trying to avoid.

My stories I'm designing on my fabric quilt is a safe way to face these feelings. It's the story of me on my hero's journey, going through the forest, into the fear, but safely, one leaf at a time. It's an ode to the things that gave me comfort back before Blaine traumatized me.

As we remade our home, I tried to remake my routine, filling it with activities I had fearfully abandoned. It started with the bold phone call to start voice lessons again.

It is a delightfully sunny day outside. I'm going to make myself vocalize to-day, which I half look forward to and half dread. I'm flung back to lessons with Blaine, leaving me in a foggy daze.

These were the moments I could actually "sit" in that "safe space inside my-self," the moments I had visualized through art.

I love watching candle flames, smelling frosty air, or touching soft fleece. That's sight, touch, and smell. I love hearing wind rustle or rainfall, and I love tasting crispy things like the burnt edge of a pizza. Those are all my five senses. I was just walking barefoot across the hall, not "doing" an actual planned "activity." I felt the smooth texture of the rug, I felt my toes, and I felt myself. That must be what just "being" feels like.

I stayed in my head to avoid the anger I could physically feel raging through my body. However, when I did allow anger to fully come into my body, anger from the abuse, from the surgical interventions, and anger for how life had "wronged" me, I transformed into an unrecognizable beast who frightened me.

I repeated my visualization, determined to find a sense of calm. But I re-alized I could never face what I was running from if I stayed in my head. The healing vortex could never be fully unleashed without my body, too.

The more anger I felt race down my legs, the more warrior traits I cre-ated.

When I'm tempted to dip back into that sizzling pool of fury, I lean on my warrior traits and stay the course, steady like a boat, calmly floating down a peaceful stream, and gently being helped along with a gentle wind in my sails. Then, I'll earn the warrior trait of steadiness.

I had to sit with this monster of a feeling long enough to let it pass. I had to dig into "anger" and it felt horrible. Still, I knew this was a step that would be worth it in the long run.

How could I trust the wisdom of my own body after years of doubting, muting, and running from my inner voice? Suddenly, I had compassion for myself as a high school senior, plagued with a secret she didn't know what to do with. Since moving to this new house, I now had a whole army of warrior tools lined up in my healing vortex, guiding me towards reclaiming myself: Home decor to make my room a shrine, my fabric quilt to remind me of the safe space inside of myself, nature, voice lessons, eating, journaling, cartooning, and sharing and expressing myself.

Every time I cartoon and share one of these secrets creatively, I feel closer to truth, and that feeling alone makes me feel so safe. In each animated story I created, I feel like I am coming clean in every sense. That's what makes me feel whole. When I doodled me exercising watching the Food Channel, and shared it with my parents, I felt proud. I felt like old Amy except with a lot of strength under her superwoman belt. That's why I wake up in the morning every day excited about cartooning. They are the epitome of the power of now.

Give thanks for a little, and you will find a lot.

I feel like a messy tube of toothpaste sometimes, making splatters all over the place when I get any hint of emotion. What is odd now is that I could not turn off those emotions if I tried. I used to be able to turn them on and off like a faucet. Now, I am unable to control them, so I can at least act somewhat civilized. I am willing to risk, and I am willing to be vulnerable. I don't have to be rock hard. I just have to be me.

But the "Thriving Amy" who wanted life couldn't help but wonder, "What *does* make you an adult, capable of being in the human world?" I realized that normal people have intuitive body cues: hunger, sleep, what they felt like doing to pass time. I had no cues whatsoever. I only knew how to operate on a regimented schedule ever since my traumas. Knowing intuitively what to use my energy for, when to sleep, when to exercise, and how to make choices frightened me. I realized what I was running from all this time: I had lost touch with myself. I had forgotten how to make decisions because, for so long, all my decisions had been made for me. Now I questioned every "decision," like, "How do you know when your body wants to go to bed?"

> *I am waiting for God to unravel me, to unwrap me like a present. But the truth is I am probably the one who must untie that ribbon.*
> *Unchanging truth: I will never ever be able to "get rid" of my energy, to just get it out of me. It is like spinning your own hamster wheel. Anxiety exists only artificially in the past and future, and there's nothing really to get angry about. Only what I can touch is what is real here.*

If all my energy didn't have to be used for physical activity, what should I do with the extra energy left to linger in my mind, heart, and soul? What did real people do? I wouldn't find the answer until I listened to my wounded bird.

> *Every day, I try so hard to stay with my uncomfortable feelings, but that doesn't make them any more comfortable. You have to keep building up tools, like muscles. Anxiety isn't an evil thing. It is like a baby that needs attention. My wounded bird just chirped up in me and wanted to cope how she used to. I'll tell it, "Oh little bird, don't worry about it. We're safe now, don't worry. I can handle this so I can grow."*

You always have the ability to find a safe place. And if you can't find it, just create it. I can't control moments. I can only allow them to color me and bring out the artfulness in the unplanned.

With trauma over and done, letting go was the only safety measure I needed to take.

"What is this feeling trying to teach me right now?" and "What gifts might I walk away with if I accept its challenge?"

I learned that rather than be frightened of emotions, I could recognize them as arrows pointing me where I needed to go next. My feelings wouldn't go away. I just had to choose which ones I acted on.

Fear is a dragon guarding our innermost treasures. When I listen to these scary feelings, they will act as pointers to who I really am.
Silence is the best teacher. If I run away from every second of emptiness, I'll never really know myself.

By giving up my rigid routines, I could look to unplanned moments as insights into myself. Courage is like a muscle. The more you use it, the stronger it gets.

My aliveness is starting to burn so brightly that I couldn't lock myself in my room if I tried.

CHAPTER 37

Reconnecting with the Real World

I KNEW THAT OTHER PEOPLE were the magic "spark" missing in my life. But…

I have a tremendous, irrational fear of opening myself up to the sea of spontaneity by leaving my room

I had only just rediscovered myself, and I was still scared of her. I needed a safe space, larger than my art studio, where I could experiment with relating, without the risk of getting hurt or alienating others. I found it in nature.

When most people ask you how you're doing, they really don't want to hear that life is hard. They don't want to hear that food freaks you out sometimes, or you have a fistula that won't heal.

As Halloween neared, I was feeling more comfortable with my new self. I couldn't wait for fresh pumpkin—the original food that had brought "emotion" back into my unfamiliar body. If creativity was where I found hope, nature was where I found happiness.

The fir trees and azalea bushes give me something to smile about; to fondly look forward to as I wake.

Every time I was scared to leave my room, I treated it like an adventure. I would venture forth as an artist, traveler, or child, pretending I'd never seen anything like what my five senses were showing me, invigorated by a passionate moment of discovery.

I didn't have a community of people yet, but nature connected me to a world larger than myself that I could belong to. Once I faced an emotion, I was able to get back in touch with what my values were. And nature was a value that had never steered me wrong.

As I was getting into bed one night, I dropped a book into my lap. Suddenly, I remembered my frustration at Columbia in the ICU bed, how my legs had to be outstretched flat on the bed, lying straight out and so awkwardly dangling there. I couldn't bend them, and all the doctors would come in and say, "Oh, you have dancer's legs." *Yeah, but I can't do anything with them!* I felt claustrophobic, with no freedom to get up, let alone sit up, strapped into bed, unable to move an inch, bound by plugs, and cords.

I was experiencing *those same feelings* in the present moment when I was safe, healthy and free. Still, my body panicked, triggered by the thud of a book landing on my lap. I became aware that so many innocent physical sensations triggered horrible hospital memories of feeling trapped and paralyzed. As I realized this mind-body connection, it was becoming clear why I would start panicking if I couldn't move around.

As the vortex of healing overtook trauma, the stronger the connection I felt to my *self*.

Getting grounded in my values coated my room in a newfound holiness. I had my symbols to represent water (a flask), fire (a candle), earth (a leaf), and wind (a fan).

I found power through these symbols, imagined from all my writing, cartooning, and art. Now my healing vortex was completely built up, surrounded, and barricaded with my army of robust, creative warriors, I wasn't alone. I hadn't known how to patch up the hope that leaked from the heart Blaine had broken years before. Now I was healing by allowing it to bleed a little bit.

I was regaining my innocence and peeling away numbness like layers of an onion: shedding away numbness to food, then to my new body. Now that I was un-numbing my heart, the real revelation came.

"Wow! Without feeling my heart, I thought Blaine created those works of magic, art, and happiness. But, look, I can feel it now—all that dynamite was in my heart the whole time! He didn't give it to me, I had it all along...and especially—NOW!"

Bam—that was who I was! And now, I started to accept myself as a normal human being, capable of finishing her journey into daylight—into the world! So, I restarted my journey back to the world with full vigor and heart. I realized real mentors were my trees. Not Blaine.

I was getting better every day if I embraced the changes that amounted from doing healthy actions.

Gratitude was now a potent warrior trait with a secret power—expanding the view of my circumstances just enough to help me reframe them.

I am grateful for the guiding voice of my tree-mentors, always telegraphing what's true. The trees have their heads on straight, and they're always with me. Everything I need to know I learn from them.

But no amount of "reframing" I did, on the canvas or on my warrior's journey, could change my physical reality: I left Yale with a new paintbrush and an old fistula. Wasn't going back to the hospital supposed to fix everything? I kept painting the days away, sometimes to feel, decorate the house, kill time, keep my mind off my leaking wound, or fill the lonely, empty space that still surrounded me. I painted to visualize hope, but with every stroke, I was losing faith that any doctor had an answer. My patience was beyond thin. The *TODAY* show couldn't have called at a better time.

No, it wasn't a radical *Medical Mysteries Solved!* segment. I was pacing circles around the kitchen in one of my "I'm numbing out to this fistula and my monotonous life" modes. As usual, NBC's the *TODAY* show was blaring, and with every lap, I heard a few cut up phrases from personalities who had grown quite familiar. It had to be 10 a.m. My mother watched the *TODAY* show with Kathie Lee and Hoda like clockwork.

"Mom! What's this segment?"

She hardly looked up from her magazines. "Everyone Has a Story." They do it once a month. Really sweet—they find an inspiring story and then write a song for that person. Who did they do this time?"

My inner musical theatre ham couldn't help but interject. "How do I get on that?"

"Oh, Amy." And then she realized I wasn't joking. "Amy, I'm already proud of you."

I just kept staring at her.

"Let's wait until you're all healthy before we start telling the world about this."

My stare continued. So did my dripping fistula. What did "all healthy" mean, and how could I ever get there?

"I'll be in the art studio." Controlling what I could, but not expecting much.

What I definitely didn't expect? A call from the *TODAY* show producer a month later.

"Is this Amy and Marilyn? We read your story, and we're happy to consider you as a finalist for our "Everyone Has a Story" segment. I'm going to put you on hold for a minute, and Kathie Lee is going to ask you a few questions."

Mom and I turned to giddy, silly putty as we nervously waited for that famous voice—talking to us! Kathie Lee actually confirmed we weren't a finalist but going to appear on the show.

"David Friedman and I have written a great song for you," Kathie Lee said. "Can't wait to meet you both soon!"

Before we knew it, my mother and I were in a cab to Rockefeller Center, actually happy that we had no idea what was in store. We were welcomed to the backstage area of the studio, for our "television prep."

My hair was being done with a curling iron for the first time in years—since I had last done theatre. My mom sat in the backstage chair next to me, nervously holding my hand as we chatted with the makeup crew. How did we get ourselves into this, and why were we being treated like queens for the day? My dad was chuckling with another friendly voice from the NBC team. As we walked past the dressing rooms, it started to sink in: "I'm going to talk about my story on national television."

Kathie Lee and Hoda rushed backstage briefly to introduce themselves. I even managed to leave two canvases I had painted for them by their dressing rooms. Each featured a woman in a cocktail dress leaping across a hill—with a wine bottle in hand, of course. (This will make sense for anyone who's seen their 10 a.m. segment!)

A commercial break started as my mom, my dad, and I were summoned into the filming area and onto a couch in its own light. Before I even had a chance to process this foreign realm, more lights came on. We were introduced, live, and I saw my mother read her letter on a separate screen. We were thrown a few questions quicker than I knew how to respond, and before could process my own answers, Heidi Blinkenstaff took the stage in front of us to sing a song from my perspective written by Kathie Lee herself and that same accompanist I had saw on this segment a month ago, David Friedman. The brassy, up-tempo song, *Still Alive*, was nothing like I expected, yet every grateful sentiment that felt real: *"Guess what? I'm still alive. I'm still here, by my will..."*

Another commercial break, and with our mouths still open, we were asked what we thought of the song. "It's so me!" I said.

Our segment ended as abruptly as we had been rushed onto the couch. My mom and I celebrated what we still couldn't believe had just taken place by browsing all the shops near Rockefeller Center. As we twirled around hangers and danced through aisles, I couldn't help taking out my phone, where I was instantly inundated with hundreds of Facebook friend requests. Suddenly, everyone wanted to know more about the "girl whose stomach exploded." *How did you survive without a stomach? How did you sustain yourself if you couldn't eat or drink for years? Had this ever happened to anyone before?*

No, it hadn't. But as bizarre as my story was, I could show them the person behind the "medical miracle." I was turning outward, and now I felt like the world was watching. I had a *public* place in the world, and I was ready for it! Just like my art show had ended and the canvases were packed away, we eventually did have to leave New York City and drive back home. I felt that same well of tears I had felt after *"Journey Into Daylight"* had officially become a memory, and the fear that once I "left," I'd never be able to rejoin the world again. Yet this time, something was different. It wasn't just that the world knew about "my story" now. I had created a path.

Before we were called onto the TODAY segment, I saw David Friedman, and immediately recognized him as the brilliant composer that had written a song I always loved singing, We Live on Borrowed Time. I had always wanted to put together a cabaret act telling a story ever since I was a teenager collecting lesser known musical theatre and cabaret songs. But I never knew what kind of story to tell. Feeling quite emboldened, I went right up to him and asked if he would work on a cabaret act with me. He was friendly and compassionate, and he also realized he was basically my neighbor in Connecticut.

Just like I had my art to keep me going, now, maybe, my singing and my story could too...I was finally out there.

CHAPTER 38

After the *Today* show— Reality Hit

THINGS WERE WONDERFUL ON all fronts except my body, which I refused to call my life. I was doing my best to be normal, and even doing hot yoga...until once again, I was asked to leave because my bags kept leaking. Living with a fistula was getting unmanageable. We were going to doctors for answers, who advised us that if I stopped eating and drinking for two to three weeks, the fistula might heal without the constant "stress" of food in the system. But, to my relief, I was eating. Taking away food now would be the ultimate stress on my system.

It had seemed like the TODAY show was my invitation back into the "normal" world. But that tiny opening where remnants of a belly button used to be was still sabotaging any attempt to keep food from leaking out of me.

My walks around our block now had two purposes—strolling around to tree-gaze and pacing in circles to ignore what was physically dripping out of me each time I tried to take a sip from my water bottle. But soon, my tears were gushing even faster. I had my nutritionist, Abby, from the hospital on speed dial. Maybe she'd know what to do.

"A typical fistula takes two to three weeks to close if we can give your system a rest from the oral input," Abby said.

"I'll try," I said with a sigh. "I'll start now."

I had tried not eating before—with no success, but I was desperate for the fistula to close. Part of me was still willing to try anything—even hell re-visited—and if two or three weeks of hell would do the trick, I was all for it. With the taste of lunch still on my tongue from just twenty minutes before, I got off the phone with Abby and called my mom to give her a heads up about my plan.

We were heartbroken as we both hung up. To this day, I can't explain to you what it's like to be feeling normal, eating and drinking when hungry, and then all of a sudden having to switch that button off and say, "I'm just going to stop everything for a month."

Once again, I was overwhelmed by hunger. But this time I was *determined* not to go numb. To mark "day one" of my famine, my mom took me to Stop & Shop, and we bought every flavor of gum. My starvation made it impossi-ble to focus on arranging my songs with David Friedman. The only successful distraction? Blogging about not eating.

I'd never have known what a blog was if it weren't for my art show just a year before. Seeing how disappointed, and once again, alone I felt after my art show had officially ended, Leona encouraged me to start a blog to keep sharing my work. She set up a simple template on Blogspot for me and gave me a quick overview of how to use it. I was skeptical, but the more I re-searched, the more enticed I was by the idea. Would people actually care about things I had to say? At first, I had no readers besides friends and fam-ily. The blog was just an unshared personal diary. But after the TODAY show, so many people had found me on Facebook that I returned to the blog after realizing this was how I could reconnect with the world!

To pass the endless hours, I'd divide my day between the furnace-room-turned-art-studio and ironically, the kitchen—a new kind of creative culinary studio. I decided to name my blog "Allspice & Acrylics" to chronicle the daily routine I had developed to cope with not being able to eat or drink. Here is my first blog entry to the world:

> <u>Amy's blog</u>: I've been wanting to do this for a long time, and this morning I finally got the drive to put together a blog! In healing from 20+ surgeries, I've done everything from starting a chocolate business, study karate, teach nursery school, star in two musicals, and most importantly, live life to the fullest despite being covered with tubes and bags. I am now 23 years old and still living at home but with dreams of hopefully soon living an independent, rewarding life where I can help other people. I started this blog to share my adventures and passion with you. Enjoy!

Once I started posting on "Allspice & Acrylics," I couldn't stop. I didn't care if anyone was reading—it was an amazing way for me to mark time, document my daily creations, and have some kind of outlet to express myself. Even sharing it with my family felt like a wonderful way to connect. Then, I used the Facebook account my friends had set up for me and shared it with my Facebook "friends." Suddenly, blogging took me out of isolation.

One morning, I woke up to my first "follower." Then my first comment. With a virtual community cheering me on, I felt unstoppable. Knowing I would blog about my daily creations was motivation to create *more*.

Now that I had chosen not to eat or drink for several weeks, I used the blog both as a chronicle of my relationship (now a sad non-relationship) with food and as a way to keep myself occupied and sane until this latest hiatus from food was over. I tried to stay optimistic as I blogged. As counterintuitive as it seemed, I needed to be around food and somehow cooking became my new daily ritual, combined, of course, with art. I cooked the best looking/smelling meals for my family (even my two dogs)!

Blogging About Food

<u>Amy's blog</u>: Day 1—Saturday, March 19, 2011

Bad Day

I've just received news that I will have to go on TPN for at least a good three weeks. That means I won't be able to eat or drink anything at all, which I've had to experience before unfortunately, but it is never fun. My fistulas don't seem to be healing, and the doctors believe that I need total bowel rest for them to close. Wish me luck…

<u>Amy's blog</u>: Day 4 & 5—*Time does* not *fly when you're starving*

I started the day STARVING as usual, so I made some pancakes for my brothers on the crepe maker.

Every day is a struggle to deny myself food and drink. Yesterday I got by on 2 pieces of gum, 1 Jell-O, and 2 ice cubes. I keep telling myself this is to starve my fistulas, and in less than four weeks, I'll be eating again. Nothing lasts forever. Stay strong.

<u>Amy's blog</u>: Day 17—*Disney World...NPO*

Well folks, I am blogging to you live from Orlando, Florida! I am hoping that this trip to Disney World to celebrate my 24th birthday will really help pass the time while I am unable to eat. For my 24th birthday, I'm entitled to have a little fun! We still had time to pass before our flight, so I did my first watercolor canvas—a swirling dancing cloud wishing us "Bon Voyage!" Here's to a good 5 days!

Maybe these weeks of oral starvation could really make the miracle happen. Had my fistula really dried up for good?

The closer I got to the glorious day thirty-two, when my fistula would magically close and the food gates would open again, the more frantic my cooking became.

Cheesy corn cakes with turkey bacon and a sunny side egg for Dad. Zucchini bread with golden raisins and walnuts for Mom. Banana cake with cinnamon streusel for my brothers to take to a Seder.

Amy's blog: Day 30 & 31—Miracles can happen

My doctor finally is starting to increase my oral intake! Besides Jell-O, I'm now starting one 6-oz. protein shake a day. Anything tastes good at this point. And for the first time in six years, my belly actually looks clear—the skin on my fistula has closed up, and my stomach area is finally dry! Spring is certainly here in all its glory as well as the rain. This is starting to slowly, as slowly as the tulips are coming up, turn into a promising season. It's a rainy day today, but I have three more days until I consult with my doctor about eating. I'm nervous and excited...

My family and I did not give up. We even took a friend to an art convention in Virginia during which my fistula reopened and leaked throughout the trip.

I had thought things were really closing up, and now it feels like I am back at square one again. But the only direction to go is forward, so onward I march.

But the marching took me past that glorious "Day thirty-two..." to forty, fifty, and beyond with no signs of improvement.

Amy's blog: *50 days of no eating and starving as ever*

I have to find a way to stay connected to my emotions, and I know that means staying connected to food however hard it is right now. So, I'm still creating daily extravagant feasts for my friends and family, and my dogs! I'm way too hungry to avoid it. Kneading the dough, at least I can feel my fingers dance. The smell of my pizza in the oven makes me cry, and the tears feel like home. It keeps me connected even though it hurts.

<u>Amy's blog</u>: Day 68—*Challah*

Since it was Shabbat, I decided to make a challah. I prayed with my family to heal this fistula. Hopefully, God will hear me.

A Musical Pause

WILL SHE EVER ONCE RECLAIM
WHAT WAS RIGHTFULLY ALL HERS?
FILL ANOTHER PICTURE FRAME
PICTURES SAY A MILLION WORDS
PICTURE DOESN'T FIT THE FRAME
DOES ANYTHING EVER STAY THE SAME?
PICTURE HANGING ON THE WALL
LITTLE GIRL, YOU HAVE IT ALL

I was using art and cooking to connect with life but they, too, were starting to frustrate me. Feeling my voice resonate physically in my body was a gentle reminder that I was still in there—I could hear myself in me. Not on the canvas or in my blueberry muffins, but deep in my body there was a voice. And it was coming from me—whoever she was. Just like my discovery of art, once I rediscovered my love for writing songs, I wrote thirty original compositions within a month. I felt like the giddy fifteen-year-old making music staff lines out of her high school assignment notebooks as I hummed intuitive melodies, wrote lyrics, strummed my guitar, or played the piano that I had not touched in years—a true relic and one of the few things that were originally from our Fairfield house.

Music took the voice of hunger out of my head and into song. Singing, I felt these words in my body, and I was getting "fed" UP! I felt like a growing giant within a cage, confined by the static, uncertain world of bags, drains, and NPO.

<u>Amy's blog</u>: Day 80—*Feeling vs. numbness step by step*

<u>Painful but forward step</u>: I expected to draw a sad picture with leaks coming out all over my body but ended up drawing a solid tree trunk through my body with fire coming out of the branches. It shows that I am really stronger than I think right now.

<u>Step back then forward</u>: I paced up and down the hallway, up and down, numbly, swallowing a lump of painful sadness in my throat.

<u>Step forward</u>: Art really helped me look my wounded self in the eye. I called it "Seeing myself as I am…for the first time."

Now that I was grounded, I could start reaching again for higher things, like a rooted, yet branching tree. I remembered how years ago the rabbi at my childhood temple had invited me up to the bimah, to watch a scribe write one Hebrew letter in the Torah. The scribe had told me, "Demand your life back. Will it to God."

Once again, I fearlessly demanded that no matter what, I would look forward to the warrior's task of facing another day.

I want to be grateful to have a life to live—consciously, not just intellectually.
But I know there is no magic switch.
How do you feel secure when constantly jumping out of a plane? You rely on
a lot of support, and eventually, your own gut instincts.

I demanded the life I wanted by creating it on my fabric blanket, manifesting it to the universe, willing it to God. And the blanket images were transferring to healthy coping actions. These were my anchors to set me straight. My fabric quilt was keeping me on track. But no matter how much you demand, all humans have limits. And I was about to reach mine.

If you wait until you feel "ready," you may spend your life waiting and never
get the real life you're meant for.

Even with healthy coping, the days were passing—eighty-two, ninety-two, and beyond. But where was the promised result? My fistula was leaking, and I was starving. So, I still found safety in a rigid routine, allowing no empty space for the cracks of emptiness, feeling, hunger, or any kind of upset whatsoever. Cooking, art-ing, and being sure to leap like a frog from activity pad to activity pad.

One Saturday, we went to our usual shopping center in Milford, where we'd be able to wipe ourselves out with Michael's, Walmart, HomeGoods, Marshalls, Staples, Joann's, and Pier 1 all in one sweep. There, I'd immerse myself in the colorful merchandise, the chatter of people rolling their carts around the store and pace every aisle in order to pass yet another day. But soon, it would be over one hundred days since I had eaten anything, which was a far cry from the two to three weeks that I was originally promised.

We were doing our usual shopping in Joann's. Mom was rolling the cart while I was zipping through every aisle determined to be the good patient and keep my mind focused, my heart numb, and my stomach free of hunger.

As accustomed as I was to being robotic, I also happen to be human. I looked around and saw everyone talking and walking with no drains taped to their legs, no IV food, no half a life. And I got angry. *Amy*, I thought. *Just try not to think about anything but...being thirsty!*

Water. It was too late to think about anything else. I allowed myself to watch a woman unloading her shopping bags sip a Poland Spring water bottle. I knew the red rush of anger's familiar whirl in my chest, filling every vein, and uncomfortably tried to stifle the frustrated fury until it felt like it was so hot, it could burn me. But before it did, I breathed over and over, and every breath that tried to contain it just fueled the fire with more anger. Then, I had it.

"Mom, where's a water bottle? I need a water bottle, just give me one!" I said, panicking with tears in my eyes.

My mom was wrought with sad compassion, haphazardly fumbling through her bag for a half drank Poland Spring water bottle.

"I'm gonna do it!" I screamed as I snatched the water bottle from her and sprinted out of the store in what could have been the ending to some drawn out melodrama. My mother ran out behind me as I stood in the middle of the parking lot and drank the rest of the water bottle, hardly catching my breath. We fell into each other's arms and cried together, feeling so many things at once. But most of all, relief. I had done it. So, I started eating and drinking again—fistula or not.

CHAPTER 39

The Show Must Go On

THE DAMAGE HAD BEEN DONE...and I had done it myself. But what would *you* do? Chugging that water bottle was my "warrior cry" that living life was more important than waiting for a fistula to close. But what did life even mean anymore? The only thing I knew for sure was that what I *did* with my life was more important than an opening in my skin I had no power to fix.

I decided to go back to working on songs with David Friedman. Fistula or not, I was going to do my show, and maybe even go back to school.

It was great singing songs with David, but what felt even better was creating a story to link the songs together. I was delighted to see how the stories behind my songs were shifting. As I figured out what I wanted to express through these songs, the backstory behind my life began to shift from victim to actress. One of the most difficult things to address was how to sing about sexual abuse in a cabaret act. Could I really do it by singing a Sondheim song? David and I thought of a million ways to divulge it: Do we write a dialogue between my abuser and me? A monologue about the moment I told my mother? Each scenario felt more and more wrong. Did I even remember the moment I "found out" I was sexually abused? After all, I had been so frozen.

David gently interrupted my stream of thought: "Why don't you just think about where you were, or the last place you can think of?"

Barnes & Noble. That was where I had discovered the book. So, I reenacted it to him.

I am in Barnes & Noble with my mom, and she is worried that I could have been molested by Blaine. I scoff at the thought and pick up *The Courage to Heal* to show her that nothing like *that* could have ever happened to me. I am reading an example of a girl who was raped to show my mom that she is wrong, and as soon as I read "and when everything familiar seems to disappear forever," I suddenly realize that this is *my* story as well.

"That works!" David said.

I relate to Mom and Dad differently now. Food has opened our world enough to have company over again, so I am really trying to be engaged with whoever's in my life. I will take any connection I can get.

I thought to myself: "If you build it, they will come. Let me just get myself back on stage, and the rest will figure itself out." Digging into the prep work for my show was like itching that tune my soul had been waiting to belt out.

As I threw myself into work that was important to me, I found myself struggling with another important decision: Should I try again to get the colostomy reversed? Was it worth the risk? Or was the bigger risk wondering whether I had missed out on the chance to have a normal body again?

I had to remind myself that whatever choice I made; I could trust it was the right one.

It was time to follow nothing else but my heart. After realizing that playing the "waiting game" with my fistula was getting me farther from making any kind of new identity, I was determined to get my life back on track.

If I could write the "story" of my life in my few twenty-five years, what kind of arc would I want to share?

I went back to the archetypal hero's journey, which had always given my life structure, but could it structure a show too?

As I reread some of my old journal entries, I realized that giving my life story a "framework" was not such a new venture. It was something I had practiced religiously for the past eight years as a survival skill. Sharing my own story through theatre was the next natural step. Now my journal entries, combined with song, would form the framework of my one-woman autobiographical musical. But where to start?

I looked at the outline I had started with and couldn't help but smile. This storyline seemed remarkably similar to the hero's journey. How we view our "story" can transform how we view our lives.

How did I pick my songs? Digging through my old audition folders like a kid sneaking into her mother's closet to play around in her mom's high heels, I rustled through sheet music in search of the "new stories" these old favorites now brought to light. There were my old Sondheim favorites, my standard musical theatre audition cuts, and the never-ending bucket list of songs I had always wanted to perform as a shameless musical theatre ham. Hours sorting through stacks of old sheet music and countless iPod playlists brought up good memories, bad memories, and a new kind of feeling: my voice ready to express them. Now trauma was pretty darn exciting—and dramatic!

Suddenly, I was relating to old favorites in entirely different ways. Every song title recalled a story I had either been aching to tell or hadn't even thought of until spurred on by a lyric. Memories that seemed fuzzy at first now boldly emerged to the forefront of my mind as I acted them out through song. I flipped through a few laminated pages of *Amy's B'way Book: A-M* (N-Z had to fit in their own binder) and pulled out "Mira," a song from the 1968 musical *Carnival!* that had always been my go-to for an open call.

Songs were like photographs; you could go to them at different road marks in your life and see your life completely differently. As I sang the next verse to myself, lines like "I have to find a place where everything can be the same" meant something very different now than at fifteen years old. Singing these songs, I was literally reclaiming my voice. And even better, it felt good! I liked pouring my heart out as I rehearsed—even the painful feelings felt exciting. After all, I always used to love belting out the Broadway torch songs of heartbreak. Theatre was proving to be yet another safe container in my healing vortex.

It was a big task to take songs I had always known and create moments to become physically present with what had happened in my life—to embody it, own it, and share it. But letting myself out of my caged mind and into my body was still an important part of my healing process.

Giving my story "creative distance" was also a way to step back, see my story like a movie, and actively change the ending rather than dwell in thoughts of what I could have or should have done. Crises were becoming stories that I could talk about for the first time with someone else, including David Brunetti, a kind, ingenious musical arranger I had just met as we sat across a piano in a New York studio, not unlike the one where Blaine taught me years before. I was replaying my life and, somehow, redoing it. Now those lessons I had chased after in my head with Blaine—mourning his loss and wanting him back—didn't seem so important. There were plenty of trustworthy people out there in the world.

I searched through my old music folders, Broadway compilations, musical theatre songbooks, jazz tunes, and my mother's old Barbra Streisand albums until a set of lyrics rang out to me as a mark on my path so far. With every lyric I read, I journaled about how it could connect to the story I was creating.

Most of all, besides continuing my theatrical career, I wanted to feel like myself again. I want to figure out what all of this meant in the big scheme of things.

Once I journaled about a song, the stories came together. These were opportunities to express the captivity I felt on an IV pole, the exhilarating feeling of taking my first walk outside the hospital, and, of course, the chance to finally belt about how starving I was! That song choice came easily: "Food, Glorious Food!"

First, I imagined who I'd love to sing this food-filled showtune to. Sometimes you want spiritual fulfillment, but there are other times that you are just damn hungry and you can't do anything tonight. What my dad would call my nightly "piña colada cocktail" was a three-liter bag of white vein food, TPN, that I would have to carry around for fourteen to sixteen hours a day in addition to a feeding tube backpack. Every night, the same old "gruel." I would fantasize about the first meal I would get to taste again.

My story was materializing before my eyes and ears...via musical theatre. As I was putting together my script, I found notes from an old song I had scribbled the year before, when I couldn't eat or drink, and was simply waiting for the fistula to heal. There had been a big power outage in my town, and now I didn't even have my coping mechanism of killing the day going from store to store, mindlessly passing the day. I was stuck in my house, standing over the table in my art room, with no windows and no light. With no motivation to paint, I sat down and lit a candle, feeling equal parts helpless and hopeless.

I reached for a turquoise sharpie and wrote one line: DAY AFTER DAY IS A WAR TO GET THROUGH

Amy, keep your mind on track, I told myself as I felt that dam of tears start to break loose. *Rhyme is structure. Just stay on track, finish the structure. Go.*

And I wrote another line: HARD TO FEEL WONDERFUL, HARD TO FEEL NEW

If I could finish a verse in that same form, I could keep myself safe. *I just have to get through the power outage. One rhyme at a time, Amy. Go.*

STRUGGLING THROUGH MY TIME RESOLUTELY

DIVERTING MYSELF FROM THE POINTLESS "WHY ME?"

I didn't know what else to write.

LIFE IS LONG

Don't give up Amy. Just write <u>something</u>.

ENOUGH TO SING MY SONG

AND I WILL GET MY TURN

I KNOW THIS CANDLE'S BOUND TO BURN

AND I WILL HAVE MY TIME TO SING

I WILL, EVEN IT IT'S ANYTHING

The verses continued, alone in my art studio. Getting my frustration out with a thick, turquoise marker allowed time to pass. I remember starting to write one verse, and once I finished, I just couldn't stop. Stanza after stanza, I was convincing myself with the empowering belief that I would not just be something forgotten, lost in the corner. And now, putting the story arc together for a one-woman musical, this was a full circle moment. First, I thought about all the situations I'd love to express these thoughts out loud in. I was finally reincorporating that scribbled piece of paper for the first time into a production that would be seen by others. I was finally reclaiming my place to at the forefront of the stage.

Now, just like creating the painting "Singing Tree" at Yale New Haven Hospital just two years before, "Corner Song" had transformed from grief to celebratory art, honoring a hurdle that was now framed in the past.

As I was making my final selections, I couldn't wait to incorporate the song I had watched one of my favorite Broadway performers sing that David Friedman and Kathie Lee Gifford had written for me: "Still Alive." I remembered sitting on that *TODAY* show couch with my parents, our eyes agog at hearing an up tempo, optimistic showtune belted out celebrating my survival.

I took the sheet music out of a sealed laminate folder, signed by David and Kathie Lee, and with each word, I realized how far my family and I had come.

I was "Still Alive" to sing about it. And make it into a story.

Every time I went back to David Friedman's house, I changed the "backstory" behind my songs. This was my chance to rewrite my narrative and to experience emotions I had suppressed for so long. How lucky I was.

Finalizing the songs that would ultimately make up this "cabaret act," Tiger Lilly, was trekking on, redefining her life by rewriting her narrative.

Music was now a safe container—a tool from the healing vortex that Blaine had once contaminated. Music was where I could always find honesty, humor, and heart.

These seemingly incoherent pieces of my life—fragments of trauma, nonsensical, illogical events, wounds opening, setbacks, disappointment, uncertainty—everything, when strung together within the framework of a musical, now made sense. Suddenly, setbacks and sidetracks were essential pieces of a plotline.

In putting together this musical, Tiger Lilly took control of her life again and spoke her truth, gutless and grateful. And that became the title of my show: *Gutless & Grateful: A Musical Feast.*

CHAPTER 40

Getting My Act Together

JUST AS MY FEAR AND UNCERTAINTY had been transformed through my paintbrush, theatre was turning my fragmented memories into a linear narrative. Music was rewiring the current of the traumatic cyclone. My story had a beginning, a middle, and an end. Now the world was going to hear about it. Years of trauma had transformed me into a cold block of dazed granite and now, through theatre, I was excavating myself, chipping away through art, song, movement, and ultimately, the power of words. Soon enough, the bare bones of the script were done. But how was I going to get my show into the world?

Jerold Goldstein was the first "real director" I ever had, directing me in his original musical, *The Three Scrooges*—a slapstick comedy that fused *A Christmas Carol* with *The Three Stooges*. I played the role of Tina Cratchit—a snarky teenage girl version of Tiny Tim. Jerold had a reputation for being brutally honest with his lovable sarcasm and tough love. By the end of the production, he won our whole family over with his love for Jewish humor and food, and from then on, he was like family. Although he had brought my parents both home-cooked Italian meals nearly every night when I was in the hospital, he and I had lost touch, primarily because my shame of "taking so long to heal" made me afraid to bare my face to the theatre community where I once felt so at home. So, it was a big leap for me to finally bring my sixteen-song cabaret act to Jerold, who was known for not pulling any punches.

Going out to lunch with my brother Matt was now a regular occurrence. We had found an Indian lunch buffet where we bonded over steaming naan and "extra, extra, super-extra mild" dishes.

"How's your show going?" he asked through bites of *tikka masala.*

"I think I'm done. I'm going to show it to Jerold."

Reading through my hundreds of journal entries and putting them together with songs, I decided to call Jerold over. I didn't know how he would react, but I was working off instinct and felt compelled to show him my work.

Binder in hand, I sang my songs, read my journal entries, and waited.

I waited for Jerold's usual "loving sarcasm" as my exit cue, but he didn't say anything for a solid minute—a rarity in our history together. He cut the silence as he sipped his coffee.

"I like it."

And so, our work began.

Little did I know that, with Jerold's faith in me, this show would catapult me back onto the stage. But for now, my living room was just fine. Now that I had a director, it was time to get serious. Performing my show for actual people was going to happen. One Friday night, Jerold sat at our kitchen table for a kosher dinner, as he had in my happy pre-coma days, and we started looking at performance spaces.

"The Triad is a nice place," he told me, as he sliced through the chicken breast on his plate. I looked it up. It was a small cabaret club in New York, and I could picture myself singing there. Physically, I was as able as anyone else now. I wasn't being kicked out of yoga class for TPN or chained to an IV pump itching to get out of the hospital. I was eating and relying only on my body's digestive capabilities.

I'll never forget the occupational therapist who told me to never give up because "one day you might even be able to walk on your own without a wheelchair." Now, as I hopped, skipped, and jumped, effortlessly grabbing snacks and meals whenever I chose, my body once again proved the medical community wrong. Now I had the goal of performing in a real, live New York theatre—larger than any community theatre or high school production. Not only did I have a clear vision in my head, it was also close enough that I could almost reach out and touch it. As that rabbi scribe had once instructed me, I had willed it to God, and now—now this was possible. I was driven—fiercely determined to create "my show."

I wasn't in school. I didn't have a job. I just had bold trust in one dream— my "show." My parents, always supportive, weren't exactly sure what I was planning on now that, digestively, I was good to go. We went for hot wonton soup at our regular Chinese takeout spot in Westport. My mom picked apart her usual chicken satay as I told her about all the latest discoveries I was making in my journal entries-turned-monologues.

"Amy, what exactly is your plan with the songs and everything?"

"I'm putting together a show about my life."

My father was skeptical. I knew his look right away. "On stage?"

"Yeah. I'll figure it out." I took one last slurp and counted the minutes until I could get home and start singing again.

My routine every day was the same: an hour of yoga in the morning, make art for a few hours in my paint-covered studio, and work on my show until I fell asleep.

With ingredients for my show coming together, I was hungrier than ever with an appetite for the stage. But the biggest leap was committing to a date.

I took a deep breath...and looked up the theatre Jerold had mentioned and wrote the theatre's manager a very nice letter about my show and assuring that if he booked it, the house would be full.

I sealed the envelope and mailed the letter. My mom and I were food shopping a few days later when my phone started to buzz. A 212 number was usually an automated voice call confirming an appointment at Columbia. I held the phone on speaker while I grabbed a cheddar cube on a sampling toothpick.

"Hello."

"Amy? This is Peter Martin."

"Oh! Hi!" I stammered as I tried to swallow the last bits of cheese.

"Amy. I got your letter. We can give you October 22, 27, 28. How does that sound?"

How does that sound? I was being offered three dates in October for my first professional run, my first show about my life, my first on so many levels!

It sounded...unbelievable. I said yes.

Now I had to explain this to my mother, picking up cold cuts in the next aisle.

"Mom! I booked my musical-in-a-binder in New York for October!" The other shoppers must have thought I was crazy—bouncing through the aisles with a new song in my heart, then bouncing right to the bathroom to deal with the various drains and bags that were still running up and down my body. Fistula or no fistula, I was taking my story to the stage.

In the meantime, my father was still investigating answers for the fistula that refused to heal. He found Dr. Kentz, a physician at Mt. Sinai who was one of the very few who didn't look at my huge folder of medical histories and throw it in the junk pile. He called my father back and, in his grandfatherly way, reassured us that things *could* turn out okay. I wrestled back and forth about the decision, but I knew if I wanted to have this surgery, I had to get it done while my father was still able help me through.

In *my* meantime, I could see my visualizations take shape...which brought me back to another dream. I wanted college. At twenty-five years old, I had never received my degree. I had never even been to a Friday night, red-plastic-cup-in-hand campus party. Sure, I had gained three resumés worth of life experience, but I still felt I was missing out. The ending of the story I was going to tell on stage was just a beginning. The real story I needed to finish was, "What now?"

The reality of my functioning but still fragile and high-maintenance body made attending college out of the question. But maybe I could work towards an online degree. I went back to the college counseling offices I had first gone to in high school and timidly approached the front desk.

"'Scuse me. I was hoping someone could help me apply to online colleges? Like getting a degree from home?" Years had passed, and the staff had all changed. A young, vibrant woman swiveled around in her chair.

"How old are you? Why don't you apply to an actual college?"

"I'm twenty-five..."

"So what?" Megan pulled me into her office and piled up brochures of places I had never even heard of. But the people in the photos seemed to be doing exactly what I craved—being immersed in a social, learning environment they were passionate about.

Despite the downward pull of doubt, I asked myself, "If not now, when?" When I couldn't give a good enough answer, I knew it was time to start browsing *actual* colleges online. Years of an "education in real life" gave me the courage and stamina to repeat the entire college application process I had gone through at seventeen. Reflecting on years of medical disappointments and frustrations, I titled my essay, "Keeping Hunger Alive."

Applications aside, I still had a show to put on. I devoted myself to emailing potential guests, publicity, and more research. For the first time, I was owning my story and telling it myself.

After years of isolation, the "theatre world" was intimidating. How was I supposed to form connections? "Networking" was undefined for me as I had no professional real-world experience. So, I did it the old-fashioned way: posting flyers on every Main Street store window, researching contacts for every news source I could find, and flipping through radio stations to see if a contact phone number was mentioned in any segment. I even went back to my high school and middle school to hand deliver invitations. My most potent weapon as a publicist was my warrior skill of persistence. It had gotten me through unimaginable medical challenges and not eating. Knowing I had the power to push through, even when exhausted or overwhelmed was my secret advantage on the long, bumpy road to success.

Every time I wanted to give up, I remembered my lyrics to *The Corner Song* and tried to keep going. For every 1,000 press releases I sent out, I heard back from maybe ten. But when I did hear back, I was immediately energized, prompting me to send out 1,000 more. Who knew what the next email might bring? And then, a trickle of interest turned into a storm. Suddenly, I had features on theatre websites, interviews with local magazines, events posted in *Time Out New York*—even a TV feature on WNBC, and New York critics interested in seeing my show.

My first interview with a cabaret site exclaimed: "Whew, Amy Oestreicher. We can't wait to see what the world has in store for you!" Seeing my show finally take shape and get attention from the press was a huge reward, but the biggest accomplishment was finding myself and feeling happy for the first time since I came to. I remembered how discouraged I was waking up from a coma and not even being able to move my toes. And now here I was, tap dancing in character shoes in a red satin dress!

As my show got closer to premiering, Jerold and I were in full rehearsal-mode, laughing, crying, and rewriting on a daily basis.

The script was coming together.

"So, who are you working on this with?" Jerold stopped playing as I turned the pages of sheet music for him.

"What do you mean? With you."

"You're not training? Lessons?"

I hadn't studied consistently with a voice teacher in years. I hadn't seen any reason to...although deep down I had a clue what I was avoiding. But now, I needed to reclaim my voice...and find a new teacher. Getting into the daily discipline of voice lessons was emotionally difficult for me at first, given what I had experienced with Blaine. Each scale forced me to directly confront the thing I felt had been taken advantage of, note by note. Just when I thought I had found myself, taking a voice lesson spurred me into a mess of memories.

I tried to remember my healing vortex. I had slowly lost touch with Rita, but I trusted I had all of the tools myself.

I realized that my voice lessons were just another exciting opportunity to face my trauma head on.

I thought about the safe space inside of myself and the visualization I had created on my fabric. As I touched each cutout that I had so carefully cut out with felt and my grandmother's fabric, my thumbs pressed against the cut-out I had made of me playing Eponine in *Les Misérables* in a professional teen theatre production—a memory that always grounded me in the love I had for nature, forming relationships, and musical theatre. I remembered all I had before Blaine.

I was the girl who forced every unwilling classmate to join me in a Les Miz medley, assigning them their designated parts to pass the thirty-minute school bus ride.

I was so obsessed with Les Misérables as an eight-year-old that I bought the huge unabridged Victor Hugo novel and intended to read it. However, I got much more pleasure bringing it to school every day and leaving it on my desk so people could think I was artsy and deep.

My babysitters were petrified of me because they knew every time they'd come over they'd be a victim of my latest skit.

I was theatre girl. I still am.

Singing these melodies was reintegrating my voice into my healing vortex, too. While I was preparing myself for the physical challenges of the show mentally, I was preparing myself physically for the surgery I hoped would follow my New York stage premiere. I had to be built up—the more nutritionally better off I was, the better chance the wound would heal as normal. That was a non-issue. I became friends with every Chinese restaurant on Post Road.

September 5, 2012: There is a chance that Dr. Kentz can reverse the colostomy and cut the fistula with ONE surgery! Nervous but excited.

September 11: I got a surgery date! Nov. 7th! His advice? "Eat as much as you can."

Because I had so little intestines left, to sustain a healthy weight, I had learned to eat an excessive amount of calories to maintain my weight and keep my high-energy routine. Basically, I got really good at eating a ton.

Because I'm a small person, it often surprises people when I eat about five dinners worth of protein within twenty minutes or leave the house for a twenty-minute errand and bring a large duffel bag filled with ten drinks, twenty bags of protein chips, three turkey wraps, and three pints of cottage cheese. So over time, I had made friends with every grocery store owner in Fairfield county. At about twelve different Asian restaurants, I had a special order that was called in daily, to the point where they'd recognize me on their caller ID, and simply say, "We got it Amy. When are you picking up your usual?"

September swept by with all-day Jerold rehearsals and Yankee games with my dad. I could relate to my dad on a new, normal level, he could breathe a sigh of relief, and we could just be happy. The High Holidays were especially sweet. For the first time in years, we all went to temple. As we got dressed in our heeled shoes and stockings, I was right back to my grandmother, and I knew she was with me through this. Everything HAD happened for a reason.

We came home to a beautiful Rosh Hashanah dinner of chicken soup, apples, challah, and honey. Life goes so fast. Savor its sweetness.

Despite my fistula, health-wise, I was vital, strong, and eating to my heart's content. I was no longer the girl on IVs, overwhelmed by her ostomy bag or a tiny fistula, waiting for life to get better. I had written a whole show on "gratitude," and although I was grateful to be alive, a part of me still wished I had a body free of any medical bags or "nuisances." But now, there was no time to focus on that. I was in full rehearsal mode. This was the first surge of relief that continuously ran through my veins.

The week before my show was more exciting and nerve-wracking than the week before my bat mitzvah. It was an odd mixture of last-minute publicity, prep, rehearsals, pre-op tests, packing for the hospital, and hoping to break a leg, but not much else. I grew more and more confident—about how I would perform on stage and in the operating room after. My family and I had talked about the idea of trying to get the fistula reversed, and Dr. Kentz presented us with the S-word once again: Surgery.

I decided it would be harder wondering "What if?" and decided to go for it. My show would close on October 28th, I had a friend's wedding on November 4, and I would be headed straight for surgery on November 7, 2012.

As I drew nearer to seeing my life blossom and bring me back to my old self, I allowed my thoughts to turn to my dream of college, and I got my application—yes, just *one* application—in. Hampshire College.

Sure, my body was fine for the stress of performing a musical three nights in a row. But what about the challenges of living away from home and maintaining my smorgasbord of medical routines? When any institution heard about everything I had been through, they understandably had concerns. My father assured Hampshire that I was medically okay to go.

I had mailed in an application to college—and booked a theatre! Finally, committed action! Was this really the start to leading a life with purpose—out there in the real world? The press releases were out, the dress was fitted, and now was time for the finishing touches to make it all real. This was something I had dreamed of doing from the hospital—a giant celebration when I was happy, healthy, where I could be on stage, look my doctors in the eye, and thank them for giving me back my life.

It was time to create the program for *Gutless & Grateful*. I was the author of my own life now. A life that people were going to hear, and see, and feel...but now, from my own perspective.

I had always remembered one old family home movie from when I was five years old. I had chased my brothers around the basement, hitting them with a ruler, to the point they were actually scared, and I screamed in my high pitched five-year-old voice, "You'll never give up, right?" That was the fighting spirit I still had within me, so I put that "kiddie Amy" quote on the back of the program.

Even from the hospital, I had fantasized about the day—someday—when I would emerge triumphantly, dressed up, laughing, and singing about circumstances that had once devastated me—showing off once again to the world who thought I had slipped away forever, and hearing them say, "Wow, she's back!" I could finally give back through doing what I loved. This magic formula for happiness was what drove me as a performer my entire life.

Jerold and I did a "soft opening" in my living room for four of my friends—the first time anyone had heard the show besides my parents. The next day, the local news was writing about it:

"Now, after near death, a couple months in a coma, two dozen surgeries, years of living on intravenous nutrition, and ongoing healing, Amy arrives at The Triad Theatre with her show *Gutless & Grateful*—Oct. 22, 27, and 28." Before I knew it, opening night was here.

CHAPTER 41

"There's no Business Like Show Business"

IT WAS 6:45 P.M. Fifteen minutes until opening night. I never had stage fright before, but even that couldn't explain the actual trembling in my fingers. I remembered how picking up a paintbrush in the Yale ICU had refocused my anger, fear and anxiety with a stroke of color. So, I picked up a pen in my dressing room, hoping any kind of grip would get my fingers to stop shaking.

I walked out on the Triad stage and sat at my desk in the downstage right corner we had so carefully marked with tape. The lights were dark, but I could see the rimmed glasses of audience members in a packed house. People had actually showed up! As the lights brightened, I recognized friends and family, who were all waiting to hear me sing.

Deep breaths, deep breaths, Amy...

The crowd was quiet. Jerold, at the piano to my left, nodded to me and played the intro we had rehearsed just the day before in my living room. The band started to play with my brother behind me strumming electric guitar. I felt support in the theatre from literally all sides. Here I was, with one chance to sing, to let the world know I was okay.

Jerold finished his musical intro, and I looked up at the audience to sing the first line of the opening song.

"I've an unrest inside me…"

And boy did I have an unrest.

But this unrest was not the stifling, shaking, fidgety fear that had kept me jogging in place, running from memories, or chained to my laptop keyboard. My voice, trembling just minutes before, pounded through the grand piano melody with a confident honesty that shocked even myself. Those butterflies I always anticipated spinning around my belly now felt like sturdy anchors, tying me deeply to that tape-marked stage and then springing me *stage right,* just as we had rehearsed. The reflections of glasses in the audience disappeared, and my eyes were enveloped by that grand spotlight, covering my goose-bumpy shoulders in warmth and safety. I had a clear view of the path ahead and I knew where to go—onto the next song!

I had thought working on the show with Jerold was life-changing, but I was in for an even bigger surprise after my performances. The publicity machine I had worked to put in place ahead of the show was bringing results.

I remembered old articles in my town news about my role in a middle school musical or a high school concert, but *Gutless & Grateful* was a show I owned as an adult on a professional stage. Now there were interviews, pictures, and news reporters stopping by my house, print articles taped to our fridge, and stories being shared online through social media. I was proud and anxious with anticipation and nervously hoping that my "show" was everything people were talking it up to be.

All my life I studied music, drama, writing, and lived for the world of the stage. It was only after I experienced the life challenges of the past eight years that I discovered just how powerful the world of theatre and musical storytelling can be.

My mother and I had been through our own hell arguing about exercise, crying with every medical setback, and fumbling our way through every uncertainty. Now, it was finally opening night. Maybe this was the true "redemption" Mom and I had originally planned for our Seder in 2005, when we had first hoped the Passover story would liberate us all from the wounds Blaine had inflicted. I remember how, just before opening night, as my mother helped me get into my red dress, she looked at me, like she looked at her "old daughter" getting dressed for a middle school musical. Looking into my eyes, she whispered, "Grandma is smiling right now..."

Mom slipped my red dress over a new body, battered, bruised, covered in scars, bags, and medical tape. But my earrings were sparkling, my eyes were stained with eyeliner, not tears, and now I had tape for my body mic, in addition to my ostomy bag. I was not defeated. This could—this would—be a new start.

As I took the bow for the very first world premiere of *Gutless*, I was inspiring others with the bizarre reality that anything is possible with a bit of resilience. Everything and anything became possible once I was willing to take on this new life on proudly.

I can't be thirteen again, but I can be the best twenty-five I can. I'll still be the performer I always wanted to be as a kid. But now, with a story to tell.

Making an Impact

When *Gutless & Grateful* premiered in New York at the Triad in October 2012, everything came to fruition. I stopped comparing myself to others and realized that I had stayed true to myself. It felt like a springboard, my bridge to the world.

I had no idea my story would not only resonate with people, but actually have an impact on them. People came up to me afterwards and told me how inspired they had been by my story. They would almost apologize, as if ashamed their own problems couldn't possibly compare, and it was almost as though they were asking for permission to heal. This always struck me odd because, as Viktor Frankl expressed, that suffering is relative. Although my situation was extreme, I experienced universal feelings that everyone goes through in life, whether it's a surgery, a breakup, or a broken heart. We feel connected by a shared experience, and this experience strengthens us just enough to keep getting through life's experiences day after day.

The Power of Stories to Connect Us

As fearless as this seemed, telling my story made me feel normal for the first time. As audience members continued to tell me about their own obstacles and triumphs, it became clear to me how we all heal and move on—when we're actually listened to, empathized with, and understood.

As if it couldn't get any better, my brother called me as I was patting on blush backstage. "Amy, William Finn is wandering around outside waiting in line to get a ticket. Should I—"

"Waiting for a ticket? Invite him in!"

I couldn't believe he had actually come! Now, I was REALLY ready!

I danced through the night, the following week brushing up my steps after hearing Jerold's long list of notes, and into the next weekend at a friend's wedding. But for this wedding, not only could I drink from a glass, I had something to say to old high school friends. I was actually doing something I was proud of—in the real world! As I wiped my entrée dish clean and shouted to old faces over blasting conga music, I didn't want the night to end. And I definitely didn't want to spend the next day with a tube shoved up my nose as preparation for the big surgery twenty-seven. But I still had an ostomy, a fistula, and the will to risk everything in order to reverse it.

I wasn't afraid. I was floating on air...and preparing to lay back down on a gurney. A gurney I had just sung about.

CHAPTER 42

Reversal of Fortune

PRE-OP FOR MY TWENTY-SEVENTH, and first elective, surgery was the worst and, looking back, clearly a harbinger of worse things to come. I remember the day before was really painful, with this huge drain shoved up my nose all day and drinking liters of gross fluid that was supposed to clear out my system. Jeff, now an official doctor, assured me that he felt really confident about this surgery going well. My vitals were great, this was the best shape I'd been in nutritionally, and Dr. Kentz had a really good plan. So, what could go wrong?

We drove to Mt. Sinai and slept over the night before at the 11 West wing, the same carpeted beautiful section of the hospital where I had reversed my neck bag years before. As my mother helped me into the bed and I tried to breathe with a tube up my nose, Dr. Kentz popped his head in.

So here I am lying on the gurney in the operating room, when the surgeon bends over me and whispers in my ear: "Now, are you SURE you really want to do this?"

My mom read to me from an anatomy textbook, and I tried to drift off to sleep as if she was reading me a goodnight story, but I was terribly uncomfortable. She looked at my father, hoping the book would allay my anxiety for the night.

She handed the book over to my dad. He explained each picture and diagram in the book, pointing to the various organs, and explaining exactly what Dr. Kentz was going to do. I could hear he was anxious, eager to make our ideal end-result become a reality, praying for our dreams to come true by the time I was wheeled back out of the operating room. I struggled again to fall asleep as he continued to lovingly explain each step to me, praying that the next morning would go as quickly as possible. After what seemed like hours, struggling to breathe with that tube up my nose, I was finally loaded onto the operating table.

After surgery, I had what I thought were the usual sensations of coming back to consciousness and waiting for my fingers to not be so numb, so I could actually move them. I had done this countless (well, twenty-six) times before. But something was different. I was hearing voices and feeling some pain I couldn't recognize. It turned out this wasn't "after surgery." It was *during*. Somehow, I wasn't given enough anesthesia, and I was awake for a good amount of the procedure—mute, paralyzed, and helpless. It was the most horrifying thing I've ever experienced. When I fully regained consciousness once the surgery was actually over, I felt stifled by the ventilator. I wanted to shout out, "Hell! I was awake for surgery! I'm not okay!" But I lay there, unable to speak for days.

In the recovery room, my eyes widened as I tried to communicate with my family. But all they could hear was the overwhelming sound of machinery and rush of medical crews swarming in and out.

Thursday, Nov. 8. I woke up panicking. I wanted to know what the outcome of the surgery was, I couldn't talk with the ventilator in, which took forever to get out. I was in the ICU, and Mom explained they found a lot of fistulas and they gave me an ileostomy, but Kentz said he could reverse it with a single stitch. That made me feel optimistic.

Too optimistic. Three extra surgeries, a few catheters, and two months at Mt. Sinai later, I went home with more problems than I came in with. The girl who thought she could do anything just before surgery could do nothing now except wait—as she had waited so many times before, for so many months and years—to see if this new, self-induced disaster would heal.

Recovering in the hospital, I was overwhelmed—wheeled into those all too familiar patient rooms and once again faced with a brand-new medical team, trying to adjust not only to my lengthy medical history but also to who I was. I would show nurses clips of the show that I had just premiered in New York, and they couldn't believe it was the same frail person, yellow, gaunt, and hardly able to walk. I felt sad watching them sadly watching along with me, in shock. They couldn't possibly understand that I was a real "person," right? I wasn't sick anymore. I couldn't be! Could they even fathom that I had starred in a musical about my life just one week before?

My medical history left doctors so floored that they usually assumed the hospital "was" my life.

Gutless & Grateful was a triumph of the human spirit—my great comeback. Now, all that work seemed to be erased in a heartbeat, as though everything I had accomplished was really just a dream I was waking up from...landing me in my own version of *The Twilight Zone*.

Putting myself out there through doing my show had finally made me feel normal. Now that I was back in the hospital with major complications, I was petrified I would have to give that up again forever. Nothing seemed to last. But now, I had a new network of support rallying around me. The biggest gift from publicizing my show and later my long post-op recovery on

Facebook was maintaining connections with old and new friends who saw the whole process unfold. I needed this online community as my way to keep in touch with the "real world" that I was more determined than ever to get back to—as soon as I was discharged, though I didn't know when that would be. I shared frequent updates of my progress and setbacks with my friends on Facebook, trying to stay cautiously optimistic.

November 13—I woke up with resilience and surrender. I told myself, I have to make this work. Kentz came in and was impressed at the drainage. He said it would be okay to sit up but not walk around because I'm tied up to everything. Damn. I drew pics of scallops.

But it didn't take long for that to shatter. It started with random parts of me leaking. The doctors reassured us, saying it was "routine drainage of the wound after surgery." But my wound kept getting bigger. Nothing about this surgery or my recovery seemed "routine."

I couldn't tell whether my fear of the fistula's re-emergence was triggered by PTSD or related to something actually happening to my body. Healing from trauma means telling yourself, "I was not safe then, but I am safe now. Now is not the trauma. I don't need to worry." But soon enough, I wasn't safe.

It started as my dad took me on one of our usual break-of-dawn walks, pushing my IV pole back and forth across the same long hallway. All of a sudden, about a gallon of green fluid burst out of me. This was *not* regular drainage after surgery. This was obviously a leak. I remember crying as my dad rushed me back to my hospital cubicle, and a bunch of doctors gathered around my bed trying to figure out what to do.

It didn't take long to take the guesswork out of whether I had formed another fistula or not.

Not only did they find one fistula, they found another, and then another until my body was overwhelmed with a giant network of fistulas and a wound that refused to close.

After my third surgery in eight days, they decided that opening me up again would probably just add to the problem. The fact that they nicked my bladder did not make things easier because now my leaking urine was even going into the open wound, which was not allowing it to heal. So now I needed a bunch of interventions and more accessories attached to various openings in my body to divert the urine from my wound. Doctors would try to raise my bed on a slant so the urine all could drain separately and bypass my open stomach, but nothing seemed to work. That's when the dreaded wound VAC was introduced, which became one of my most traumatic memories.

The wound VAC was exactly what it sounded like—a machine that was hooked up to my wound, literally vacuum packing it, trying to suck all the liquid out of the gaping hole in my stomach in order to dry the wound.

Every time I had a fistula, this clumsy machine left me more traumatized. For the machine to work, not even a single molecule of air can get through. "Hooking me up" was an arduous process that could take up to a full hour, putting enough layers of specialized gauze into the large cave of the wound in my belly, making sure everything was completely airtight. The repeated layering was painful, cumbersome, inefficient, messy, and a huge waste of time. Once all the layering and taping was done, the final step was actually attaching the vacuum. If we were successful in creating an amazing or tight seal, instantly I'd feel a pull on my stomach, and those layers of foam, initially towering inches tall on my belly, would shrink down to nothing in an instant.

I was like Sisyphus, pushing the rock up the hill. Except I had no physical strength whatsoever, and my mental fitness was wearing thin as well.

Now, not only did I have an ileostomy, I had a massive, open, gaping wound that was developing into an intricate network of fistulas. Even worse, in the third attempt at surgery, the surgeon had nicked my bladder in the process. I came out of surgery with another fistula in my bladder and was told I'd have to have a catheter in for "at least several months."

I wasn't home in a week, but I really did have the best parents ever. They slept with me in my hospital room every night, and my dad, just as he had done in Columbia, Bridgeport, and each of the other seven hospitals I had been at, worked tirelessly to make sure I could get better. I was sad watching my father check with nurses and doctors to see what could be done to rectify this, worry, fear, and stress visible in his tired eyes. I felt such overwhelming guilt that I would have nightmares and wake up screaming, feeling as though I were drowning in hopeless darkness. I mostly felt guilty about my dad.

"Dad?" I cried out in the middle of the night. "I'm sorry for making this awful decision. You shouldn't have to suffer too."

He firmly responded, "Stop. It's not your fault."

But with my decision to have this stupid surgery, my father was back in sleepless savior mode: taking scrupulous notes on every doctor's move, making sure my wound dressings were changed correctly, setting constant alarms to make sure he didn't fall asleep, and taking me on IV pole walks constantly up and down the hallways as I mechanically stared into space.

The week before Thanksgiving brought some progress, but my body was still, to say the least, uncooperative.

November 17, 2012—I can walk today! Hey, baby steps (pun intended). No word on the food or drink though. Weekends are so hard in the hospital. No one is here. Time goes so slowly. I can't believe I was just jumping all over the stage a few avenues away. I just want pizza back!

I could walk after ten days, but I ended up staying in that hospital for almost three months, once again unable to eat or drink indefinitely. The surgery was a complete failure on all accounts, spiraling into three emergency surgeries within the first eight days. The surgeon kept saying that a few more stitches or quick interventions could fix things efficiently, but he kept cutting out more and more intestines, to the point where I believe my father actually asked him to stop trying to operate.

Every day, nurses tried to dress my wound with some other apparatus so I wouldn't be soaking wet every minute.

I was connected to more drains than I could count. Nurses were constantly packing gauze into me. They would try to put a large bag over my wound, but nothing would fit over the gash since the opening was basically a giant cave in my stomach. Each day was filled with painful dressing changes that made me cry out not only from the pain of the sutures being pulled out so roughly but also the fear of what was lurking inside—the idea that this "wound" was more than just a wound but something I was all too familiar with.

As it became clearer that I was not getting discharged from the hospital as I would after a "routine" surgery, I waited for each day to pass, trying to block out of my head the idea that I didn't know what I was passing them for. There were no answers, and the final outcome was unknown...Over the next few weeks, malabsorption caused me to lose thirty pounds and an immeasurable amount of spirit.

I struggled to keep any kind of hope with a massive, new gaping wound in the middle of my stomach that was scary to look at and even more frightening to think about. As more days passed in the unit, it was still just as difficult for me to wake up, see the ceiling, and know and accept that I had chosen this surgery, and now I was here.

This guilty thought echoed the feelings of shame, blame, and self-hatred I'd felt lying frozen and helpless as Blaine molested me for months. In both situations, the thriving life I had known felt just within reach—like I could literally reach out and grab it. I was just on stage singing about all of this in an upbeat musical. The number that brought the house down every night was called *The Physician*. I joked about all this stuff.

Every day, the doctors would try some new procedures as a way to start bridging the huge gap across my stomach. I would be taken to Interventional Radiology or the Endoscopy Suite for an x-ray, extra CAT scan, or ultrasound. Somehow these were not as fun as the field trips I remember from Columbia. Maybe that's because now I had a real life and had been going on real field trips just weeks prior—to Rockefeller Center to do an interview on NBC for *Gutless*, for example. Now, rather than taking a taxi, I was transported by stretcher.

Thanks to the wonders of the Internet, I discovered: pickle, bacon, and cupcake flavored floss, toothpaste, and gum. I was so excited to unwrap it and feel the quick burst of overly sweet artificial bacon explode in my mouth and then vanish. And I must say none of it tasted like the real thing, not even the turkey-flavored gumballs.

The more the doctors treated me like a patient, the more even I was starting to believe it.

The constant leaking and discomfort from the stitches and tubes attaching me to three walls, sleeping was impossible, and getting to bed was as difficult as it had been waking up from a coma. My nightmares kept getting worse and worse, and now I not only had vivid memories of my happy pre-coma life, but also of my post-coma happy and fulfilling life performing *Gutless*. I now had newly created memories to miss—going out with my brother to the Indian restaurant and getting tandoori chicken before a show rehearsal, then driving together to the theatre, where he would be playing guitar behind me while I sang. Once again, my voice was the first to go from being intubated. This was so devastating, yet it was also the least of my worries—or so I heard at morning rounds.

I'll never understand doctors talking negatively or even impersonally about the consequences of a disastrous surgery right in front of a patient. While my body was doing the impossible work of trying to heal from my disastrous surgery, my father did the impossible work of making sure I got through. Besides his regular job, I was now his full-time job—again. He was commuting from his private practices in Connecticut then heading straight to Mt. Sinai after work, then leaving to go back to work at the crack of dawn. I listened to my father ask the doctor thousands of questions and propose hundreds of solutions. His words and constant ideas were the only thing that offered me hope because even if I had lost faith in all of the doctors, my dad was smart. If anyone could find an answer, it would be him.

When he wasn't taking me around for the walks I insisted on—I was getting antsy and frustrated with the lack of answers and needed to get out of bed—he worked with every nurse and doctor on my case. He would get up at 4 a.m., take thirty minutes to help me get ready and then would push my pole back and forth down the hallway from four-thirty to five, and I would feel that same agony waiting for the sun to rise that I did pushing my IV pole in circles back in the days of the Yale oncology unit.

Then at 5 a.m., he'd rush back to Connecticut after taking me for as many laps as he could. Restless, depressed, hungry, and bored, I would continue to push the heavy pole back and forth, back and forth on my own until around 7 or 7:30 a.m. when I saw the doctors heading to my room for their morning rounds. My father didn't find an immediate answer to my problems, but he did catch many mistakes that could have set me back even further.

Throughout my time in the hospital, we continued to fight day-to-day battles that the outside world knew nothing about, and these unknown secrets drew my dad and I closer and closer.

My bladder fistula was a catastrophe we hadn't expected. While healing my large gaping stomach incision and multiple fistulas was the biggest concern, now I had doctors from urology assigned to my case, trying to figure out this new hole in my system. Having two teams work on me at once caused even more breaches in communication, even more poking and prodding, and even more stampedes of faceless doctors who treated me as the patient who had always been "the patient." The bladder fistula was showing no signs of healing, and I soon found out that the catheter was something I would have to take along with me after I left the hospital—something I never even dreamed of.

These were the day to day realities of Mt. Sinai, the monotonous feeling of no answers, constant leaking, bandage changes, and quiet, unending hospital time. This was shaken up every now and then by an occasional disaster, conundrum, dilemma, or bit of bad news that had to be broken to me. In a way, these setbacks were more reassuring than the constant hum of nothing because at least I knew a doctor was still interested in the fact that I was there at all.

Soon, my nightmares grew more and more horrid. I dreamed of ghastly prisons, gruesome murders, being chained up in isolated fields, or the worst, being awake during surgery, which had become something I had now actually experienced. My life frolicking in the real world felt like a dream—something that was hard to visualize anymore. It didn't feel real. In my half-sedated state, I posted on Facebook: I'M NEVER GETTING OUT OF HERE. THIS SURGEON SCREWED UP EVERYTHING. MY LIFE IS OVER. My parents finally took away my cellphone.

As always, my family was there for me. My mom stayed at Mt. Sinai with me the entire time, as she had for every hospital stint. I never forgot how fortunate I was to have never spent a night alone. She had picked up her hobby making jewelry when we were stuck at Yale years before. So, this time she was well-prepared and brought her jewelry kit. While I made clay sculptures of hot dogs and pasta, she spent her days making beautiful necklaces and taking a break to get out when my dad was there.

One night my brothers came to the hospital and showed me how to play Angry Birds on their phone. I remember thinking as I saw them, "Wow, this feeling of 'being human,' sitting in a chair and casually playing games on the phone, will I ever get that back? Even my own brothers live in a world so separate from me." I stared at them from my bedside, feeling more paralyzed and alienated than ever before.

On the upside, being connected to social media this time, I had people rooting for me throughout. It felt nice and so different from any other time before. My friends would post pictures of me performing *Gutless & Grateful*, telling me to stay strong and resolute. I knew in my heart that they really had no concept of what that meant and what reality I was facing, but it was all they could do at this point and anything they could do meant the world to me.

Even though I hated my circumstances, there was a small glimmer of hope. Even after a surgery that went terribly wrong with a long list of complications, I found myself making a gratitude list in the hospital. I'd make myself list things I was grateful for—from A to Z. Even on some of my hardest days, I found that by the time I got to "Z," there were at least a few things to smile at and be thankful for. My life had not changed dramatically, but my *thoughts* had. Soon my alphabetical list turned from "Almost walked, Better heart rate, Coughed less" to "Awesome walk outside, Best afternoon ever, Cheerful spirits today." I was gradually claiming ownership of my world again.

Finding gratitude was a way to make "sense" of my story. If I could be grateful for things happening, they could fit into my life. I could own what happened to me and make something from it. These gratitude lists were my life story being spelled out night after night.

I remember always loving the book *Harold and the Purple Crayon*. I loved the idea of a little child being able to create his own world. It made me feel like I could, too. That's the beauty of a metaphor: Through a larger vision, we can relate to our own unique stories.

I had now made the transition from reclaiming my story—a more inward process done through journaling, making art, and putting together *Gutless & Grateful*—to sharing my story with the world—a more outward process. Also, as I shared updates on social media about my recovery from surgery, I realized my story wasn't just my own—it was an inspiration to others. I felt that what I was going through could offer something to others, just as in the hospital, I had felt the biographies my mom read to me of heroes who had been through adversity had something to offer me. I thought a one-woman musical would tie my story together in a gloriously finished bow. But this story was unraveling, and now had to be refashioned.

Throughout my hospital stay, another doctor would get an idea of how to "fix" things, and I'd be taken down to another unit to have a different wire, tube or drain inserted, which would usually fall right back out or spring a leak hours later, after it had taken hours to put into place. This was the first time I had a central port coming out of my neck, making it even more uncomfortable to make the slightest movement. Doctors tried pigskin plugs, stents, mesh, skin grafts, and many tricks and experiments to name. The more accessories attached to me, the harder it was to try to go for walks. I couldn't let that stop me.

Even attached to dozens of wires plugged into the wall, I would use those wires like a leash and walk the farthest radius I could, chained to my bed like a pit bull to a fence.

It didn't take long for me to a get fed up, along with my mother who would often ask if I could stop stepping all over her space as I tried to navigate my way around the bed, walking back and forth, bound by kinking wires. We were all getting a little stir crazy, even for people who had grown used to this kind of life. The wound VAC remained stuck to me, and if the airtight seal had the tiniest gap, any and all kinds of drainage would spill right through the carefully packed layers of gauze. I felt closed in on all fronts. And like Prometheus after a day of unbearable torture, it started all over again the next morning.

We asked the nurses on the floor if there was any kind of portable wound VAC. We were sure they had to exist, but they could not find one. So, my dad and I actually constructed our own kind of machinery and hooked it up to this big battery pack. After we had meticulously attached everything together, he was able to carry this huge machine that almost looked like a suitcase. I was finally able to get free for a short time, but the vacuuming was only somewhat successful and mostly ended with a lot of leaking and a lot of tears streaming down my face.

And just when I thought I couldn't take it anymore, December 11th, I was released. Not from the problems I caused for my body with my surgery but from my confinement in the hospital. As with my stay at Yale, there was nothing more the doctors could do except send me home to wait and see.

CHAPTER 43

Put a Bag on It

MY DISCHARGE SHOULD HAVE BEEN a happy occasion. But once again, we knew it was because the doctors had done all they could, and now the hardest part would be living at home in uncertainty with no answers—the only certainty being that I was definitely worse off than I had been coming in. I had spent enough time feeling different from everyone else, and now I had more physical "differences" than I could handle. Once again, I had been unable to eat or drink for months as doctors tried to reconcile an open wound that turned into a fistula. On top of that, I had traded my colostomy for an ileostomy. But despite all the setbacks—or maybe in response to them—something changed within me after that surgery. The damage that the surgery had caused could not take away from the woman I had become. On the way home from the hospital, my parents took me to the mall to try to make me feel "normal."

But with an unpredictable wound, I ended up barely making it through one store before I started to leak everywhere. Upset, frustrated, and overwhelmed, I ran to the bathroom and stuffed dozens of paper towels into my t-shirt, trying to stay dry for as long as I could.

Once I got home, I managed to get from day to day as a twenty-five-year-old wearing layers of diapers, packed to the brim with hand towels. And what was waiting for me in the mail when I got home? My acceptance letter to

Hampshire College. This was beyond bittersweet. Hadn't I been in this same situation ten years before? Receiving my first college acceptance letters just before landing in a coma? Now, I was coming out of the hospital, receiving another letter about a future that seemed beyond my reach. The idea of me living independently, comfortable, healthy, and energetic was a distant fantasy. Moreover, the doctors had permitted me to eat "a little," but really just for my own sanity. I was controlled by TPN nutrition again. Back to square one.

One afternoon I tried leaving my house for a walk. Every time I opened the door, my pants would become drenched as my wound let out another unexpected burst. This felt like such maniacal torture that I actually started laughing. Was this how it was going to be for the rest of my life?

What I couldn't control and had to accept was that this wound was not going to heal. But wound or not, I needed to live my life—a full life, doing the things I loved to do: eating and drinking, performing on stage, and getting my long-awaited college degree. Now it was up to me to figure out how exactly to make that life work.

One of the hardest things I ever had to do was decide that I needed to put a bag over my wound. The bag meant acknowledging that I would never get my smooth, "normal" stomach back. It meant facing that I had made the decision to get this twenty-seventh surgery, and it had failed on all accounts. But did I really want to admit to myself that this elective surgery was a mistake?

Tina was the visiting nurse who first suggested a bag on my fistula to "make life easier." "It will heal," I told myself. "A bag can wait." So, I ignored her. That didn't stop Tina from dropping off new bags in my mailbox daily, determined to help find a solution.

Finding that solution took almost as much trial and error as Thomas Edison's attempts to invent the light bulb. It took dozens of bags, ideas, creative brainstorming, Googling, nurse consults, and literal cutting and pasting. I had to rely on my skills as an artist—a hobby I had actually picked up in hospitals—to snip, glue, rearrange, and create some kind of apparatus that could possibly hold my insides inside of me.

What complicated things more was that this surgery had taken out even more intestines. Now, I only absorbed about 20% of what I ate and the other 80% came right out of my wound. I was a leaking mess. This was going to have to be a heavy-duty bag.

Creating the perfect combination of a bag and adhesive cut to the perfect shape was more work that an artist does preparing for an art show. It was tiring, frustrating, discouraging work as each bag seemed to leak or fail in a certain area. It took months of leaky experiments before we actually managed to invent a bag solution that worked—at least most of the time.

Dr. Kentz and his team still had no medical answers for me. But every few weeks, Dr. Kentz would ask me to try a charcoal test. I would drink a disgusting cup of chalky liquid black charcoal and see what happened after twenty-four hours. If at the end of a twenty-four-hour cycle there was no black coming out of my wound, it meant the fistula had really closed, and I could eat and drink for real. After weeks of dread, false hope, and more charcoal than any one human could ever want to drink, I made it through an entire day. Finally!

I was able to shop with my mom and not feel anything stain my gauze. It felt like the happiest day of my life. We went home, and I started to let myself dream again that even though I had an ileostomy, it was okay. At least I didn't come out of the surgery any worse. It was just a little "adventure" I was having, and now I could at least go on with life functionally. That night, almost at the end of twenty-four hours—we had almost made it—I was lying in bed getting ready to sleep when I saw a tiny hint of black coming out of the gauze.

"Dad? Can you check out the wound for a second?"

My dad unpacked all of the gauze carefully and he got out the glasses he uses for his dermatology practice. I saw him squinting again just as he squinted at my fistula years ago when we had never heard what one was.

"What's wrong?"

Sure enough, there was a little bit of black.

"Okay, Amy, don't worry about it. It's just a little bit."

But then, as he kept unpacking the gauze, all the black charcoal started coming out at once.

We had to repeat this same test with my bladder fistula. Weeks later, I finally didn't have to carry a catheter pouch stuffed into a purse. I took what I could get. At this point, I didn't even want a normal body. Just one that didn't keep re-opening.

I went back to cooking. Smothering my senses with the hodgepodge of aromas in my spice drawer was all I could do not to slip back into my old, well-worn habits of numbing out to avoid the nightmare my life had become.

Jan. 30—I woke up this morning crying. Then cooked minestrone.

Feb. 12— Doctor appointment. He tried to "restitch" my fistula shut. Leaking out of wound worse than ever. Don't know when or if the answer will come.

My body was still stuck in an excruciating holding pattern. Something had to give.

Feb. 27—Left there drenched. Have to get a hold of this wound.

Feb. 29—Finally found a bag to fit over my wound. Now that I see how much drainage is collecting in it, I can't believe I tried to go out in the real world with just gauze stuffed into diapers. As emotionally difficult as it is to accept another bag, it's better than being wet every second.

Mar. 1—Dad tried to take me to a movie theatre. My bag exploded all over. We're at our wit's end right now.

After several more unproductive and frustrating weeks of bandage changing and leaking all over the house, I was ready for a change.

Mar. 3—Nurse came to give me new options for bagging my wound. I broke down crying. It wasn't the magic fix I hoped for.

Not long after, my Dad's cell phone rang.

"Dr. Kentz, Hi!"

Dr. Kentz had proposed a "deal" to my father. I would come to stay at the hospital for two weeks max, so he could try to find a better solution. I didn't want to be Kentz's surgical guinea pig once again. Why would I subject myself to another two weeks of hospital torture? It was a big decision to go back to the hospital and work with the same surgeon who I felt had failed me and my entire family. I grudgingly packed my bags and told myself it was just two weeks. My optimistic mother packed up all of her usual hospital go-tos—popcorn, iPod, jewelry-making supplies, and tons of catalogs, then said, "At least we might find answers this way." So, we hoped for the best.

Once we got there, the "fun" immediately began. Every day, Dr. Kentz ran a new series of tests and experimental interventions, while I grew more and more fed up and emotionally drained. Each new procedure was a bigger blow to my spirit.

One day, I had been lying in radiology for three hours where they had tried to put a stent in. As soon as I sat up, it fell out of place. I couldn't take it anymore. When they were done, I slipped off my hospital bracelet and was surprised at how easy the tracking chip was to remove from the plastic band. After leaving it in my room, I ran away, out from the hospital and down 90th street. I was a furious fireball of energy that eventually dissipated into a frustrated girl wandering around and window shopping, pretending that none of this was happening. Knowing that my mother was probably freaking out, I picked up my phone, which had been ringing and ringing. It was the head nurse on the floor who knew our family antics quite well at this point. In a timid voice, she kindly asked me to come back. I couldn't bring myself to vent at her, so I didn't say anything and ended the call.

My phone kept ringing as I kept walking in and out of stores trying to believe my life had not sunk to this point—escaping from the surgical floor at Mt. Sinai and going window shopping on the Upper East Side. I finally picked up my phone, and this time it was Dr. Kentz, sounding like a hostage negotiator trying to make a deal with me.

"Amy, you don't have to come to your room. I can meet you in the lobby."

I thought about this. It felt safe enough. "Fine."

So, I headed back towards the hospital, which was quite a ways away at this point. Dr. Kentz was in the lobby, waiting for me. We sat down and stared at the table together, and it felt like we were playing a high stakes game of poker. I looked angrily at my hands, clenching the table with frustration.

"I'll tell you this," he leaned over to me. "I have one other idea...a wire we can thread through the fistula a different way. I know how fed up you are, and I feel awful. And I know this must be really difficult for you, but just give me this and let me try one more procedure. If it doesn't work, you can leave."

I felt like I was talking to a crazy old man, telling me about his latest inventions. I could see in his eyes that even he was stretching for an answer.

I tried it. It didn't work. We left. I went home, defeated.

How was I supposed to be okay with the idea of not eating? It was more "efficient" for the fistula to heal, in their eyes. But it was also destroying me.

A month later, Dr. Kentz had another idea for us—fibrin glue.

It opened at Bloomingdales.

Finally, one of Tina's bags helped me get the leaking under control, at least enough to start getting out of the house with a little more confidence and a little less fear. I could walk, but I couldn't run, and run was all I wanted to do. I wanted to run away from everything, from the hell my life had become.

Do you know the feeling you get when you run? The harsh pounding of the wind against your chest, your legs jolted by the bounce on the pavement, the endless expanse of clouds swallowing up every other thought in the world? At that moment, nothing matters but the feeling of flight. I'm not a runner, but I have run away from many things—emotions, feelings, and circumstances that have made me feel uncomfortable. It was how I thought I was surviving fine when really I was merely getting through.

One morning, I woke up with such a fire in my gut, an anger so overwhelming the energy frightened me. I didn't know what to do with it, and the emotions were too overpowering to try to numb them. My thoughts and feelings were threatening to swallow me whole.

With not a rational thought in my head, I ran out the door and just started running. I didn't know where, for how long or why, but it was the adrenaline of panic—a red hot high through my legs and tingling in my chest. Tears caught in my eye sockets that I hoped the wind bashing across my face might dry up.

I was too scared to kill myself, and I didn't think I wanted to either. I wanted a middle ground—just to exist in another world, and if I ran long enough, I'd get there, somehow, somewhere. I ran for three hours before I found a highway, and without thinking, I started running onto the shoulder of it. I thought, "The farther I go, the further this will all be behind me." Of course, of all days I decide to run for my life, it starts to rain and thunder. Suddenly, the highway was flooded, I was drenched, and I had cars beeping at me, wondering what a frail girl in a soaked T-shirt was doing running on the shoulder of the highway.

It was only a matter of time before a police car pulled up and asked me to get inside. I was shaking, angry, embarrassed, and nervous like I had just gotten my first detention in school. He said, "I've gotten about thirty calls in the past twenty minutes saying this girl is running on the shoulder of the highway. Where did you think you were going?" I was upset that my escape had been halted and suddenly very ashamed. Wiping away tears, I stammered, "To the mall."

"You thought you could get to the mall on the shoulder of the highway?"

"Yes."

He turned around and looked at me for a brief pause and said, "I can drive you."

I refused to look at him, pressed my elbows into my sides, and barely whispered, "No, I'll go home."

I didn't want to kill myself because, in my heart, I knew how much I adored life. But I needed a break. I was sick of living in fear, wading in uncertainty, and reflecting on a former life that I was never able to get back before my coma at the age of eighteen, a time when life is supposed to open doors. Then I remembered times in my life post-coma that I was happy. I tried to remember what the circumstances were, what I was thinking, who was around me, what I was doing. And they were small moments. They were moments I felt connected. As I ran on the shoulder of the highway that rainy April day, I laughed at my circumstances. "I'll show the entire world that I don't care anymore! I'm done!" I ran and ran, feeling the wind against my legs, my shirt getting soaked, and the horns of concerned cars that passed me by.

When the police brought me home that day, I was furious. I spent the afternoon pacing around the kitchen screaming that I was going to take every knife in the house. I didn't know what I meant by that, but I wanted a reaction—from others, but also from myself. I wanted to see how much I still cared. I had no proof that things would get better, but I did have a few solid things at that moment that I could stand on and anchor myself to just to get me through. In that very moment:

1. I had my mother and whole family.
2. I had my body with a heart that was beating strongly.
3. I had the rain on my skin.
4. I had life. Whatever it was, I had it in my hands.

I started with that tear and realized that my tear was not a death-sentence of depression or everlasting sadness; it was a sign to start grieving and mourning my losses. I started putting my thoughts together through song, art, and words that, over time, I was able to share with those I loved.

The next day, I woke up and ran outside again. But this time, I knew where I was going. Instinctively, I ran outside to look at a tree, and as I realized what was important in the world, I felt my eyes enlarge and my frozen heart begin to expand. Suddenly, I felt aligned with Earth, the world, with life, with the thousands of people who have come before me and have been tried and tested, some perhaps who had also given up hope—people like my grandmother who had survived Auschwitz at eighteen years old. I felt roots coming up through the earth, and I stopped thinking about a situation I felt trapped in and started to think about what "values" I could trap myself in— values that could guide me through a very uncertain time. When life is shaky, your values keep you anchored.

So, I spent the day walking down my street singing to myself, noticing the cars that passed by, gazing down the path ahead, staying curious to see where it led. That was my new runner's high. It may have left me winded, angry, frustrated, panicked, or overwhelmed with sadness, but it's the high of being alive.

Gutless and Grateful was, as Winston Churchill said, "not the end, nor the beginning of the end, but the end of the beginning." As always, I had a long way to go. And the world needed to hear.

CHAPTER 44

Three Big Gambles

I'm throwing darts at a towering pillar of trust, trying to see what sticks.

I'VE SPENT A LOT OF TIME waiting in my life, and as a born go-getter, I've never been great with patience. I had to seize the moment because I wasn't sure what else there was. So, I took three big gambles: I decided to go to college; I called two theatres (still in my hospital gown) to book another run of *Gutless & Grateful*, and I entered the world of online dating.

When finally discharged from my disastrous twenty-seventh surgery with a wound refusing to heal, I felt like I had lost all connection to the outside world again. How was I supposed to clean up the mess I had made of my still gutless, once grateful life? Even the trees were losing more leaves by the day.

Blind faith. No fear, just faith. If I'm lonely, if I can't stand my medical situation, I'm just going to tell myself, "I'm healthy enough" and start remaking my life. The time is now, as good as any other time.

I used the same mentality that had helped me endure everything else: If you act healthy, you'll feel healthy. Fake it till you make it.

One day, a childhood friend of mine named Sara called my mother. She assertively stated, "I just moved here from the city, and I don't know anyone. I grew up with Amy, and I'd love to get together." Still wearing hospital pajamas and barely able to get out of bed, I was in no mood for company. But I reluctantly agreed. Sara popped right over, and in the course of our conversation casually mentioned that she had met her boyfriend online. At first, I thought nothing of it. Dating anyone, much less finding a friend online, was the furthest thing from my mind. Or was it?

I'd never had a boyfriend before. I'd never even been on a casual date. My only "experience" was with a predator three times my age. At twenty-five, I may have been a bit naïve in my romantic experience, but my life experience certainly made up for it. Online? Was that how people started dating now? If not interested, I was at least curious.

As a teen, I was a busybody with her hands on a million projects at once and was more excited about auditioning for the next musical than flirting with the guy whose locker was closest to mine. I knew I'd have the rest of my life to date, find love, and eventually settle down. However, after this last blow, I felt wise beyond my years, and an infant discovering the world, regaining physical strength and suddenly having to be taken care of again.

I took a risk that felt, in the moment, even bigger than deciding to have my fateful twenty-seventh surgery. I put myself out there, in the dating market, for real, on OKCupid.

I had made a career for myself as an artist by being fearless, shameless, and bold, ignoring my inner critic and just expressing whatever I was feeling. Why shouldn't dating be the same?

This guy Ryan sent me a message, and we clicked! He's smart, funny, and cute. I wish I was 20 pounds heavier, but I am motivated!

A real guy? I had the power to respond. Right? I didn't understand why I had to wait. I had been waiting long enough. That's why I decided to go for it. Why wait to start a relationship. If not now, when?

March 4—Texted with Ryan all day, emailed all night. I am so excited for my date on Friday!

In the meantime, I was still tending to my new professional life as an actor. When I called to book another run of *Gutless & Grateful*, I was thirty pounds underweight and just recovering my voice from being intubated. I wasn't sure how I would sing and dance connected to TPN for twenty-four hours a day again, or while toting a purse around with a catheter in it, but I did know that I needed to get back to doing what I loved. Now that I had experienced the hell of surgery twenty-seven and its aftermath, I decided to use what had happened to me as more material. It lent itself perfectly to extra comedy for *Gutless & Grateful: A Second Helping!*

Friday November 2—William Finn called. He said, "I figured out what your show is about." He said I have to reach my "breaking point" with a really angry song, then realize midway that I can't stay mad at the world, that's just not who I am. He said, "That is your lesson for the day." And just hung up. He's the best. Had hibachi for dinner.

I remembered that a huge part of my healing process was unleashing the anger I had kept stored up in the healing vortex for so long. I had felt so much anger in me at one time that I even tried to get it all out by running down the shoulder of the highway. Maybe this was missing the piece I needed to discharge this angry energy still frozen inside of me. Playwriting granted me creative ownership, and writing this monologue, maybe I could launch myself back into the works after Surgery 27.

Ryan had messaged me the day I created my dating profile. By the end of that day we were writing novels back and forth to each other. We had all the same likes and dislikes, had visited all the same places, and had the same quirky sense of humor. He made me feel like a person again and realize who I was before the medical ordeal—and who I still was now.

I was filled with confidence when I realized, as I wrote these notes to Ryan, I was actually a person, and an interesting one, too! Maybe I wasn't just the medical patient the doctors made me feel like all the time. Just like I said in my script for *Gutless & Grateful*, now my life had a richer purpose. Maybe I did have something going for me.

March 6—Emailed more producers, got great feedback! Friended Ryan on Facebook. I'm so excited for my date this week!

March 10—Each day gets better. Amazing rehearsal with Jerold. He sees the glimmer is back in my eye. Ryan wrote me all day.

Life, which had seemed to drag by for the past few months, was now zipping along on a track of normalcy. It was a life so normal that it seemed completely exotic. During the day, I was hard at work rehearsing with Jerold. It felt great to discipline myself and work on what I loved. By night, I was dating!

Despite my excitement about my newly energized self, I tried to put off meeting Ryan in person for as long as I could. After my satanic twenty-seventh surgery, I had lost so much confidence in my body, how it looked and how I managed it, that it was hard to imagine meeting a dating partner, much less getting intimate. But I kept up my "nothing left to lose" mindset and agreed to meet him at Tinto, a restaurant that he suggested.

Tinto was in the basement of some kind of building complex that was impossible to find. Of course, my parents drove me there and parked a block away to ensure they had a clear view of an online potential serial killer (my mother's neurosis about the unknown world of online dating) and that I was in safe hands.

I nervously headed into the restaurant and found Ryan just as he described—in a black dress shirt, sitting at a high table by the bar. He immediately stood up when he saw me, nodded like a gentleman, and pulled out a chair. "I'll worry about the leaking later," I told myself as I scooted myself into the seat and picked up a menu, firm and heavy in my hands. This was a real date! I could tell Ryan was as nervous as I was as he tried to grin and tell me about their great selection of Tapas, whatever that was...

"Tap-ass? What's that?"

"It's like a tasting menu where you can order a bunch of appetizers at once—the little beef tacos are my favorite."

"Okay, cool. I'll get...whatever you're having!"

I didn't have the heart to tell him I'm a wimp when it comes to spicy food. Or that I had just started eating again after months (again) of nothing. Or that most of it came out a hole on my belly. I just made sure the nearest bathroom was within cyesight.

The plates came, and as we both nibbled away at the little dishes, served like miniature pieces of art, we awkwardly asked each other follow up questions on the mutual passions we shared online. The bartenders looked at the only two diners, quickly catching the cues that we were meeting for the first time. I felt like I had a friend I could laugh with and perhaps a growing romantic feeling inside that I'd never felt before. My heart had never fluttered like this. The adrenaline butterflies I'd get on stage couldn't compare.

The news covered my story once again. I was the girl who got sick and now was performing a show about it. As I ran all over town posting flyers and leaving brochures, one retail clerk remarked to me, "I just read about you in the paper—you're doing that show again!" Yes, I was!

I wasn't scared to put myself out there for my show, now that whatever I put my heart into was actually happening. And for the first time, I was putting my heart into romance—and feeling the rewards. After Ryan and I met at Tinto, we were inseparable.

It was hard to know what "feelings" felt like anymore from all the numb years of being forced to deny my body food or water, while nutritional IVs mechanically streamed through my veins. Now, love flowed through those same veins. Ryan put me back in touch with my vitality.

When I first premiered *Gutless & Grateful* at the Triad October 2012, it was my first real dive into the musical theatre pool after what seemed to be a lifetime of medical intrusion.

Rewriting my show was the perfect way to find more closure after surgery had left me—literally—with so many open ends.

The third thread of my journey was Hampshire College. I had applied before my surgery, and never expected to be in such poor medical shape just months before the semester started. But if I was capable of setting up an online dating profile, I was capable of going to college. If dating could open up my heart, I knew Hampshire could open up a world of possibilities.

I envisioned the world of higher education was going to be a magical world of "independence." I could finally live on my own, have a social life, go to the kind of parties I saw in teen movies, and feel like a real-live adult. I dreamed of getting a degree in the arts and becoming a teacher, a writer, artist, actress—anything I set my mind to, really.

The month of March flew by as things started heating up with Ryan, and I went into full preparation mode for my show.

Threading through the aisles at Barnes & Noble to unwind after hours of singing through *Gutless* (dreamy-eyed and heart tap-dancing on air), Ryan finally burst through the double doors, and I let myself drown in self-indulgent "I have a boyfriend" bliss as we wrapped our arms around each other. It was way too early for a "meet the parents...and Jerold," but I didn't want to say goodnight. The bookstore was closing.

"Would it be weird to ask you to come over now? My parents are home."

"That's okay."

"And Jerold." I wasn't sure if Ryan knew what he was getting himself into.

"I can go get a bottle of wine or something."

I hoisted myself into Ryan's truck, and I couldn't tell who was more nervous as I gave him directions to our home.

Jerold was his usual sarcastic self, but I could tell that even he was impressed as Ryan nervously acted like his best gentleman self. I was beaming as Ryan trembled, making nervous conversation with my father. My mother quickly joined us at the table, making sure the salmon was the only specimen being "grilled," and it didn't take long before we were all tossing lighthearted quips like hot potatoes. It was starting to feel like home, after a surgery threatened to turn our house into hospital zone again. Our home was brimming with health, laughter, joy, light...and the intoxicating smell of grilled salmon. Meet the parents was a success.

March 31—Awesome day! Went to design invitations for my show, then the best Passover ever, great time, no one left until 11pm! Definitely a new Passover—much better off than '05! I feel so connected with my friends. Ryan picked me up for a lovely hibachi dinner. Feel like such a couple now.

April 10—Best birthday! Whole family and Ryan went to see Matt play at Apollo. 88 friends wished me happy birthday on Facebook. Yay. Bag was acting up all day. I hate being me sometimes.

April 19—Our one-month anniversary! I can tell Dad is sad I don't spend as much time with him anymore.

April 27—Hampshire Accepted Students Day. Today really affirmed that this is the right place for me. Everyone is so passionate about learning, and I really see myself growing there.

We arrived on the Hampshire campus early in the morning, as I put makeup on during the long three-hour drive. I got out of the car and took one expansive look across those beautiful New England Hills, which reminded me of the lush, Berkshire landscape that had always brought me back to myself. The campus was just gorgeous as I had remembered it. I ran through the grass like a little kid to the big tent in the center of the beautiful greenery, where hundreds of first-year students were now sitting with their parents, like the college experience I had always dreamed of.

Every student here seemed to be enthralled with the idea of making your own program from scratch. This kind of resourcefulness and creativity was my life force already. How could I go wrong here? The Dean of Students then ran through an entire list of the eclectic interests of this year's class. People were into all sorts of things from equine therapy, philosophy, marine biology, clowning, and everything in between. It didn't even matter how old everyone was. Passion exuded from every seat, and I could not wait to meet everyone, with their purple hair, and eccentric outfits, and very established sense of identity. These were people who half knew who they were and half yearned to discover themselves. And I was, too.

For the first time I couldn't wait for my parents to get out of there. I was twenty-five and going to be independent for the first time. I was accepted. I think I was actually accepting myself now. I did belong here.

CHAPTER 45

Life!

LIFE WAS MOVING AT A RAPID pace. I was psyched to do my show in three different venues by the end of the summer. May was packed with Yankee games, long walks with Ryan all over town, and trying every new restaurant in the area. I was living a life unlike one I had ever experienced.

Being with Ryan was a combination of childlike discovery and suddenly accessing the woman in me that I had never even dreamed of being. The days zoomed by with our hikes, geocaching, food shopping (I never met anyone who loved Stop & Shop as much as I did!), posting flyers for my show, rehearsing with Jerold, voice lessons, and grabbing any free second to journal about it.

I was also filling out the remaining paperwork for Hampshire College, telling myself that I should go, even though I was conjuring up fantasies of domesticating myself as a housewife for the rest of my life. I also pictured myself telling Ryan my college plans but thought maybe that should wait.

Interspersed with the excitement of tech rehearsals, interviews, and flyer postings were frequent appointments with physicians my father had researched who might have creative answers for me. I still hadn't given up on healing the fistula. But every new appointment only brought frustration, tension, and tears as my dad recounted my medical history to each "specialty" doctor for the umpteenth time while my fistula continued to deplete my hydration, nutrition, and hope.

But somehow my new life circumstances—love for Ryan, being social with friends, and engaging with others in new ways—took precedence over my leaking fistula or the lack of answers. I truly felt the power of companionship overpower my medical circumstances.

At a pivotal point, where I was trying to transition through this precarious phase and reclaim my life, Ryan came at the perfect time with the essential survival skill that I didn't know I had needed all along. It was the missing piece that neither my art nor my writing could provide—people. I was able to get out of the house, independent of my parents. How else would I have gone to trivia night at a bar, danced in a club, strolled romantically through parks, and uncovered my ability to have actual feelings?.

Now I had Ryan to share this all with me. After I rehearsed with Jerold for our five-hour marathon, Ryan and I would sit in our kitchen stuffing envelopes with show flyers to send out. We celebrated the end of a long day by boiling spaghetti and laughing as we washed dishes together. After walking Ryan outside to his truck, I came back in with more than a song in my heart. Facing out the window, my mom said, "Wow, he really adores you, honey. You should see how he looks at you when you sing."

The park was so gorgeous with the blaring circle of sun setting behind gigantic tall trees, and the moon already appearing at the other end of the sky, waiting in its dressing room for its showtime. Can't wait to take this spirit with me into my own dressing room this June!

In June 2013, I got to come back "home" in two respects. I brought *Gutless & Grateful* back to where to all started—the Triad Theatre in New York City. But now, after surgery twenty-seven, I was on a completely new playing field with a long medical journey of questions to answer ahead of me. I was now on TPN and had a sock on my bicep to cover up my port. I still had the energy of a racehorse, which had taken much time and effort to regain. The bag on my wound allowed me to do what I love. And I had shared the "updated" version of my story.

I had also brought *Gutless* back "home" in another sense. I was bringing it back to my hometown, where local people who had followed my story could now see my great comeback. And the third aspect of coming home? Coming home to a relationship!

I adored Ryan. Still, I was worried that my first healthy sexual experience might trigger some unresolved feelings from the abuse I experienced at the hands of my voice teacher. If a stimulant as simple as a French fry had conjured up such frightening emotions, then why wouldn't having someone to hold, caress, and care about me so affectionately remind me of a time that these actions were manipulated by Blaine in such horrifying ways?

This was the first time I was required to express feelings openly. For years, I had mainly spoken to my parents and doctors who understood my antisocial, awkward ways of functioning when I was in "numbed out mode."

I finally had a sense of what my life should look like—who I was supposed to be, what I was supposed to do, and who I was supposed to do it with. I realized this was about me taking care of me. I had to be in good shape myself, physically and emotionally, so I could be there for others.

This was a new feeling of life, far different than the manically mechanical months of chaos I created in order to *not* feel anything. Meeting and trusting Ryan gave me back something that I truly wasn't sure I would ever recover—myself. I accepted that I would have to stay dead inside as a result of my traumas. "A small price to pay for everything," I said. But this relationship was proving that assumption wrong, day by day.

I didn't think feeling like the old, bubbly Amy who giggled in school class-rooms was possible, or that I could discover an actual woman burgeoning right under my skin. Was this the third, higher, and more objective self that I had always discussed with Rita, or another evolution of me?

Whatever self was emerging, I was beginning to like her. She sprouted from having other people in my life—and Ryan. No self-help book or jour-naling could have prepared me for that.

My parents, though naturally overprotective of their daughter who had been sick, worn, and removed from the real world for so long, were happy I was getting out. It meant they could take a break from malls every weekend and begin to live their own lives more fully. But they were naturally wary of Ryan at first—some guy from Arizona who had popped up and suddenly be-come a staple in my life. Ryan's upfront certainty that we should get "serious" right away had initially alarmed me, but one night out at a time, my feelings shifted to a confident knowing that this WAS my time to be happy—to be in love.

I trusted the instinct within me to trust—that same trust that was once shattered by Blaine. I had now spent years working to reassemble that trust and reground it in myself, so I could feel and listen to my heart again.

At this point, my ostomy was a secret I was determined to keep to myself and not an easy one to keep from Ryan. My emergency bag, an oversized purse crammed with every medical accessory required if my own bag sprung a leak, followed me wherever I went. In this "top-secret bag" I kept six dif-ferent kinds of tape, four ostomy bags, four wound bags, three different kinds of scissors, three packages of gauze, a diaper, tons of hand towels, and a few other "craft" supplies. I also had a hairdryer to seal the wax in place once I had gone through the elaborate process of attaching the wound bag.

Finding the right bag to cover my large wound—and not fall off—required a lot of creativity. But try going from store to store in New York and not only finding a bathroom, but also finding a bathroom with an outlet for a hairdryer! And on top of that, finding a private bathroom. (I had learned the hard way that people freak out when they see you putting a bag on an open wound in a hotel lobby restroom.)

Long before my twenty-seventh surgery, I had bought tickets to see Brandi Carlile in concert, now one of my favorite performers after I discovered her song, *The Story*, and used it to end *Gutless & Grateful*. Now in a relationship, I invited Ryan to come, and we made an adventure out of spending the day in the city, strolling down winding pathways in Central Park holding hands, sampling from exotic food kiosks, and praying my wound bags taped underneath my dress would behave.

"What the heck did you bring with you?" Ryan playfully joked as I yanked my purse-turned-emergency-bag from getting caught in the door of the theater.

"Oh, it's just all my stuff!" I joked as I tried to stifle the sharp clang of the metal osto-bond container against the suture scissors.

I often thought about what would happen if we were out and about or on vacation and I depleted all of my supplies. Would I be stranded? Forced to go home? Unable to eat or drink? Since most of what I was eating was malabsorbed and came right through the wound bag, if I ran out of bags, I wouldn't have a choice.

Of all days, the day I was out in the city with Ryan, both of my bags leaked. I finally found a private bathroom in a nail salon, but of course, no outlet. I did my best to bandage my skin and press my fingers down tightly in lieu of heat, but as soon as I packed up my supplies, the bag leaked again. By the time we sat down for the concert, I had run out of bags, and now was left with a diaper and some paper towels to stuff in it. Not the most glamorous night out.

About twenty minutes into the concert, the leaking got out of control, and I regretfully told Ryan we had to leave. He didn't question it and immediately looked up the next train while I scrambled to wipe off the drainage-stained theatre seat with my coat. It was clear I couldn't keep my secret from Ryan much longer.

To this day, I have a difficult time sitting down because of where my bags lie on my body. Even people who know me sometimes forget and innocently ask if I'd "like to take a seat." It's difficult trying to introduce the concept to new faces without them thinking I'm overly nervous or too fidgety to sit. I try to silence this with, "I have medical circumstances," but it tends to confuse people even more. I frantically scout out an electrical outlet in every bathroom, and which high-top table are the closest distance that restroom door, marking with each bite and sip, how many steps I am away from it. Jerold called it "doing the bag dance." I called it "the ticking time bomb."

As much as I tried to tell myself that my ostomy and wound were just things *on* my body and not *who* I was, they constantly preoccupied me. I was worried that my difficulty being present with him would make him think I was pulling away. Leaving the concert early was another reminder of how trapped my medical circumstances could make me feel. And now that affected someone else.

I decided I had to tell Ryan about my ostomy. My mom disagreed; she didn't see that this was necessary so early on. She thought it was too much. I had only known him for a month. But in my heart, I knew that though I wasn't my ostomy, it was still a part of me, enough to affect me, and I knew what keeping secrets did.

It took a while for me to "stomach" up the strength to tell Ryan, but when I finally spilled, I was shocked to find him unfazed. He even responded, "I think I am taking this better than you are."

By June, I was living a fast-paced life—a far cry from the days of waiting for doctors to come by and tell me I still had to "wait." My days were filled with band rehearsals, being hospitalized for blood infections, and Ryan and I taking long morning walks all over different neighborhoods. He had been house hunting even before he met me, and I couldn't help thinking that he was accelerating his timetable now that he had fallen hard for me.

I was falling too, yet I felt safe. I was imagining a future shared with another person...and I sensed Ryan was, too.

One day, we took one of our lengthy wandering walks, passing through three towns, stopping in a few grocery stores along the way for snacks, and bouncing over topics from 90s pop culture trivia to politics, art, philosophy, and Ryan's attempt at schooling me in "technical coding." The conversation came back to us, and just like on our second date when I blurted out, "I think you should kiss me," I impulsively said, "I'm starting to think I'm going to marry you."

I didn't realize what came out of my mouth as we kept walking, his grip on my hand growing tighter yet softer. I was more shocked than he, but I trusted the love I felt for him—a love that connected me to the Amy before Blaine.

Soon enough, I was performing *Gutless & Grateful* in New York, once again at the Triad Theatre, followed by a run in Connecticut at the Bijou Theatre.

Throughout all of this, Ryan was by my side. I'll never forget, as we were packing up to leave the Bijou, an older woman saw how Ryan cared for me so affectionately. She said, "You're lucky, you've got a great guy." Ryan beamed, "No, I'm the lucky one." I wasn't sure who was luckier. As Ryan wrapped his strong arms around me and we celebrated at our favorite date spot, buying snacks at Stop & Shop, I thought all I needed was him in my life, and I was so thankful.

I now knew we were going to get married. But when?! He'd often tease me, saying, "I'm gonna propose to you..." I found a jeweler in the city who was willing to make custom rings. Unbeknownst to me, he went into see her while I went into New York and headed just a few blocks away to rehearse for my show. As soon as we met up afterwards, I was met with the taunting "I have a *ring*."

I was enjoying the playfulness, the innocence, and for once, I felt carefree as we slipped down Fifth Avenue hand in hand, he with a ring in his pocket, me with the joyful ache of love pounding in my heart.

My health, however, had still not recovered from my surgical hit in November. Although my shows went great, I was still severely underweight, and this time, had to wear a sock (red sock, of course) over my arm to go over the TPN PICC line. I couldn't believe that just in October, the last time I had done the show, I had been thirty pounds heavier and able to sustain myself with food alone. Moreover, I was saddened that Ryan didn't know what I looked like as my full self before the setback and longed to feel pretty again.

My wound got more unmanageable, losing more and more fluid. But I was determined to conserve my strength and be in the best shape I could for my final performance of the summer at Barrington Stage Company, thanks to the invitation from William Finn. So, I decided I had to get a PICC line in again, not for my health or the sake of my show, or because my parents insisted, but for Ryan. I was thinking long-term.

I came out of the usual "poke wires around until one fits in a vein" procedure, but that night Ryan hugged me, and I realized it was the first time I had been hugged in this romance-filled way with a line in my arm. This was a sign that from now on, everything I did would be buoyed by this kind of support. My parents were with me no matter what, but Ryan was the new addition I didn't know I needed.

So, with my new PICC line, I ventured forth to the Berkshires, to perform my show as part of "Mr. Finn's Cabaret Series." I was performing *Gutless & Grateful* in three different states within two months—my first official "tour!" Ryan and I decided to make a trip out of it, hiking the same mountains that Jeff had talked to me about as he sat by my bedside in the Columbia ICU years before. I had truly come full circle.

Three days after we came home from the Berkshires, we packed our bags and headed for Ryan's childhood happy place—Arizona. My parents were concerned. I had never gone on a trip like this, successfully at least, and I was going to be staying with a family I had never met. The week with Ryan's family blew by.

As we made our daily drive back from the local grocery store, Ryan took another route, past the geysers he had told me about—and there they were, shooting off in the distance. I could tell Ryan's sweat wasn't from the dry heat as we got out of the car and he led me around in circles, weaving past trees, lampposts, mountains, and that gloriously lit up fountain spurting into the air.

He let go of my hand to fumble in his pocket, got down on one knee, and asked me, "Will you be my wife?"

I was suddenly "out-of-body," except this time I wasn't numb but overwhelmed with feeling. Was this really happening?

"Yes!" I screamed. "Yes, I will marry you!"

We celebrated with slices from Pizza Hut, and I basked in a happiness I had never felt before.

CHAPTER 46

Being Engaged Changes Everything

NOW THAT WE WERE GETTING MARRIED, I had to tell Ryan about my upcoming college plans. I could still barely believe it myself. Everything was happening so fast. Conflicting about staying home for love, or leaving for college, I decided to tell Ryan.

I was ready to throw Hampshire out the window as soon as I decided that I was living with you. Deep inside, I knew that would only be cheating myself. Love opened up my eyes. Now I am even more ready to take on college. I can't cheat myself out of the life I deserve to live.

Just as he had reacted when I anxiously told him I had an ostomy, Ryan acted like he had known all along. I couldn't help feeling that he was happy for me and ready to take this journey with me. For a few weekends, he said he'd even be able to stay over.

With three successful runs of *Gutless & Grateful*, a ring on my finger, and college around the corner, my future had never seemed brighter. The rest of the summer was packed with domestic adventures, daydreaming, college planning, exploring, lots of cooking, and even more eating! After a few blissful days of being a fiancée, I found this note waiting for me in my email:

I read your story and am blown away by what you have gone through and how you are handling everything. Your very special WOC nurse, Tina, couldn't be more proud of what you have accomplished. After reading about you, I would love to speak with you if you get a chance. To refresh your memory about who I am please go to www.greatcomebacks.com. Thanks. - Rolf

Apparently, Tina, the nurse who had been so patient and compassionate with me at such a difficult time in my life, had nominated me for this award.

When Rolf and I spoke, he introduced himself to me as a former NFL linebacker, as well as an ostomate doing great things. Rolf had been a football player his entire life, and then found himself suddenly in pain, unable to do what he loved. In his second pro season, he learned he had ulcerative colitis and that he would have to make some hard choices about his health and career. Now he was the national spokesman for the Crohn's and Colitis Foundation of America.

Each year several ostomates who have shared their stories and inspired others are eligible to receive the Great Comebacks awards.

Even more exciting, he told me about ostomy support—a group of young, thriving people just like me who happened to have ostomies. As we talked, I realized that Rolf would soon join the growing community of people around me—an army of warriors—to support me and make sure that even with an opening in my abdomen I still wouldn't fall into the gap.

Now that I was actually going to college, I spent the summer trying to get my body in shape for what I knew would be a physically challenging time once I got to Hampshire. I was open to trying whatever the doctors thought would give me the best chance of healing my fistula. Doctors still had no answers, but even the worst things didn't seem "terrible" because I had someone to talk to about them with.

"Go figure. Having someone to tell your troubles to could make life that much easier," I thought to myself as we strolled past the beautiful High Line greenery.

As the start of Hampshire approached, my father and I went into a last-minute panic. We visited any hospital that would have us for tests and even flew out to a transplant clinic in Houston to look for answers outside the box.

Even on TPN, my family worried that I would not be able to maintain my health in college. After all, trying to manage my TPN at Northwestern University had put me in the hospital with a near fatal infection. Was I crazy trying this again?

During back-to-school shopping with my mom, I grew increasingly nervous about the medical supplies and special accommodations I would need. I hadn't sat down in years because of my bag. What would happen when I went to my first lecture or first meal in the dining hall?

It was a summer of adventure, food, family, joy, and growth. We did more in that summer than I had done in eight years. Restaurants, food shopping, cooking, family, new family, friends, performing *Gutless & Grateful* in three states, a Berkshires vacation, a Great Comebacks nomination, introduction to the bar scene (we quickly gave up on New York clubs after no one let us in once they saw me with my thigh-high bright red socks, neon Asics sneakers, and a backpack filled with pounds of cheese and gallons of yogurt), Yankee games with my dad, cheering Matt on at the Apollo Theatre, and most importantly, waking up with someone who was now instantly part of my world and every pulse-racing moment.

But my body did not want to keep up. Even on TPN, I was losing more fluid from the draining wound every day, and it was starting to show in my appearance. I hated having no control over by body's stability, and suddenly being dependent on TPN when I had managed so well without it before. The day before I went to college, I chewed and swallowed every bite and hoped for the best, although there seemed to be no clear rhyme or reason to what stayed in and what came out.

We packed everything up and managed to cram all of my medical supplies in five big cartons along with three more taped-up cardboard boxes of my protein-packed shakes, bars, frozen meals, and several pounds of cheese blocks.

I knew Ryan was happy for me as we fit the last huge box of medical supplies into the backseat, but I could sense a wave of sadness come over him as he drove me closer, watching me giddily put makeup on (which I usually never did) in his rear-view mirror as I tried to settle my bated breath.

Adam and Dad arrived in their cars shortly after to unload even more heaping piles of medical equipment, books, and standing-height tables for me to work on, and with all our arms balancing towering stacks of supplies, we found our way to Prescott 172. It was now time for the four of us to strategize: how they'd fit all my food, standing supports, emergency medical supplies, and everything else into the small space. Knowing that once my bags were in place and that I couldn't bend down on my own, my father tried to map out the best design he could and tried to cram every piece of medical equipment needed for my daily bag changes on my bathroom shelf.

Could I really do this on my own?

By the time we all finished unpacking, the boys were exhausted, and I was running off to the Hampshire cafeteria for the first time, thrilled to pile my plate miles high and meet as many new faces as I could. But Ryan! I couldn't just run off, although part of me wanted to numb my ever-burgeoning heart as he returned the embrace I hurriedly gave him before dinner.

"So, I guess I'll leave now?"

"If you want to...yeah, I guess you have to. Love you."

It was strange watching him go to his truck, start the engine, and drive off, but this was my chance to achieve my long-awaited dream of an independent college education.

Day one at Hampshire College was a zealous invitation to immerse myself in knowledge, engage with other people, and be a real live person! I was even invited to go to parties. I was psyched! I had been surviving for so long with an all-or-nothing mindset that it felt impossible to find middle ground. Just like hunger cues, social cues had to be learned with practice.

Meeting new people is like one enzyme reacting with a variety of catalysts; when we meet new people, we open a world inside ourselves that we might never know otherwise where every encounter produces a different outcome, like an instant immersion in the magic of living—a jolt of happiness, a glimpse of what could be.

One afternoon, I felt my ostomy get obstructed. Within a minute, I was squirming on the floor, crying and clutching my stomach, waiting for Adam to drive three hours to my dorm with emergency fluids. My parents then decided it was best to take me home for the weekend to recover. Would Hampshire be another Northwestern when I had come so close to college, but my body had betrayed me?

Fortunately, the fluids quickly cleared my obstruction and soon I was anxious to get out of the house and back to Hampshire. Within no time I caught up on my classes and was back to being a kid in a candy store. Signing up at every booth in the HampFest activity fair for extracurricular clubs was even more exhilarating than completing my usual supermarket sweep at Stop & Shop. I didn't even know what I was signing up for—I was signing up for life! Judaism groups, art clubs Shake and Bake (reading Shakespeare while baking pies), farm collectives, improv groups, karate clubs...I was stacking my shelves with friends, courses, and meals (although I did get a few looks at how much grub I piled on my plate). On top of all this, I was still engaged.

Sept 12—Ryan came to visit. We went to Stop & Shop. Then I remembered that people *are now important in my life, not just food shopping, so we went back and had dinner with friends and caught an improv show. I love that he gets to see how happy I am here.*

My excitement notwithstanding, the pace of college was beginning to wear on me.

Sept 18—Met with the Dean, who said I looked tired and should maybe go home for a while. I got upset and ran back to my dorm and slipped around 4 p.m. I woke up at 7 p.m. lying in a pool of blood. I got stitches at the ER. My head is throbbing and sore and in pain. Came back to the dorm to rest. I am sad I missed the dance party tonight.

But I pressed on, determined to get everything out of college that I had come for.

Thinking of my own "mythical warrior gods," I designed my study unit around Mayan art with confidence...until I learned that the following week, we'd actually be using our lesson plans—with real live children!

I nervously went through the standard fingerprinting, skeptical looks from fidgety eight-year-olds, and the vigilant watch of their teachers as the kids proceeded to throw the supplies at each other and roll on the floor. Thankfully, art had already taught me to love the messy surprises that show up along the way.

I also had the opportunity to take a playwriting course, which meant writing a play of my own. *Gutless* was all about my journey, told from my perspective. Hampshire was opening up my healing vortex of creativity.

I was so engrossed in (finally) being a college student that I had left everything that I had completely forgotten about the Great Comebacks Award phone call with Rolf. So, when he called with "news" for me, I was stunned.

While I was bouncing between Hampshire's new experiences, I was also being bounced from one health crisis to another. My fistula was making it very difficult to keep my health up, and as much as I hated TPN, I accepted that it was the only way I could keep myself medically stable. As dangerous as TPN was, right now, I needed it. I had to make two "responsible" decisions:

1. I needed to use the PICC line to maintain my nutrition.
2. Daily use of the PICC line was only feasible if I stayed home.

Reluctantly, I said goodbye to campus and moved my things from my dorm back home where I would pursue independent studies.

Although TPN did not cause pain, it did cause worry and aggravation. I had to time everything so the bag could be changed at the proper intervals. The more "normal" I felt, the more I resented my "special" circumstances. I was still relatively numb, but Ryan kept poking through. Now that I was in love, I needed to keep myself alive. Ryan was the anchor I needed to stay calm and the pull I needed to keep moving forward.

Stuck at home, playwriting became my escape. Every day, I conjured up my prized memories, like my pre-coma trip to the Berkshires with Matt. I could almost reach out and touch that picture-perfect memory. So, I grabbed a pen and wrote a scene.

All of my courses were adding to the tapestry of my world view. My long-delayed college student status had turned out to be a gift—far better, in fact, than if things had gone as I had originally planned. In my poetry course, I had been known for waving my hand fanatically to ask or answer as many questions possible.

"Hey class, Amy isn't the only one that needs to volunteer..."

At Hampshire, I had been sneaking my hand into a big jar of candy, reaping the sweet rewards of learning from inspiring professors, students, and ideas. As a teen, would I really have cared as much? Real-life experience was coloring in my textbooks, so I could turn each assignment into actions to enrich every day. Studying from home seemed to give me the best of both worlds—for now.

CHAPTER 47

Home Schooling

MY FAMILY HOME HAD BEEN a makeshift ICU, an art studio, a business headquarters for chocolate, and now it became my own personal college campus. Now that I was home, I was even more motivated about my college studies. I wrote scene after scene for my "play," which was granting me permission to remember and reflect on happier family times, abuse, moments in the Columbia ICU I didn't even think I had been awake for.

I was also unexpectedly thriving in another class: The Science of Stress—a science I was about to "officially learn" but felt all too familiar with. I had never set foot in the science building and tried to not let the lab setup or hieroglyphic-like charts plastering the hallways intimidate me. But one poster of a prokaryotic cell filled me with nostalgia.

My science mind was definitely put to the test, as well as my acting skills, as I pretended I knew exactly how to use equipment on those dreaded lab days.

"Class, your final project is going to be a very involved research dissertation on anything we've discussed in class you'd like to explore further."

What did that mean? More labs?

I thought about my own stress now and the stress I had felt since high school. What did I want to "investigate further?" We had learned how stress and the sympathetic nervous system interact with the digestive system to increase the risk of ulcers and involves the circulatory and cardiovascular system.

I remembered one line written in a review of *Gutless & Grateful*'s New York premiere:

"Although there is, of course, a connection between mind and body, it was somewhat hard to swallow that the source of her illness could be blamed on being raped, which was implied at the beginning."

I had felt hurt when I read this on my phone on the way to the final performance. Was she making jest on the theory that even *doctors* were leaning towards? When people heard about my crazy story, the first question they asked was, "Well, what caused your stomach to explode?" I wasn't sure. But something in this science course pulled me to investigate it.

I started researching everything—PTSD, parasympathetic nervous system, ulcer, stress, sexual abuse, digestive disorder, cardiovascular system—but nothing seemed to click.

Who else would write a paper on a theory that their stomach exploded from PTSD? It took courage and commitment to decide to prove that the body-mind connection explained my body's violent physical reaction that led to a coma, immediately following being sexually abused for months.

Stress affects the nervous system in various ways. There is significant data to show that a sustained stress on the system, such as in PTSD, can create severe health problems, particularly in the digestive tract. When someone is traumatized, they go into a fight or flight response. In this time of panic, the heart rate increases, and the digestive system stops activity.

My eyes widened as one study I read began to discuss the freeze response: *"However, in trauma, the body never returns to homeostasis, as it believes that it is still in a threatened state. When the HPA axis is activated in trauma for a prolonged period of time, it can lead to digestive malfunctions."*

The more I researched, the clearer this was becoming. Maybe my instincts were right all along. It was startling yet liberating. My duty as both science student and playwright was to illustrate what appeared so clearly to me. My playwriting professor and I delved through every study side by side.

"Elly! Do you believe now trauma can affect you like this? That *has* to explain—"

"Amy, for a playwright, this is GOLD!"

I was addicted to researching this "science of stress"—for arts' sake and my own. I discovered another book, *Why Zebras Don't Get Ulcers*, after being struck by the back cover:

> *In a fascinating look at the science of stress, biologist Robert Sapolsky presents an intriguing case, that people develop such diseases partly because our bodies aren't designed for the constant stresses of a modern-day life—like sitting in daily traffic jams or growing up in poverty. Rather, they seem more built for the kind of short-term stress faced by a zebra—like outrunning a lion.*

I remembered those same panicked feelings outrunning my imaginary "hitmen" in high school. Keeping secrets had made me sick. *Storage*—yes, that would be the name of my play! My Science of Stress class inspired newfound confidence in my playwriting and my own healing process, fueled by science and psychology. I was unlocking secrets in storage and writing them outward, into the world.

I wanted to come to terms with all the parts of me that had gotten "cut off"—the innocent teenage girl who had "left her body" after being molested by a trusted mentor and the unrecognizable shadow of a former self that awoke from a coma several months later. I thought it might be interesting to explore the idea of being "frozen"—how when I was molested, I did not fight or flee. Freezing was the only way I could protect my innocence and once mellifluent world.

Gutless & Grateful brought key moments of my medical recovery together to share a hope-filled story of resilience. That resilience now readied me to write a play which could set those stored-up pains and losses free.

I tried to recreate the experience of how my memories surfaced—in images and sounds—for the stage. Through my characters, I could play out accepting my abuser's betrayal as well as my physical body's sudden change. Scene by scene, I could grieve what was lost. Creating the characters, I could orchestrate the two parts of me which had ignored each other for so long, making amends and moving forward together, into the future.

Midway through completing *Storage*, I came across my brother Jeff's journal that he had written on my laptop while I was in the hospital. A day-by-day account of the first seventy-two days of my coma, it was hard for me to read. But I couldn't stop. I went back into my notes with Rita, all of my typed up journal entries, and even interviewed my family on where they were that awful first night.

Every line I wrote brought up more memories. The more uncomfortable I felt, the more I realized I needed to face them.

Thriving Amy: I trust myself. I have a vast amount of resources hidden inside. My trees keep me safe in their enchanted forest community.
Wounded Amy: I need someone to keep me safe.

It wasn't long before I discovered a problem in the script. Thriving Amy was a powerful, woman, while Wounded Amy was a neglected child. Thriving Amy and I needed to have a little powwow.

Imagine you are talking to a two-year-old. Would you really expect her to know things everyone else does? Just cradle her in your arms. Just listen to Wounded Amy. Reassure her that she isn't alone.

As these script problems came to light, they revealed the holes in my own healing, and through each careful revision, I was learning how to take care of myself.

Thriving Amy: (now facing the truth)—What happened Amy? What happened to us?

Wounded Amy: I don't know. It was too much for me. I had to ...leave you I guess—I couldn't face it.

In just acknowledging the presence of these various parts of me, I was touching a part of myself I had avoided for years.

After my first college term ended, I continued working on my play.

Armed with a thirty-page thesis for my Science of Stress class, I "unstored" my inner knowing that trauma had a physical aftermath. I added the final "confrontation scene" between my pre-coma and post-coma selves which brought everything to a head. As much as I despised certain physical and emotional aspects of my coma self, I had to accept her.

While my play was helping me resolve the split inside me, I had to move forward as "engaged Amy" because Ryan was the man I wanted to be there for. With that frightening trust in my heart, I pushed myself to write a scene for myself that ultimately would not make it into the final script. Thriving and Wounded Amy finally learned to accept and embrace one another— something I was, as Rita always described, dipping my toes into.

I had finally finished my first college term, albeit at home. I missed the friends I had made and felt isolated not being on campus. But I was still bursting with creativity. Ryan and I cooked up a storm for Thanksgiving. This time, I could actually eat all thirty-two food items on our menu!

November 28, 2013—Nice Thanksgiving. Woke up with Ryan and went to Whole Foods, met Jeff at the diner, then went home and cooked up a tornado! Minestrone, pumpkin pie, and mashed potatoes. So grateful to share it with Ryan. Watched old home movies and then we went upstairs and read a Jewish wedding book with Ryan.

Family was back in my life, and I was doing school from home. The days were for coursework, and at night Ryan and I would have our silly fun, writing food parodies to sing at our favorite restaurants. I was loving my life.

As I dove deeper into my play, I continued unearthing traumatic memories. As hard as it was for me to read, I kept going back to Jeff's journal, imagining what it was like for my entire family to sit with the minute-to-minute uncertainty of my near-fatal condition. That led me to imagining my brothers' own reactions when my mother finally told them I was abused. Writing this play became my new healing process. Just like crafting the arc of *Gutless* helped me reach the next threshold in my life, this play was going to do the rest of the work.

CHAPTER 48

Turning My Life into a Story

I WAS RECLAIMING SO MUCH happiness that now, I had to give some back. Performing *Gutless* had seemed to inspire people, but I what could I do now consistently to have a positive impact on people? Blogging, which I had started after my *Journey Into Daylight* art show, became my new way of journaling and a way to offer something to the public instead of just writing pages and pages in a private notebook.

What mattered to me most now? Wedding planning. Like everything else I did, I wanted this to be a creatively out-of-the-box celebration. I started brainstorming right away. But there were still medical questions that needed answers. Although I was "functioning" in spite of my fistula, I didn't want this leak left unresolved, so my dad kept writing to medical professionals across the country until a doctor in Georgetown agreed to see us. Ryan and I spent the entire Amtrak ride studying Jewish prayer books.

At the appointment, we once again endured the exhaustion of chronicling my entire medical history and trying to brainstorm a plan that might make things better for me. The doctors started talking about small bowel *transplants*, stopping eating and drinking, ramping up the TPN IV nutrition, and everything else I didn't want to hear.

Having Ryan there was my way of showing the doctor that I was a real person who deserved to get better. We left the office with no answers—just another stomach obstruction, so the train ride home was spent in more pain. But the search for a medical miracle continued, taking us from DC to Houston Medical Center, where there were even fewer answers for us—at least ones I wanted to hear.

At any medical appointment, no matter how far I had come, it was always hard not to feel like a faceless, weak, useless patient again.

To pass the days that seemed to whirl on perpetually with no medical answers, and savor each moment leading up to my wedding day, I started keeping a line-a-day journal.

After ten days, I looked back at my daily journal and with each entry, I had to wonder if I was rushing into things with Ryan. In that moment it didn't matter. I was so happy with our life together that I pushed right past it.

I had once Googled in the hospital, "How do I find myself?" Now, college was the new searching ground to find my "calling."

January 17, 2014—I've submitted Gutless & Grateful to the United Solo Festival in New York for next fall. I got my final evaluations back from Hampshire and passed my first term of college! I submitted my story to a bunch of magazines and to Katie Couric. I hope something comes through. Ryan and I went to temple at night, and then we watched Comedy Central.
January 20, 2014—Ryan and I started to pick out our registry.

After an adventure-packed winter holiday, the transition back to school would prove challenging, especially because my fistula kept getting obstructed. Because my digestive system did not work on peristalsis like an intact system, I would eat food and it would sit at the bottom of my make-shift stomach and not move through me unless I moved around.

Now that I was eating out at restaurants, sampling different foods, and sitting down every now and then, I was getting sick more and more. I had yet to gain the thirty pounds I lost after my surgery, and I knew going back to school would be a struggle, especially with stomach aches at least once a week. I had to be practical, so as much as I wanted to be a college kid, I couldn't stay on campus all the time—not for my body and not for my en-gaged lifestyle. I crammed my courses into three days so I would be able to come home for part of the week and be with Ryan.

Despite my best efforts to stay healthy, my draining wound continued to deplete me, causing my weight to drop even on IV nutrition. As I got weaker, I once again had to make my term an independent study. I still came in once a week for my Teaching Art to Children class, where I went to teach an art class at a local Amherst elementary school. These brief visits to campus were bittersweet—tiny glimpses of a life I badly wanted. On the flipside, as much as I would have liked to throw myself into being a college student, I couldn't imagine life without my future husband. No longer isolated, I felt the pull that people had in my life now—in both directions.

I also wanted to start reclaiming ownership over my own situation. I had to learn to take care of whatever body I had at the moment. Ryan wanted to know everything about me, and while I didn't tell him everything I did share a lot. Part of me was relieved that I could unload all these memories, but part of me was also surprised because I hadn't realized I had these memories un-til I started to talk about them. I knew healing could not exist in a vacuum, but I also realized that having someone to share with openly was another layer of healing.

Now that I was feeling more like myself, it felt safe to get back into the theatre world. Every Wednesday, I'd jump on a train to Harlem to catch my brother, Matt, play piano for amateur night at the Apollo Theatre. Once in a while, the emcee would ask me to come up on stage and tap dance, much to my brother's embarrassment. This Wednesday night was Broadway-themed, where all the contestants were required to sing songs from musicals. What could be better? I never expected to be triggered by the first musical theatre song a contestant sang. I burst out in tears from flashbacks of old voice lessons, shattered trust, and a life forever lost, all because of a Broadway showtune. But then I realized, with a fiancé, a sense of self growing by the day, and firmer footing in the real world, that maybe being "triggered" by certain childhood memories wasn't such an uncommon event. Don't we all come across childhood photos and wish things could be as simple as a fourth-grade talent show, or a polaroid snapshot of a family dinner?

I got out a pen and started to map out the past ten years on a newspaper lying out on the table. It started with a dot—my first emergency surgery on April 25, 2005. The dot turned into a shaky line following a tumultuous path as I recalled doctors fighting to save my life. The wobbly line gradually branched into different directions as I recalled people I met, experiences I had that happened as a result of my life's detour. My line grew thicker and bolder as I pressed my pen harder onto the newspaper, realizing the strength I acquired, the wisdom I gained, and the maturity I grew into because of my experiences.

Suddenly, this line turned into a splatter all across the newspaper, as I saw one "unlucky" event unfold into millions of tiny little branches—more people I had met, places I had been, things I had done, lessons I had learned, feelings I had experienced, all because of one initial breaking point that separated the life I had "planned" from the life that followed.

I stepped away and looked back at the newspaper, now a mess with frantic scribbles, lines, and arrows. In the past ten years, one event had snowballed into a whole series of experiences that have made me who I am today. And then it all became clear to me. Looking back on the "unlucky" events in my life, I still wouldn't have it any other way. And it's not because I'm "happy" with everything that has taken place. If I hadn't gone through A, B, and C, maybe I wouldn't have all of these scars. But would I still have met the amazing people who have come into my life?

I had officially finished my first year of college, and I was determined to finish all four years! Before this milestone, every goal had seemed like a pipe dream, but this time, my body—even though it wavered—didn't let me down. I was capable of following through.

But now, this summer was going to be all about celebrating our wedding, only a year away. The first way to celebrate? Engagement party. Maybe there could be a happy ending.

Flying with Medical "Exceptions"

We were getting ready to fly out to North Carolina to see the Convatec plant and celebrate the Great Comebacks Eastern Regional ceremony, where I would speak publicly about having an ostomy for the very first time. I knew this would be a powerful experience, but nothing could have prepared me for its impact. The problem was getting there. Flying was always an ordeal, not only for the medical supplies that always stopped the TSA, but also the gallons of food and drink I had to take with me even for a three-hour plane ride. New York Presbyterian Hospital even made me take a note for TSA agents that included a line about "a history of gangrene" in my stomach.

Luckily that letter did what it was supposed to do and I made it to North Carolina.

"Lights up" for Great Comebacks

The schedule for Great Comebacks included a video shoot handled by Town Square Productions. Great Comebacks described them as "a heavy hitter in the film industry." I was beyond excited. The other ostomates at the ceremony were young, bold, fearless leaders. I knew I was tough, but there's something to be said for meeting other people with similar conditions, and knowing you're not doing this alone.

Being the Eastern Regional Recipient changed my perspective on any kind of "baggage."

I met a beautiful fashion model, a dancer, a teacher, a nurse, inventors, and warriors, all of whom were enthusiastic, vivacious souls. And they were so proud of their ostomies and grateful that their ostomies enabled them to lead such happy, healthy, and full lives.

So much of my own story was unknown to the outside world. Nobody knew I had spent hours in the bathroom changing my bags every morning. Nobody knew how I had locked myself in my room and journaled obsessively to avoid being exposed to the outside world where normal people could eat and drink freely. It felt wonderful to share what coping with my medical situation was like for me. It also felt wonderful to gush about my father's tireless efforts to advocate for my health and save my life. When I got home, I was ready to start doing press for my show at United Solo Festival. Everything seemed to happen at once—school, wedding, vacations, *Gutless & Grateful*—and I wanted to make sure that I was still present enough to absorb and appreciate it all.

After Greensboro, it was my dad's turn to have surgery—for long-standing back pain. Instantly, my PTSD kicked in as I worried about the outcome. Surgery is always risky. Even worse, I didn't want my father to be on the patient side of what I had gone through. As hard as my surgeries were, it is equally hard—in a different way—for the family that sits by your side watching you.

I had made it. But neither Ryan nor I could have anticipated such an incredible vacation. To our surprise, I even gained some weight while I was there. And I got to show Ryan my world by having him join me at my speaking event for National Convention of Wound, Ostomy, and Continence Nurses. Maybe all my digestive system needed was for me to be happy—body and mind were finally connecting.

My body couldn't do all the things I wanted it to and most likely never would. But thanks to Great Comebacks, I had a new perspective on my condition and a new, positive present—so positive that I wanted to stay in it. Great Comebacks taught me to be proud, to be honest, and to love myself.

I had made it. I had made the great comeback. And with our wedding exactly a year from now, I knew that everything would do exactly that— COME BACK.

CHAPTER 49

Enchanted with Life

I WAS NEVER A GIRL who had dreamed of a magical wedding day in a fairytale ball gown, but I allowed myself to indulge in the fantasy. Was it possible to want something you never thought you'd care about? I realized that rather than just a celebration of two souls united as one, this was actually my own homecoming, coming home to the life I had fought for all along—I just hadn't known exactly what it could look like. Maybe this was it! This wedding would connect me to family, my roots, legacy, and with Grandma. I envisioned myself raising a family as my parents had so lovingly did, bringing us to temple, lighting Shabbat candles, celebrating Passovers, and cooking dinners from scratch. In a life that had changed drastically over the years, where I had questioned faith, trust, my body, my purpose, and life's overall plan for me, marriage was stability.

I also used my wedding as an opportunity to feel feminine again, to reconnect with long lost friends and to really feel like I was coming into my own as a woman. Old acquaintances were reaching out to me with their congratulations, and I constantly reimagined my future and the woman I was meant to be. My self was changing as quickly as the days—from survivor saved by the world of creativity, to finding independence as a college student and dating, and now a wife with a new sense of family. But with each day medically, I was dwindling, still unable to stabilize nutritionally or to get a break from my outpouring fistulas. I wanted to be the picture of health on my wedding day and be momentarily free of the constant worrying, empty-ing, guarding, and changing of the two bags on my torso—just one day unburdened by even the thought of them.

The idea of wedding dress shopping was exciting at first—after all, I had walked past my mom's television enough times and overheard the squeals of brides to be on TLC's *Say Yes to the Dress*. Admittedly, I did feel some girlish excitement scrolling through Pinterest pages, flipping through magazines, and ripping out ads with the latest backless dress designs. But I quickly be-came discouraged as I looked at gown after gown and wondered how my medical equipment would fit inside a tight, beaded bodice. Each photo I looked at seemed to promote skin and shape. How would a backless gown look with a colossal surgical scar down my back? And how could I wear six-inch stilettos after going through severe neuropathy, which I experienced after being left on my right side for six months while I laid in a bed, coma-tose?

Walking into my first bridal store and trying to fit my body—bags and all—into those tight little dresses was a rude awakening. In the real world, beauty comes in all shapes, sizes, colors and circumstances. In the wedding world, beauty becomes much narrower and free of ostomy bags and fistula bandages.

It wasn't my future husband I was trying to impress—he knew my white Asics were my "dress up shoes." It wasn't my mother who did everything she could to make me feel like every other bride. It was me. I had done more in these ten years than most people do in a lifetime, and I still wasn't happy with myself. I was angry at my body—frustrated that I couldn't just be like everyone else. As a bride, I had longed to feel as feminine as a life-size Barbie Doll complete with voluptuous, womanly curves. Now I was wishing I had chosen December as my wedding month just so I would have an excuse to bury myself in a furry, winter white cape.

I basically wanted to look like a giant wedding cake. The dress had to have enough give for my ostomy bags, which expanded whenever I ate. After a snide comment from a bridesmaid that I could "always just not eat that day," and a brief pity-party, I told myself that the dress would look as beautiful as I felt in it. Call it my "Why not?" mindset, or maybe my excitement trumping over "thinking things through," but I even threw in an application to my mom's new favorite TLC show, although they didn't go for it. With my medical situation in mind, a local dressmaker and I created the perfect fit.

My dress was not "skin tight," but it fit me in all the right places and embraced the medical bags that were still saving my life.

Now, I had my wedding dress, a performance that October, a second year of school to start, a fiancé to enjoy the summer with—and not enough time! Even my body seemed to be catching onto the infectious joy. I was actually starting to gain weight for the first time in the two years since my surgery! Or maybe it was just all of the Yankee game buffets that my dad was treating us to.

With my health improving, Hampshire was able to work out an attendance plan where I could even live on campus part time for the upcoming semester.

But with every positive trend came the downward plummet as my nutrition unexpectedly wavered again. Living with a fistula meant constant worry and wonder if my body would choose to cooperate and absorb everything I was eating. Back in Connecticut, Ryan and I spent one August afternoon running through Norwalk's Cranbury Park jumping over fences, skipping down rolling hills, and chasing each other behind an endless expanse of trees—it was probably the most fun you could ever have doing an engagement photo shoot. But by the time the photographer had finished all the pictures, I started to feel lightheaded. Crisis escalated quickly and that night was spent in Bridgeport Hospital where, for the next week, I would be treated for another terrible PICC line infection—my twelfth.

The infection was treated and it wasn't long before I was back to my punchy self, restlessly pacing the hospital hallways ready to dash out of the unit. Because having a PICC line exposed me to potentially deadly infections, my family would look out for symptoms that overtook me all at once—fever, shaking chills, a racing heartbeat, confusion, change in behavior, skin rash. I was discharged from the hospital, and rushed to meet Ryan with our wedding planner, where she remarked that I (still on IV antibiotics) had more energy than he did.

It was a difficult transition to school. My open wound was getting unwieldy to maintain and trying to keep up my health and maintenance in a college dorm was becoming more of a stretch as my fistula worsened. Changing bags was now taking me a full ninety minutes every morning, and with every slight tweak or fidget, the bag would leak and swallow up another hour. I was spending hours running back and forth between my classes and the bathroom. I was also getting a monthly overgrowth of bacteria which would instantly obstruct my system and leave me cringing in pain for forty-eight hour stretches.

Because Hampshire grown familiar with my work ethic, the administration was willing to discuss how they could accommodate me so I could finish another year.

My mind bounced back and forth between classes and my soon-to-be-husband. Study hours were filled with both writing term papers and composing quirky love songs I'd send him on his work voicemail.

As my wedding approached, my relationship with my father was changing by the day. He was happy for me, but I could sense his concerns as he tried to find more answers to healing my fistula. I had reached a place of acceptance long ago that my parents couldn't fix everything. Yet, there was still a glimmer of hope in me that Dr. Dad would come to the rescue, and maybe if he called the right doctors, we would be on our way.

Gutless & Grateful was back in my life, old hat by now but a big spark to look forward to and a distraction from the inescapable fear that my body would never fully heal.

October 10, 2014—My show is tomorrow! Bonded with Dad today. I love how we can be on equal footing now and talk about adult things. I love how proud my parents are of me. After everything I've been through, I still just want to make them proud.

And every time I performed it, I was sharing my story from a different place—sometimes with an IV, sometimes with my parents in the audience, sometimes with my fiancé waiting backstage. The show had taken so many forms and reached so many different people already.

After my show, I went back to school with a twinkle in my eye. My mind expanded with Hampshire's tagline "To Know is Not Enough" and my heart was engaged (in every sense!) with each tiny stimulus I encountered. I had never felt more open to the universe.

My first "psychology" course was a whole new language for "Self"-education. Now, I was reading in a textbook exactly why and how creativity had carved my own path to healing.

Like clockwork, by the end of the school week, I was overcome with chills, my fever spiked, and by 2 a.m., my parents drove three hours up to Hampshire to drive me back home. The next few days were filled with antibiotic

IVs, and within a few days, I'd be restlessly pacing the hospital hallways, ready to start from scratch again. The thrill of "doing it all" wasn't helping my body. One week I was sent home with what I thought was another PICC line infection. My Hampshire committee had already warned me that if I had to do any more independent studies, I would be forced to take a medical leave. I desperately didn't want that to happen.

Gutless & Grateful had meant so much because with great effort, I had actually finished what I started. Yet, even in pulling off my one-woman show, I had taken a forced "break" when doctors persuaded me to try going NPO to heal the never-healed fistula. If everything in life was so exciting, then why did I have to take a "time out?" I was so used to going endlessly like the Energizer Bunny as a way to mark time and cope, but now, I really did want to keep going. Life was getting too good to miss anything!

December 12—I WILL graduate! Just push through a bit more, Amy.

I had thought throughout these years that my life experience was enough of a college education. But Hampshire was pushing me to seek beyond my own experience, giving me the courage to invent my new normal. And the confidence to know that the world needed my unique new normal. By the end of the term, which I managed to get through, I was asked to tie everything together into a formal plan of study.

Having finished another year of college, I was getting close to a new kind of "real" life. It felt okay to "dream bigger!" I took my very first business class—Social Entrepreneurship.

I had never used these two words together before, but when my professor defined a "Social Entrepreneur," it sure sounded a lot like me: "An individual with innovative solutions to society's issues, ambitiously offering new ideas for wide-scale change."

Starting a business and making a living for myself would mean I was a "person"—that magic "role" that everyone else seemed to have in nine-to-five jobs. My own journal entries took a new, business-oriented focus.

I've gotta use what I LOVE and make a real sustained calling out of it, something with a larger reach that might actually help people! I want to make the arts a universal means for expression, communication, and release. I'll learn more about the psychological aftermath of trauma to explore how difficult experiences change our brain chemistry and rewire our thoughts.

I even wrote an article: "28 Lessons Learned in 28 Years Turning Passion to Business," which I was now submitting to other websites besides my own blog. I discovered that I was more confident than I believed when it came to starting a business. Just as I was once intimidated by the thought of getting a college education, I realized that my survival skills were helping me get through anything and make something of myself—as a college grad, wife, artist...and a businesswoman!

CHAPTER 50

Unfinished Business

RITA WAS A FACE FROM THE PAST, but she was speaking to me louder than ever through my play. As my draft passed four hundred pages, I realized how much healing I still had to do. There was a message I was trying to understand through the ongoing dialogues, a still wounded part I didn't want to hear. Would I ever be happy with it unresolved? When I had wrestled with uncertainty at Yale, art had been my savior. So, I turned back to painting and added blogging back into the mix. But this was the first time I was creating not from a place of desperation but from one of love.

Hey everyone! I know it's been a while since I've updated this blog. But now that I am painting, cooking, and having adventures again, I figured now would be a great time to pick it back up!

I was back into art full force. I immediately reached out to every gallery in the area that I could Google. Back in my studio, I covered every jacket and finger in paint, banging canvases against the walls for hours. Yet, this art came from a calmer place than in years past. The trees I continued to paint were flexible, malleable, and changing with the seasons. I was no longer making art as a way to hide from the world, distract myself from not eating, or mark time. I was making art to celebrate feeling in sync with the rhythm of life. Maybe this was art's true purpose all along.

Blogging was connecting me to the world in a way it hadn't before Ryan. I wanted to share what I had been through with a purpose—to empower others to get through their own obstacles and thrive in spite of them. I tried to end each blog entry with a question—a "call to action" to my "audience" and a helpful tip that had inspired me along the way. People were starting to catch onto my message now. I was thrilled when I started getting comments from people who were actually affected by what I was sharing.

Continuing my blog where I had left off years ago was a way of rewriting my history and heading for a bright, new triumphant finish. Suddenly, past, present, and future were aligned. When online readers started to comment daily that I was helping them, or even that my art inspired them to want to try painting themselves, I was hooked.

"Your story is moving, scary, and exciting all at once. You yourself are a miracle in action."

Guiding people through a journey that I was still learning how to navigate myself gave art a whole new dimension. I could make my mark on the world not just by making an artistic contribution but also by helping other people. That was my "aha" moment. The flipside of gratitude was being able to give back.

"Your strength is so beautiful! I connected completely with your story."
"I am inspired by how you continue to show up, no matter what life has offered you as a challenge."

I would go through my day taking nature walks and running down to my art studio waiting for the lessons to come to me that I could share with my followers on the web. Every post strengthened my connections to the world

I wanted to belong to. As I went from survivor to warrior to role model, I still couldn't leave a painting without adding teardrop somewhere.

Studying Art?

By now I had painted hundreds of canvases, exhibited my work, and won prizes at juried art shows, but I had never taken an art class. College was the place to try new things, so I enrolled in Painting Into Abstraction. Until now, I had managed to make art by banging around a canvas covered in smears of paint. How would my toilet paper collage art look when compared to actual art students?

I seemed to be the only student who couldn't namedrop twenty artists in a row or critique the newest postmodernism exhibit at MoMA. I became good at smiling, nodding, taking notes, and chiming in after I'd done a quick Google search to make sure I knew what everyone was talking about.

I set up my studio by the sink, and within minutes, I had saturated the sink, countertop, and my clothes with an acrylic set I'd brought from home. My professor stood behind me as I engrossed myself up in non-stop brushstrokes and smears.

"Amy, what if you just...stopped?"

"Here?" I hadn't filled the canvas yet.

"Just see what happens."

I sadly dropped my paintbrush and stared at my "devastatingly bare" canvas.

"That's art." He smiled and walked away.

I also continued to bring scavenging into my art, a trick I first learned in the hospital, where my finishing touches were always whatever scraps, wrappers or "garbage" I could find.

"Amy, you seem to use excess gleefully."

"Um. Thanks!"

"Rather than compress your polychrome, complex ideas on a flat canvas, how about giving sculpture a try? Have you done sculpting before?"

For my debut as a sculptor, I visited HomeGoods, the place where I had once purchased tchotchkes and home furnishings to make my home "sacred," and picked up a $10 globe. Ryan had gotten me so fascinated with spackle that I covered the globe in it along with crumpled paper towels and acrylic paint to create an actual "singing tree."

Somehow, I had made it through my first art class. With flying colors...and painted trees.

Finally, I heard back from one of the many local galleries I had reached out to. The reply came from a total stranger who would become a life-changing friend. Jeanine had written back with genuine enthusiasm. She actually wanted to read my never-ending stream of consciousness journals! She insisted on coming over to my house, where she looked at every painting with such curiosity. What would she, someone with an actual art background, think of my work? I felt nervous yet giddy that I was about to receive a kind of "validation" I didn't even know I wanted.

At one point, the wet oil paint (I hadn't known oil paint never dries) got all over Jeanine's designer cashmere sweater. She mentioned casually that it wouldn't wash out (maybe I should have paid a bit more attention in my art class at Hampshire), but she left laughing. And that's how a true mentor came into in my life.

The eclectic mix of people filling my days created a safety net where even when life grew shaky, I couldn't fall. Even though, at times, numbness was a more comfortable choice, Jeanine reinforced my trust that loyal relationships were always possible, and once you found them, irreplaceable.

Jeanine's hardest piece of advice echoed what my Hampshire professor had said.

> *I have been advised by some real painting pros, that I should stretch myself and try to be more minimalistic with my art. WHAT?! And let me just say that it's harder than it looks! (For me.)*

Jeanine coined me "AmyWhirl" to describe my constant rush of busy creativity. Creatively my mind was flourishing but there were still no answers for my fistula. As a result, I was becoming dissociated again, as I tried to bridge the gap between the two worlds of a fulfilling creative life and one of endless medical uncertainty. No matter how hard I tried, I couldn't find the right ending to my play because I had not gotten to an end point myself. How would Thriving Amy and Wounded Amy unite? After Blaine's betrayal, I learned that *you* are the only person worthy of being placed on an all-trusting pedestal. How could my characters express that difficult lesson? I remembered how art expressed what was too painful for words. I needed images to write what even dialogue could not.

Certain images that had pervaded my nightmares were now emerging in my play. I remembered the stark lights in the hospital, how paralyzed and devoid of feeling I was. I remembered that one idyllic pre-coma Berkshires trip with Matt and how I would build up the majestically dreamlike qualities of those rolling hills each time I revisited that memory. I contrasted the grimly sterile hospital to the Berkshires, always bright and full-of-life, until a wolf, Blaine, preys on the play's protagonist, now, "Patricia." When the wolf finds his prey, the Berkshires dissolve into a dark, haunted forest.

Playwriting was now a safe container to explore these awful memories again, another powerful tool in my healing vortex, and the anchor I discovered when I needed it the most, especially with marriage on the horizon.

As every form of creativity helped me continue to reframe my circumstances, I realized the anchor I needed all along...was just me.

CHAPTER 51

Artists *Talk?*

MOUNTING MY FIRST ART SHOW, *Journey Into Daylight*, right out of Yale, was a personal milestone. I had amassed just as much work, but my art had grown, reflecting another turn in my detour. After reaching out to basically every gallery in Fairfield County, I had found a local café, interested in displaying my work *and* having me give an "artist talk."

Making art sparked many self-revelations, just as performing *Gutless & Grateful* had been years before. Sharing my art was another great discovery, but now—I had to talk about it? Art was always my way of expressing exactly what I couldn't put into words. That was the point! What was I supposed to say about what I was too vulnerable to express in actual speech? When I nervously made my way to the lounge, where I would be "speaking." The café owner approached me casually, "Just talk a bit about your art, and what it means to you..."

Trees had always been a strong presence in my art. So that's where I started. I began to describe what I liked to paint and why, and how I discovered painting in the first place. Jeanine came to watch and pulled me aside during the reception.

"As soon as you get into a room, people think they know your story right away—okay, she's anorexic, and this is how she recovered. Then, you drop the bomb about your stomach and their mouths fall open—they're not really sure what to say. But then, just watch the shift in awareness that washes over the crowd as you transcend your story and explain your ideas, and how you healed. By the end, you win them over with your spirit and they are completely in love with you."

She was right. Once I started telling my story, infusing my words with the passion that overflowed into everything I did, I seemed to be opening up their hearts and their minds. I learned that it's very human to want to judge one another, or to throw a label on something, but the wonderful part of being human is knowing that we all have the capacity to open our hearts once we listen.

Painting was Tiger Lily's new warrior routine. As canvases filled, so did my hopes for what lay ahead.

I couldn't get enough of connection in every respect. While my blog was my forum for sharing and connecting, my art studio was my space for continued self-discovery and reinvention. Every day, my canvas taught me another lesson about coming into the world.

Today's blog: The words "I Will Be Free" came to me after seeing how I felt after painting this. It was so liberating dancing around juggling three big canvases in my hands. This was my manifestation for every remaining moment of my life—to constantly seek more freedom from the limitations we place on ourselves every day—even limits we don't know we are setting.

Once I left the studio, whatever I had created stayed with me and set the groundwork for what I needed to learn for myself that day.

Blogging gave my days a refreshing lightness. As I shared my experience with an unknown audience, I was drawing a healthy distance from it. Especially as the ten-year mark came nearer, I couldn't wait to dig into that secret bag of goodies from my past every morning. Each blog sentence was followed by an exclamation point in this virtual show and tell. The greatest excitement every morning was waking up to total strangers' responses:

"The more I check out your artwork, the more I fall in love."

Although I was struggling, as always, with nutrition, still on TPN, and corresponding with Houston doctors to try to get a hold of this wound, my weight was slowly improving. By now I had realized that everything eventually comes back, but sometimes it takes more time than you'd like. I was determined to feel beautiful on my wedding day. I had to gain back all I had lost after this awful mistake of a twenty-seventh surgery.

By now, Jeanine and I had developed a close friendship. She had been the first person to discover my art and take me into the world of real artists, where now I was more than the girl who collaged with toilet paper. Jeanine told me I had finally outgrown the kiddie craft paints I had used in hospitals, and refined me, while still encouraging my spunky kidlike spirit.

"AmyWhirl—I'm putting together an art salon. I think you'll really like these people. It'd be amazing for you to meet other artists using what they do to heal."

"That sounds exactly like me! So, what is this called?"

"Resilience."

It was the first time I'd thought about that word as an artist, and my initiation into the healing that can only come from community.

As the group gathered together for the first time in one room, it was uncanny how many similarities united us. The biggest struggle for me, as we all discussed trauma, art, resilience, and shared our own stories, was not bursting into, "Oh, me too, I felt that same exact way!" I was only used to rambling for hours in long pages of journal entries in my room. I was still learning the art of engaging in conversation!

It was a whole new energy and awareness learning how to "take in." After months of planning, the day had finally come to perform the Art & the Transformative Power of Resilience Salon. Baking for the post-show reception, I could actually prepare the recipes I had created when I was starving for real food. I wrote a series of monologues, "Five Windows of Resilience," using the five windows surrounding the space to share how creativity had moved me through each hurdle so far. Jeanine introduced me to the crowd as I waited in the back of the room.

"She is an inspirational figure to be sure, but her creativity expands well beyond her story."

Jeanine sat down, and with long windows ahead of me, I started at the first "window" of my journey. As I finished circling the room, I looked at the crowd with the final line, "If I had to do it over again, I wouldn't change a thing."

CHAPTER 52

Recreating... *Me*

I HAD NOW STUDIED PSYCHOLOGY and was seeing post-traumatic growth in action. It was clear that arts could heal what conventional medicine could not. After all, what was conventional medicine doing for my fistula? I was still at a medical low, but my spirit was as high as ever. I had now come out of my story enough to talk about it. I had to help others do the same. I went into my all or nothing mode, Googling speaking opportunities and applying for any conference I could find.

I had performed *Gutless & Grateful* as musical theatre in four states. But ever since its 2012 debut, when people started lining up to tell me their own story, I knew there was something to my show that could teach other people to thrive. Couldn't education be entertaining, too?

During one of my Google binges, I landed on the Transformative Language Arts Network website. I didn't know what calls for "papers," "abstracts" or "proposals" meant. But if I saw "submit," I pressed it. I worked like a dog on the application.

I got in! I was actually crying when I saw my name on the schedule. I don't know why being accepted hit me so much. It felt like, "Wow, I've made it." It's surreal that people are paying for a weekend to take a class with me on the power of words.

For the first time, I was going to be a leader! Passover was approaching and so was the ten-year anniversary of my world changing forever. How was I supposed to feel? A sentence in the Passover Haggadah is, "All who are hungry, come and eat," which starts off the big feast. So, I asked myself, "What are you hungry for?" The Passover Seder is for asking questions and sharing the ancient tale of exile and redemption with people who have not heard it before. Telling this story is a way to pretend like you yourself are escaping from your own personal slavery. I was, in a way, exiled from the life I planned, and now I was finding redemption by creating a new one.

Anniversary Syndrome

Just as I was trying to get my bearings, the ten-year anniversary of my actual trip to the ER was upon me.

Like everyone else, I was growing up and bittersweetly moving on. What I didn't anticipate was that my weight would quickly spiral out of control. Over my birthday weekend, which we had excitedly planned in New York for weeks, my speech got slower as my energy dragged. By Saturday, I was walking on flat concrete to a museum with Ryan, and I had to stop because I was so winded. Even at my worst, I still had the energy of a racehorse. My PICC line was out, and I thought I had been doing better. This had to be the outcome of a bad night's sleep.

As Ryan and I headed to the Guggenheim Museum, I fainted in the middle of the street bruising my face as strangers rushed over to me and asked if I was okay.

Because my wound was draining so much of my nutrition, now my electrolytes were so low that I was in severe danger. I was rushed for another PICC line and a heavy dose of TPN. My body suddenly felt fragile. My voice was gone, and I couldn't even move my fingers. My body had crashed seemingly overnight.

My birthday weekend had turned into a week-long stint at Bridgeport Hospital, but I was not going to let being a patient take me back to the trauma vortex.

Blogging in the Hospital

Yesterday at sundown brought the very end to Yom Hashoah, and even though I was in the hospital, I needed to pay a tribute to my grandparents in some way. So, I set an empty canvas on my hospital bed and filled it with their faces. Thankfully, my labs are back to normal, and the food here ain't bad!

In Bridgeport Hospital, where every admission felt like déjà vu, the bed became my studio desk, and instead of being ashamed of my "setback," I took pride in the lessons I was learning.

Hey, I am truly thankful I am blessed with the miraculous gift of life after such a crazy medical ordeal. What comes with that is the understanding that my body's not a perfect system, so every now and then I need some up-tuning.

Seeking Balance

When I was discharged from hospital this time, I had an awakening, perfectly timed with the spring. My limits had been tested once again, and I came out okay. With every setback in my life—including the big "explosion" exactly ten years prior, I tried to reevaluate how life was going. Maybe this was some kind of sign that I was supposed to slow down, although it was very hard for me to do that, especially with new opportunities popping up every day.

After a week of boosting my nutrition intravenously, Ryan picked me up from the hospital, held my shaky hand, and slowly walked me to the car, as my dad helped him unload all the canvases that I had created during my stay. Ryan guided me up the steps, then surprised me with a planter he pulled out of his truck. Later that day, we sat at our kitchen table together, my huge IV pole towering over us, planting new seeds for spring. As I colored in labels for "azaleas" and "green beans," he tenderly tucked each seed into the fresh soil.

I was planting seeds for my new start.

Being in love was just that—an opportunity to BE and stop obsessively pursuing the next big thing.

But I was also angry. With my wedding only two months away, I looked thinner than a skeleton, I still could barely talk, and my father had to help me up the stairs every night. I just wanted to look beautiful on my wedding day and now I had so frighteningly far to go—at least forty pounds.

I went the next day to the radiologist to get another PICC line inserted. As he did his usual stabbing in my arm trying to find a single vein that wasn't shot, I was sobbing hysterically. He figured it was from the pain of sticking needles in my arm, but I was crying because I had almost made it, and this was *not* going to happen to me just as I was getting married. I would have my wedding day, and my medical crises would not screw this up. When I got in the car with my mom, barely able to move my arm, I screamed at the car roof, shouting at God that he was not going to take away my wedding day.

I was trying, as that rabbi had told me so long ago, to "will it to God," but my cheeks were hollow, my eyes were sunken in, and sitting upright left me winded. I couldn't believe how my body could be so powerful, then lose everything within a few hours. Was I pushing myself too hard? And even if I admitted this to myself, would I ever behave any differently?

I didn't even want Ryan to see me because I was so ashamed of how I looked. My mom would try to take me out of the house for a quick trip out to "lift my spirits," but I refused and stayed in my studio at home because the looks I was getting were sharper than daggers. Once again, I was back in the body where I was perceived as anorexic or too "sick" to be treated as an independent entity, free of pity. Whatever it was, I was not feeling like a bride.

Bachelorette Party...Amy Style

I was never one to party at a club or play drinking games in high school. Besides trivia nights with Ryan, I had never been to a bar. So, I knew my bachelorette party was not going to be like the ones I'd seen in romantic comedies. Besides, I had just gotten out of the hospital and looked like it, too. But sometimes all you need is the love of your mother and some dear friends to make you feel beautiful.

For my bachelorette party my mom and my maid of honor, Sara, planned a full day of surprise, jam-packed with karaoke, a West Village food tour, an "escape the room" mystery game, and Chinese food for dinner. I wasn't in my full body yet, but I was on the way. My cautious parents followed us by car throughout the entire day.

Others Were There for Me—I Was There for Others

At a time when I wanted to hide behind closed doors, I showed up through my blog, where I breathed in the courage to come forward with this setback and my frail shape.

Sometimes I received notes of enthusiasm, condolences, and courage. Sometimes I received no comments at all. But just through the act of coming to my computer, getting these thoughts out, and somehow heard in the universe, I was manifesting the good faith that this setback would lead somewhere.

Just as my mom had made comments in red Sharpie on my printed-out journal entries years ago, her new kind of virtual commenting felt much healthier!

Marilyn Oestreicher April 22, 2015 at 1:32 p.m.— How brave you are to share such personal feelings knowing that you might inspire someone else and their healing!

Ryan and I continued to study the rituals of Judaism as our wedding day got closer, and our talks with the rabbi were transitioning from Jewish philosophy to the practicalities of a Jewish wedding. Everything was coming to fruition.

What I Learned from Being Engaged

With my wedding about two weeks away, I found myself looking back on a three-year whirlwind. Who knew that a little online tinkering could lead to finding the love of my life? I had never had a boyfriend, dated or even gone to a bar. Setting up an online dating profile was more of a creative writing exercise for me than a mission. Yet there was a pull in me to connect, a yearning to feel, to reawaken that "happy carefree" part of me I had as a kid, and ignite a wiser, mature woman in me, a part of me I knew I had to acquire eventually.

The wedding was almost upon us. Prior to the ceremony, we signed a marriage contract, called a ketubah, in the presence of our closest family and friends. Centering myself back in the traditions of Judaism helped re-anchor me in the faith that by the time the wedding approached, things would somehow be better. I took it one day at a time.

And with the TPN, I was looking better and better every day.

It had taken me ten years to reconfigure, reclaim, and re-establish my-self. Now that I was ready to start a new life with a husband, what from my family did I want to take with me?

From my mother, I learned compassion and hope.

From my father, I learned determination and loyalty.

From my grandmother, I learned faith and wisdom.

From my grandfather, I learned humor and creativity.

And I wanted most to show that to my father. I just wasn't sure how. I decided by finding lyrics for our father-daughter dance that could express that sentiment somehow. But where to start?

Down to the Wire—Literally!

The IV nutrition had slowly improved my weight, and although we were all nervous, I got my PICC line taken out the day before my wedding. I wanted to be as free as I could, and with a wound bag that constantly had to be emp-tied under a huge dress, and an ostomy bag that threatened to leak all over the many layers of tulle. I wanted my arms to be just my fair, newlywed skin.

On my wedding day, I felt beautiful. I had gained mostly all my weight back, and I had more bounce in me than the howling rain that night. I man-aged to jump around in my Asics sneakers, in my huge dress with red Swarovski crystals sewed into the bodice, wishing the night would never end.

I wasn't used to holding onto time. As my brothers proudly hoisted me high above the crowd in a chair for a round of Hava Nagila, I realized I wanted to hold onto this moment forever.

As our rabbi brought the two of us together, I looked at my parents—would they cry, would they smile? (And of course, did I win favorite child for getting married first?) My father and I had chosen to dance to "Who Will Love Me As I Am?" from one of our favorite musicals, *Side Show*.

Our rabbi spoke with tears in her eyes, saying that we had taught her much more than we would ever know. As we stood there beneath a chuppah I had made, conducting the ceremony we designed ourselves, I trembled in "fearful awe," as Abraham Heschel—a leading Jewish theologian of his time, would put it—of the power of joy, presence, love, and feeling in the world. I had found that safe space inside of myself, and finally, in the universe.

My mother had brought my grandma's old kitchen robe to the ceremony, which she would always wear in our kitchen in Fairfield, as she'd yell at us to put socks on while cooking us egg noodles. Just before the ceremony, I wrapped her old robe around me and my mother. Wearing my wedding dress, with Grandma's robe, I felt her spirit glimmering as I prepared to say my vows.

I vow to always be the joy dancing in your heart, like the singing flowers I paint, to be the food in your soul, as long as you always replenish it with your stroganoff.
This wedding day is our new beginning as husband and wife, and I can't wait to travel it with you.

I had never felt more "in" the world. And most importantly, after my wedding, I was feeling my grandmother with me more and more every day.

For years, I had stared at that very last picture taken before my coma. Passover 2005: I'm hunched over the kitchen table in pain, and my grandmother is touching my shoulder with that knowing look in her eyes. Now, with her kitchen robe draped over my chair, her unwavering love was guiding my way. And it turned out to be the only guide I needed.

CHAPTER 53

I #LoveMyDetour

CONNECTION MEANT EVERYTHING to me, but I was relieved that my phone was off and tucked away in my room that day. I could actually be present in a situation—a personal milestone! But my no-phone bliss period didn't last long. Even "connection" was all or nothing Amy-mode. I thrived (obsessively, as with everything else) on connection to my blog readers and social media followers.

The day after our wedding, Ryan and I celebrated by doing what we did best: getting food. We pulled up to Subway, and I chowed down on my regular sandwich-—"four times the normal amount of turkey, please"—only now I was wearing a ring. We witnessed two of our friends' weddings over the next month and held each other as our special day was already fading further into memory. The day after my childhood friend married a man she'd met by accident on a plane to Switzerland, we took a honeymoon of our own.

Traveling was never a casual matter for me. We had to ship three huge boxes of medical equipment and another three boxes of my special protein chips and power bars I couldn't get overseas. It wasn't easy eating 8,000 calories of entirely low fat, low sugar nutrition, and it was even harder finding my "staples" in a different country—which is perhaps why my parents had asked if we could "just honeymoon in Disney World" (which would have been okay with me).

But I wasn't going to let my physical limitations narrow my desire to see the world. We considered Thailand, Italy, and a cross-country road trip. Then we both got the idea—although neither of us had ever been—for a cruise! I had heard there were endless buffets all day, my idea of heaven. After ogling travel brochures, we found a Royal Caribbean cruise setting sail from Puerto Rico to a handful of U.S. Virgin Islands.

With my dad the dermatologist, I grew up thinking beaches were skin cancer waiting to happen, so any tropical place was foreign territory to me. At summer camp, I'd been nicknamed Casper—the ghost-like girl who sat at the waterfront with a towel draped over her head.

It was Ryan's idea to spend time in Puerto Rico. He had been participating in Revolutionary War reenactments, and every April he went to the city of Old San Juan and stayed at The Galleria, a rustic inn filled with old sculptures, talking parrots, and stairs of stone. He couldn't wait to take me, and I couldn't wait to go.

I had survived years without a drop of water, but I started to panic as I realized I would be in areas with no cell phone service. What about connection? Wasn't I supposed to be blogging and sharing the exciting and crazy experiences and places my husband and I were exploring together as newlyweds? Before I knew it, my thoughts had spiraled into...

I can't believe I'm sitting here under a tree on an island doing nothing, calling no one, with a perfectly good phone in my hand, a full battery, and no service! What is the point?!

Was I really questioning the meaning and purpose of my honeymoon? My week of nothing but time with the man to whom I had just vowed my life? I was building moments and memories with my husband—memories that no one else needed to know about but us. As much as I felt pulled to stay connected to my tribe and always be a "spokesperson" for all survivors at all times, I tried to remember what my role was at *this* moment. I didn't need pictures, texts or emails. I needed ME to be in those moments. I was the one creating and collecting these memories, not my mobile device. And my heart had infinite room for storage.

When I locked up my phone that night, I unlocked the ability to be present. I had made a life out of escaping all physical sensations. So not only did I lose touch with my physical hunger cues, I also lost touch with my limits. I knew how to either lock myself in my room all day and type in isolation, or incessantly blog, post, and tweet. Balance was as terrifying to me as using my own judgment, and I was still slow to remember how to make choices and trust them.

On our trip, Ryan and I had taken a tour of the rainforest. As we stood atop the plateau and gazed at the greenery below, I was able to gain perspective on the ups and downs of my journey and get a glimpse of the excitement that lay ahead. The journey to love and marriage had been long, but now I was vulnerable and beginning to share my feelings intimately with a trusted friend. I had to let down my guard and lose a layer of numbness that, honestly, I missed at times.

We spent a week taking moonlit walks by the beach, dancing at salsa clubs, and sightseeing. I was *doing* all the things I had watched in movies to pass time in Bridgeport Hospital! But no matter how hard I tried, I still had to deal with bags stuck to my body and needing a bathroom all the time—pretty inconvenient when you're exploring a historic village. It was hard to accept that I no longer had the freedom of a healthy teenage girl. I wondered how, as Ryan and I started leading a life of intimacy in marriage, I would rectify the fact that my body was something I was afraid of.

When our ship made one of its final stops in Aruba, my digestive system became obstructed. Ryan had gone out parasailing that morning, and I was stuck in bed with the same awful pain that had threatened to sabotage my college career. The emergency room in Aruba wasn't equipped for me, so I was flown home. Our honeymoon was over.

Back home, Ryan and I were a couple now, no longer two individual people. The idea of returning home different reminded me of my own personal medical journey. Love had cracked through my numbness, and I was broken open, ready to take everything in.

After the honeymoon, everything in my life seemed to be about finding some kind of closure. I had proven the doctors wrong. But I didn't want to be an exception. I wanted to be proof that miracles can happen, and although doctors may be hesitant to give a patient "false hope" if they don't have "proof," sometimes false hope is the best medicine. If it's all we have, then that's more than enough to stand on.

In addition to being a visiting performer in hospitals, I was now taking *Gutless & Grateful* not to a theatre, but to a conference—the one I had applied to back in April. I booked a flight for me, my parents, Ryan, and Jerold to Kansas City, Missouri to perform my show in a small classroom for participants attending the Transformative Language Arts Network's Power of Words conference. I hadn't known that speakers could get paid for talking to people.

I started overthinking everything. Did I have to make a PowerPoint? Buy a laser pointer? At one point Jerold, my Broadway veteran musical director, rolled his eyes. "You're trying too hard. Just do your show and let it stand on its own." Would that really be enough?

At the last minute, I second-guessed everything, and *Gutless & Grateful* was a sham that had no place in a healing arts conference.

Attendees couldn't learn from musical theatre, right? "Recognizing that we each hold a piece of truth." Those words on TLAN's "About" page resonated with me as the lesson learned through my own experience, which now was my duty to share. My story perhaps only had a fraction of insight in how we bounce back from trauma. I recalled the old Hasidic story about carrying shards of holiness within us.

When we break open, our light not only has the power to come out and be expressed, but to touch, interact, and engage with the light of someone else.

There had to be a sliver of everyone's individual story that could resonate with someone just at the precise time they need to hear it.

So, I added one question to the beginning of my show: *"Have you ever felt something that was too painful to express in words?"*

An astounding four people finally showed up in that classroom, and although it was not exactly a full house, I was thrilled. I was officially a "workshop presenter." This "presentation" proved theatre could inspire others to share their story through their own expressive outlet—the secret that saved my life.

Flying home from Kansas City, I came away with a new sense of confidence. My one-woman show was now a gateway to a new world of opportunities.

Treasured childhood memories were now coming full circle, too. I had my own art exhibit in the Discovery Museum—my childhood go-to place right down the street from my old house in Fairfield. The title? *Tree Dreams*.

My art had moved from healing me to making others happy. Just as the hero's archetypal journey takes an individual out of his society, through hardship, undergoing a transformation in the darkness, and coming back to society with a gift to give, I was repurposing, refining, and developing my own work at these final stages in my journey—or at least, for now. Now married, I was on the "road back" section of the hero's journey, returning to the ordinary world.

By happy accident, my career as a writer and public speaker was off and running. People kept reaching out to me after seeing my show or stopping by an art exhibit. I took advantage of every possible online forum—probably not the best thing for someone who seemed to be addicted to the "submit" button. Before I knew it, my name and my story were all over the Internet, and I was freelance writing for dozens of websites and blogs. I started receiving comments from others who were looking for insights and advice.

These comments motivated me to use my show for something deeper. I rummaged through my old "Social Entrepreneurship" notes from Hampshire and recognized the next step of Tiger Lilly's journey.

My life had changed enough over the past ten years and had actually transformed so much that I could no longer say my life would be "something else" without this "interruption." My mother, when going through the worst of times with me, told me that my medical crisis would someday just be a "blip." Now, the blip had turned into a big, beautiful detour.

Detours have the power to change us through an alternate route, leading us to experiences we could have never known about. But most importantly, on a detour, anything is just as possible—even starting college at twenty-five!

I remembered how driven I was in high school, with a careful plan and a determined focus to carry me through it. Who knew all my college apps would be for nothing? When life suddenly flips on its head, what is the healthiest way to cope? I realized college students going through the transition to adulthood were the audience I needed to reach out to and help them navigate their own detours.

I got home from Kansas City to start my first week back at Hampshire and my third year of college, cramming four classes together in two days, then jumping in the car and heading home to Ryan for the rest of the week. Now, the biggest illness I suffered from was FOMO—fear of missing out. I wanted to be with everyone, go everywhere, and do everything. My body wanted otherwise.

My fistula was at its worse, and my bag would constantly leak when I tried to sit down or even twist to raise my hand in a classroom. And if I wasn't anxious enough about missing interacting with students as a result of zipping back and forth every week, I also had to run back to my dorm multiple times a day to fix leaking bags—the worst kind of "breaking open."

The only hope I had was knowing my father was still occasionally looking for new doctors and my mother's blind optimism. But I had a mission. I knew college could be a stressful time, even for perfectly healthy kids. I saw students all around me who were flustered with the many options, conflicts, and obstacles that college presented.

"Your show's not right for colleges." Jerold told me. "They won't get it. Your show is for theatres."

But I knew college kids would relate. I was technically still a college kid myself!

The more statistics I read about college students dropping out for mental health-related reasons, the more urgent I realized my campus concerns were. Getting the lead role of Nancy in *Oliver* after being discharged from the hospital had saved my life. It gave me a role in a group and in society, reintegrated me with community, and gave me a purpose, a passion, a connection to my aliveness, and a gift to give back to my community. Theatre had revived me. I couldn't think of a better vehicle in which to create a college mental health program!

Just as I had created the warrior's backpack on my own medical journey, I came up with a regimen to help students create their own resiliency toolbox—a must-have to deal with stress and navigate life's detours. In the final component of my program, I introduced students to a panel of counselors, faculty, and wellness resources on campus, opening the channel of communication between the student body and staff to create a more compassionate campus.

How do you learn to love your detours? You follow the path and see where it takes you—that makes you a DETOURIST.

Now that I had that energy within me, the world was going to hear about it. I went to Wikipedia, looked up every college in every state (I kid you not) and found the directory of every college I could. From that directory, I emailed ten relevant contacts, explaining a bit about my "program." For a while, I got radio silence. Then I got a few "warm wishes" and kind words on my "incredible story." Then I got suggestions for people I "should reach out to." I also got "I've forwarded your message to this department." And then, one glorious day, I heard from a college who thought my program "sounded great" and wanted to have a phone conversation with me. As I waited for our 4:30 p.m. call that Tuesday, I was more nervous than I would be at any musical theatre audition. The phone rang, I picked up and enthusiastically told the Student Activities Coordinator about me and "my college program," quickly brimming over with excitement at the confidence I was gaining. As I spoke, I realized how passionate I was about this message reaching the college community. And by the end of our conversation, I felt that *Gutless & Grateful* was perfect material for any college event. Apparently, they didn't.

But that didn't discourage me. I went on to reach out to hundreds and hundreds of schools. And I started getting more replies back, more emails, more phone calls, and more interests. As I corresponded, in a way I was re-framing the narrative of the show and its purpose. I was discovering the mental health messages behind *Gutless & Grateful*.

And by the time I booked my first college, BOY was I ready!

My first "test college" was my own Hampshire College as a "run through" for my big business college program debut. I got together with the Wellness Director and jotted down some ideas:

With my detour mindset, I was able to manage my challenging journey and turn it into something that enhanced my life—an essential coping skill for any college student/student of life. I call people who navigate their detours, "Detourists."

As soon as Jerold played the first few notes, the show came and went in what felt like a minute. My classmates and professors were all seated close to the small stage, laughing as they experienced my journey with me. After the final song, I ran behind the piano, where I had stowed away my carefully typed "presentation outline," and then thought, "I'm just gonna talk." How had gratitude, creativity, and telling my story helped me process what had happened to me? How could what I learned about resilience help others on campus?

I wasn't sure exactly what was going to come out of my mouth, but by the time I finished, even Jerold was impressed. I had proven to myself that my story could empower a college community. I could help students recognize their own set of needs, and their right to be heard. I proudly invited the Wellness Director to join me on stage and we conducted a Q&A on student mental health. This had suddenly fashioned itself into a program that could make a difference. And then I booked my first colleges.

Boston College in February, Haverford College in March, to Clark University in April—this detour was not a dead end. All I needed was me, my laptop, and a red dress—my lucky color. Meeting these students afterwards and swapping stories as we laughed through our shared struggles, I realized that each campus could teach me just as much as I could hope to teach them.

I had only decided that I wanted to turn Gutless & Grateful into a mental health program in September, and a thousand hours of emailing later, I had booked myself for the rest of the year at eleven other schools, while finishing my third year at Hampshire!

With my medical situation I still wasn't sure what the endpoint of my recovery was. Perhaps that's why I still was stalling working on the play I had started at Hampshire. I was uncertain of the ending.

CHAPTER 54

From Hashtag to Mission

RYAN AND I HAD POKED fun at hashtags as silly exchanges wrecking the English language. But hashtags had the power to create positive labels and bring people together. #LoveMyDetour never seemed more right.

Sometimes we feel bogged down because we let the "uniqueness" of our struggles make us feel victimized. Instead, we should find the uniqueness not in the specific obstacle we are facing but in what that obstacle forces us to do. We confuse our circumstance for a character trait or for "who we are." But on detours, we are still us, plus whatever we choose to reap from that new experience. Any kind of detour could be a treasure hunt for those hidden rewards. Detours keep us on our toes, keeping our eyes, hearts and minds open.

I wanted to inspire people to flourish because of rather than in spite of their challenges. So, I started thinking of more reasons to love "life detours."

#LoveMyDetour Takes Off

#LoveMyDetour quickly became a fun way to get people enthusiastic about any sidetrack in their path. After a decade, it wasn't my story that was important to me anymore. It was time to pay it forward.

After a presentation at a Hebrew high school, which I called *Hope as Spirituality Builds Resilience*, a teen girl came up to me in tears, telling me about her friend who, at seventeen, was stuck in hospitals with a chronic condition. She hugged me and told me I reminded her of her friend, wishing her friend could have been there to hear my story. At that moment, I could remember exactly what it felt like to have lost everything and be sure I would never get anything back and life would never change. The idea that I'd be talking about it, with space around and behind me, was a fantasy that I never would have even considered. I was more driven than ever to get this message spread. I was still in awe that I had made it this far.

Maybe my survival strategy wasn't that complicated. Maybe it really was four of the most commonplace words and you might find on a Hallmark card. I came up with my ultimate recipe for resilience: Four Hardcore Skills for Detourists:

1. Gratitude: When you know what you're grateful for, you know what your values are. Your values act like arrows telling you what direction you need to take on your road.

2. Hope: Is a job. It has to be created as a rope to hold onto in difficult times. It's the fuel that propels us down our Detourist path.

3. Creativity: We can create a safe container to be present with experiences we are still coming to terms with. Creative expression gently engages us with emotions that may be too overwhelming for words. You don't need to be an artist to create. You just need an open heart and a mind willing to take a backseat.

4. Stories: Telling our stories helps us process them. We gain confidence through our shared experience, and traveling is always less scary with a partner.

Even if you're not ready to share your story, read a book. Hear about the courageous adventures of others. We learn by example, so when that detour surprises you, you'll be able to pull those heroic stories out of your back pocket to guide your own hero's journey. I also reminded students that long-term mindsets come with baby steps:

1. Find one thing what makes you grateful.
2. Be willing to fabricate hope when you can't find it.
3. Get creative and express yourself with a quick doodle.
4. Swap some stories.

Thinking back, I realized that these four strategies were intricate threads woven throughout every peak and valley of my journey that had kept me afloat. Gratitude, hope, creativity, and stories could transform our struggles into gifts that would make life worth living again.

I had already presented *Gutless & Grateful* at a conference on storytelling and healing. Now that I had picked up an interest in mental health, I was ready to apply to the big guys. I looked up PTSD and mental health conferences and kept on submitting proposals, even for highly rewarding and mostly unpaid gigs. I applied to dozens of conferences and received rejections as well as acceptances. But in each proposal, I was once again rewriting my narrative.

I treated each conference application as a writing exercise by listing key objectives and the gifts of traumas for myself. And then the idea of delivering a workshop to others to share the gifts of what I had learned made everything seem worthwhile. Maybe that is what the psychic meant when she said I was to be a "wounded healer."

I got my first mental health conference and started presenting on art therapy, psychology, PTSD, post-traumatic growth, yoga, music, and storytelling. Even better than presenting was being able to go to these conferences and meet people who were as passionate as I was about making an impact. This was a new way to feel a part of the world.

I had searched for a definition of "happiness" for so many years. Finally, I decided I was happy because I was present. Learning to find the beauty in the detours was learning how to be alive, how to find the miracles in whatever path I took. Post-traumatic growth was the most thrilling detour of all.

CHAPTER 55

Coming to Terms with Abuse

TALKING TO STUDENTS—and in particular sexual assault survivors—about "finding the upside of trauma" was energizing, but it had an unexpected side effect—bringing up flashbacks of my own abuse. When students came up to me, relating their personal story to something I shared, I remembered scenes from high school, which felt like a far off, castaway world. After my performance at Russell Sage College, a student shyly approached me and shared how she was struggling with an eating disorder on campus. Hearing my story, she said, gave her a new appreciation of the value of food in her life. I hugged the girl tightly, and as she walked away, I found myself in another world, eleven years earlier.

* * *

My teenage self was walking out of my pediatrician's office. "Ninety-one pounds?" I burst out crying hysterically. What was going on?

I had gone for my routine physical and expected it to be just that—routine. A few weeks earlier, my English teacher had commented, "You've lost a bit of weight." On my actor resumé, I listed my weight at 118 pounds, average for my age and size. I never weighed myself at home, and now the scale in the doctor's office told me I had dropped nearly 25% of my body weight.

My first thought, after drying my tears, was "I just have to eat more." And I tried. But surprisingly, it was hard. This was the first time I became conscious that, since Blaine started abusing me, I had nearly stopped eating. My mother hadn't noticed, but now the doctor's scale revealed the truth. Blaine had caused me to avoid any emotion or physical feeling in my body. Chewing was the most emotionally painful thing I could do because it involved all my muscles and organs—my teeth crunching up the food, feeling the mush ooze down your throat, and of course, digesting. Chewing reminded me that my body existed. I was so resentful of my body, which held feelings of guilt, dirtiness, and denial, that my shoulders shuddered with disgust any time Blaine's transformation from mentor to monster crossed my mind.

What Blaine had done was too much to digest.

My family was concerned after my visit to the doctor, but Blaine quickly offered a reason for my weight loss.

"She's anorexic," he told my mom. "Typical at this age."

Me, anorexic? The girl who had loved every part of her body as a singing, dancing, fireball of energy? Blaine had me just where he wanted me. To my horror, my mom fell for it, and believed that I, not Blaine, was the crazy, disordered one. Now she was calling him every night for advice on what to do with her troubled daughter. Blaine told her to get me to a psychiatrist, which she did.

I told the psychiatrist I wanted to gain weight as quickly and efficiently as possible.

"Oh, really," she tested me, barely looking up from her notepad. I could tell she had already made up her mind and was stereotyping me, assuming I was terrified of being fat.

"Yes, really." I didn't know what else to say. I just wanted to feel normal and healthy again.

"Well, food won't be efficient. My recommendation is to do a strict diet of just Ensures. Four thousand calories worth. Can you do that?"

I didn't know what an Ensure was.

"Okay. How many of those do I drink?" She took out a calculator.

"About fourteen...and a half. So, fifteen. Can you do fifteen?"

"Uh...sure."

So, all my "food" would come from a can? If it meant getting my body back, I was up to the challenge. After the appointment, my parents and I headed to a restaurant for my last "food dinner" with Blaine. Then we all went to CVS, where he cheered us on as my dad bought endless boxes of Ensures. Afterwards, I went to Blaine's apartment for comfort. As soon as he went upstairs, I burst into a mad fit of jumping jacks. I felt stuck and restless. I couldn't be with myself and I certainly couldn't be with *him*.

As much as I had grown to hate Blaine, we did invite him over for Thanksgiving. I convinced myself, "Blaine is just like that nasty relative you're supposed to invite."

I hated him as much as I hated myself, but I clung to him because I wasn't sure of any other option.

Everyone in my family was concerned about me, but I couldn't tell them what was literally eating away at me because I wasn't consciously aware of it myself. If I had let the truth surface in my mind, I would have been smothered in shame.

For one fleeting moment of that Thanksgiving, I found a way to escape the mess I felt. I designed a colorful board game based on the Oestreichers, where the trivia questions were facts about each family member. After dinner, I took it out and asked Blaine if he would leave just our actual family to play. I needed my family back, more desperately than they knew. And I got them for the hour we played the game.

The next time I would feel protected, cared for, and heard would not be until I woke up from a coma, with Blaine gone, and my whole family by my side.

The Ensures weren't helping, but they *were* causing stomach aches. My dad told my mom, "This isn't real food." But now, drinking was far easier than eating. The less I chewed, the less I felt. So, I got the idea to gain weight through making giant smoothies. By now I could barely use my mouth at all. I hardly spoke. Blaine had stolen my voice. Worse, I couldn't form the words to tell anyone what Blaine was *still* doing.

It started with Blaine's suggestion for a smoothie powder he used, what he coined "the ultimate meal," which had nutrients and vitamins that theoretically could replace what you were missing by forgoing real food. But I knew I still needed more calories. So, I made my smoothies with whole milk. Then I started adding protein powder. And yogurt. And eventually baby food. Then—wait for it—*cans of beans*. I was so numb I didn't care. I just wanted to gain weight and burst out of the victim cage Blaine had stuck me in.

Years later, after food was taken away from me, it was especially ironic that when I was finally able to eat again, I would have to face my traumatic associations with food all over.

* * *

Even as the flashbacks haunted me, the more I shared my story with college students, the more I felt myself blooming as I dug into the roots of trauma. Yet I still felt uprooted since Ryan and I had returned from our honeymoon. I was ready to start our new life together, but things didn't feel fully in place. Most of our wedding presents were still in boxes, and with Ryan's new promotion and his "on call" schedule (apparently engineers had those, too), we were missing the "couple" time that had drawn us so close at the beginning.

As I ran towards my new life as a wife, an artist, a college student, and a conference speaker, life was rich, and every door was opening at once. The more offers I received, the more opportunities I seized. But part of me felt like I was still running away from something. I had turned obstacles into opportunities, and now the opportunities were looking more like obstacles I was setting up for myself. I needed to slow down, but slowing down was not my strong suit, and I was scared. I could talk trauma, backwards and forwards, but I still felt a disconnect that I knew would hinder me as I went on into the world.

I decided to see a therapist.

The truth about trauma is that it never goes away—you just create a stronger healing vortex.

I did an online search to find a therapist who "had experience working with PTSD." I set up an appointment and walked into a roomy office clutching my *Waking the Tiger* book to my chest, reading highlighted sections and rattling off what had happened to me so I could get to the "therapy part." The therapist, like every other person before, was floored by my story, and I could instantly sense how sorry he was for me—not exactly what I was looking for, but understandable.

"Were you in love with your voice teacher?" he asked.

My initial reaction was to fire back, "Of course not! That's ridiculous!" Followed by an almost subliminal thought, "Well, he is a therapist...and I was seventeen. Why didn't I do anything?"

I had come so far in speaking about what had happened to me, but there were still words, sensations, or random moments that made me feel uncomfortable. When I mentioned that my abuser was sixty years old, and that I was seventeen, I thought to myself, shouldn't I have known better?

Sometimes, when you think you've broken open, you've only cracked through the surface.

When I learned that animals actually "freeze" in the wild as a survival skill, and I had, too, suddenly the answer to my question was clear. I never told the therapist, but I knew who needed to hear my answer most.

Of course, I wasn't in love with Blaine. How can you assume that just because I didn't fight back right then and there?

Students needed to understand the confusion over how what may "appear" as consent could actually be a freeze response. And I could help them by relaying my own story. What else would have explained me walking numbly like a robot up and down the hallways of Fairfield High School? Even my own abuser had called me a space cadet, a label that confirmed the guilty thoughts in my head.

Telling the story of my abuse happened in layers over ten years. It took a while for me to no longer feel ashamed, apologetic, or self-conscious that people would think I had been in love. After all, I was seventeen, and students have crushes on teachers all the time. But no matter how old I was, Blaine took advantage of his position of power over me. Now, he was long gone from the picture. Right?

I'm confused what's triggering what—the broken open parts of healing from sexual molestation or the parts of me literally broken open, leaking on me day after day, night after night, and a constant pull to zip as far out of my body as I can.

These confusing threads were weaving a complex tapestry of trauma that were threatening to stall the progress I thought I was making. Trauma sometimes felt like a deceiving, never-ending hall of mirrors, where it was hard not to feel like anything would ever change.

"Your body responded, but you didn't."

Rita had once told me this when I talked about being uncomfortable with the physical sensations of feeling good eating pumpkin and then talking about the physical sensations with Blaine. *You were brainwashed to believe you were worthless.*

Where was all of this guilt and shame still coming from? I was freelance writing for dozens of sites about being open, sharing your truth...but were there still ideas I didn't want to think about?

Curious, I went back through my old cartoons of the "wounded bird with the bleeding wing" and the caption I had written:

Poor wounded Amy, you are so mean to her! What is that? How about practicing a little loving kindness to this girl that's so scared, vulnerable, and has been through hell? She needs you. Show her some compassion.

While I was getting ready for marriage, self-compassion had helped me conquer any fears of intimacy that I had related to the abuse. Part of me still felt like I was chasing happiness, but I had to remind myself that I *did* have everything I needed right now. I had love, others, and myself. There was only the need to be present.

My e-mail inbox could wait. Nothing was practical except appreciating what I had all around me. If I got caught up in the little things in life, or found myself in a "being productive frenzy," I could always just remind myself to tune into what really mattered.

Eager to clear out any last remnants of shame and Blaine from my system, I allowed myself to explore my memories further.

The first tiny inkling of discomfort I felt with Blaine was after a lesson when he went to show me some music. This time he smoked his pipe on the couch. And I got so excited thinking, "Awesome, he really is starting to see me as an equal now. I feel so sophisticated!" I didn't want to say anything that might ruin the moment and make him realize I was a teenager unaccustomed to chatting with impressive esoteric people!

The next week he said, "You know, Amy, I realized I was wrong last week in smoking my pipe with you because even though I love sharing this beautiful music with you, I still need to show respect for our student-teacher relationship. In taking out my pipe last week, I crossed those boundaries."

Disappointed, I thought, "I guess I'm kidding myself assuming that a grownup like Blaine would ever actually consider being friends with a kid like me, especially when he teaches famous actors." But then how did it become okay to sleep with me? I guess smoking your pipe is different? Blaine had an excuse for everything.

I started to feel like Rapunzel trapped in her tower—a wounded bird now subjected to staying at this old man's apartment every weekend, closed off from the outside world, and held captive in a situation I felt powerless to escape from. I lost trust in myself, in anyone, and anything. I had given up all of my friends for Blaine. Now, I felt I had made a rash move. I was stuck with no one but him.

Blaine's apartment was at street level—out in the open—not hidden in some dark basement of a building or nestled on near the top of high rise. Pedestrians walked right by, yet they had no idea what was happening inside. His studio had a sliding door to a porch, which he had turned into a garden. But stone walls and fences surrounded all four sides, closing us into a claustrophobic square of nature that made no sense to anyone in the outside world. His world became my prison.

In that garden space there were creeping vines and flowers crawling up the walls. There were little fountains and plaques shaped like sun and stars to decorate the stone. The world knew nothing about this space. Only we could access it through his sliding door. The apartment had everything you needed—a porch, a kitchen, an upstairs—you never had to leave.

It started to rain. He was playing me those stupid art songs again, and I couldn't contain my sadness. I missed having fun—the stupid, silly, teenage kind.

What happened next remains one of the saddest images in my mind. Blaine was so desperate to show me he could be fun.

"I'll show you fun! Look! Take your shoes off!"

He took my hand, in our bare feet, and acted like a kid, kicking up rain with his old, wrinkly toes, and trying to have "spontaneous" fun. "See? We can do anything!"

But it was a lost cause. As I numbly kicked around the rain, those raindrops felt like the tears I couldn't cry yet. It was hopeless. Blaine the teacher was forever gone. And now I was forever stuck, kicking up my tears on his splinter-ridden wooden porch, while my friends had real fun in the real world.

How had I gone from always feeling so confident in myself, knowing and loving who I was, and feeling safe, to suddenly hating every part of me, hating life, hating each moment, hating eating, and turning to exercise to numb my pain?

I came to hate Blaine with a passion. When he, my mom, and I were together, I would freshly talk back to him, which would embarrass my mom. Once he called my mother and said, "Quite frankly, Amy was very rude to me today." Of course, he neglected to mention that he had kept me up the entire night before sexually abusing me.

I had never resented myself or Blaine more. Or my family for thinking I was the one who was messed up.

When my show premiered in 2012, part of me had been nervous to mention that it touched on sexual abuse. I was now a speaker for RAINN, (Rape, Abuse & Incest National Network) where I learned that each year, tens of thousands of college students become survivors of sexual assault.

Knowing you're not alone can change everything for a survivor. I needed to use my own voice to make an impact.

So, I went back to *Gutless & Grateful* and expanded on what that felt like for me. The sexual abuse was no longer a quick "mention and be done with it" portion of the show. Now, I was going to say something about it. Freezing (unable to take action in the moment) was probably the biggest aspect of abuse that most people didn't fully understand.

It also took me years to accept that a mentor in my life had violated his position of authority. I blamed myself, convinced that no one could take advantage of me if I hadn't invited it.

Instead of sexual abuse being something I stuck in my show almost as an afterthought, I used my show as a platform to speak out. *Gutless & Grateful* be a mental health program, as well as an invitation to speak up against sexual assault.

CHAPTER 56

Slaying the Snake

I WAS HEALING, BUT THE MEMORY of Blaine was still poisoning my mind and filling my body with anxious energy. At the same time, I was married and wrestling with forming a new identity.

I couldn't go back to who I had been, but I didn't want to lose that Amy either. I didn't want to change. Remembering how I always saw Blaine as a snake, I created another visualization:

A slimy snake enters her through her left eye which traps her into a frozen ice cage which she cannot escape from. The snake lives inside of her, slithering around her body while she is frozen solid, incapable of being herself, until she sings the snake to sleep, skins it, and creates beautiful snake shoes. She clicks her heels and begins to dance in the bright sunshine, breathing in life again.

In biology, the definition of entropy states that things are either alive and moving or dead. When they stop moving, they die. To be alive, things have to always be changing, growing, healing, and manifesting different aspects of themselves, and when this stops, you die. The healing process is a part of life. You don't leave that to move *into* life. You *are* doing life right now.

I don't want to get stuck back in victim mode. If it takes giving up my numbness companion, then I'll do it. I don't think I am going to say, "I can't wait to get my life started." Maybe I'll say, "I can't wait to heal all of me." Because I'll never stop healing. I want to heal my heart. Then I want to heal the world...and wear high heels!

For me to live, I had to embrace change fully. Change was and is a form of creation. My creativity had a new purpose—sharing my story with college students and conference goers, hoping they might be inspired to confront their abuse in the ways I had.

With each presentation or workshop, I grew more comfortable with my story. The more creative outlets I could use to explore the abuse, the less attached to it I felt. Trusting myself required a magical balancing act of forgiving myself for not fighting back in the moment of abuse, while at the same time, acknowledging that I had the power all along.

I have the power to bring myself down to the floor. I have the power to bring myself gloriously back up again. I have the power to make my own choices. I guess this didn't sink in when I was numb with Blaine. Now that I am mastering my memories, I am coming into my own, but different. Amy, the warrior. Back into Amy's old body, but different, maybe with a few scars, maybe with a fistula for a little bit. But those are my tiger stripes, my warrior medals.

I was no longer blaming myself for what happened. With that mind shift, I was able to support myself much more effectively.

Blaine is not here anymore. He doesn't deserve anything that he took from you, and that is why he doesn't have it. He is the one who is empty inside, not you.

I had to dive back into the most unpleasant memories of abuse to let go of the voice that declared I was responsible for what had happened to me. I used the negative hateful words I had once blamed myself with and gave them to Wounded Amy, now a character, outside of myself. I wrote a new script for the woman I was now, ending with just one line, "It wasn't my fault."

Once I felt these words resonate in my body and in my soul, I liberated myself. I had nothing to be ashamed of. And I had every right to reclaim my life, my aliveness, move on, and experience the world in all of its radiant colors once again.

I had already written one angry letter to Blaine. Now I was ready to write a new one and finally let him go.

Ten years have passed since my stomach exploded, and a burdensome secret has become the fire to illuminate my path. I don't think of the abuse as a secret anymore. Just because I haven't confronted you in person doesn't mean the universe can't hear it. I've shared my story. You are my art, my theatre, my growth, my lesson learned. But you are NOT my secret. I've learned that secrets make us sick. And yours will keep you sick.

After giving the keynote speech for the "Take Back The Night" ceremony in Phoenix, Arizona, I scribbled out my letter, folded it, and threw it away.

Endings and Beginnings

I have to shift the image that I have of myself so I can take in new things and be okay with it. Trauma changes you. Life changes you. If you cling to rocks while you are floating down the river, your knees will just get scraped by the current.

I can't get back who I was but the good part is, I CAN create it, and I won't let Blaine, or anyone else, do it for me.

I WAS TEACHING OTHERS ABOUT hope and trust, trauma and recovery, and how to rebuild your life, while my life was still under construction. It was time to trust I could develop my own blueprint for the future.

Meanwhile at Hampshire, I was working with my professors through independent studies, so I could manage my continuously unfolding health saga and still be able to complete my third year. Being at home also gave me the great opportunity to observe my family and take note of how trauma had impacted us and still had its effects now. My interactions with my family were now my field notes, which were becoming clues on what was is going to be the most important theme in this play. How does one person's trauma affect the family and communities? And why is trauma so important for everyone to understand?

Writing and rewriting my play, which I titled *Storage*, was one way I worked through the challenge of framing my story when I didn't know how it would end—like framing a house without the benefit of the architect's drawings.

One thing was clear from my play: I was now able to frame my story in terms of my family and the effect it had on all of us—not just me.

Creating the Universal Detour

I started with something I could say confidently: What happened to me may not have happened to anyone else, but my story and the tools for recovery I discovered are universal. Anyone can apply them. And with that as my foundation, I began to reconstruct the presentation I was giving on campuses.

> *People don't turn to "self-help" books until they face a problem. We need to be more conscious of the need for self-care, not only in times of crises. We are constantly healing and improving ourselves. It's the nature of being alive on this earth.*
>
> *I want to take the stigma away from "healing" and "trauma." The people who typically purchase PTSD books are those directly affected by PTSD. I don't want to make trauma an "exclusive" club anymore. Not everyone will know what the emergency room is like. Not everyone will be sexually abused. But we all go through something we feel "nobody else can relate to." When we can validate that we deserve to heal, we are freed. We get a glimpse of a stronger version of ourselves—a self that we all deserve to know. Healing is a natural maintenance process, like a snake shedding its skin, or a broom brushing off dusty shelves.*

I could answer endless questions from people about the story I had already lived, but I couldn't yet answer the question of where my story was going next. How exactly should I assemble the new me, the Amy of the future?

No Right Way Meant no Wrong Way

Once I realized there was no "right" way to frame my story or know where to go next, things got easier. I just had to make a choice. I couldn't control the outcome, but I could control my willingness to move forward.

We have all the choices in the world, plus the capability to decide! We'll never know what choice is right or why things happen the way they do, but we've got our instincts.

If I couldn't predict how my story would end up, I could try imagining how I wanted it to end up.

Imagine a world where every day we are healing and striving to better ourselves. If we approach life like we need to heal from the "trauma" of the everyday—without making that seem like a bad thing—then every day we are making an effort to delve inside and rediscover ourselves.

When the trajectory of my life changed, I had to find my new arc. My life now was the one I was creating—and constantly recreating on my ever-shifting journey.

People love talking about the temperament of the tortured artist, how Van Gogh was "mad," etc. Maybe we need to start thinking of this in reverse. Instead of seeing artists as suffering from madness, we need to access our inner Van Gogh and embrace the tortured artist in each of us to heal.

When you've experienced trauma, life seems to look much better in the rear-view mirror. But if you keep your focus there, you can't see or even appreciate what's right in front of you or set your sights on what's to come. The lens of trauma makes us see the simple pleasures we took for granted as everyday occurrences in a new light. Gratitude becomes the filter through which we experience the past, the present, and the future. With an aerial perspective on my journey, I went back to my childhood memories, and realized that being present was the key to what filled those moments with happiness.

As I wrapped up my third year at Hampshire college, I realized that even my studies had taken a beautiful detour. Now that I had studied psychology along with the arts, I was understanding the drive to create when facing trauma. These new ideas were being shaped by the business skills I was learning at Hampshire, turning my studies into a career I could take beyond college, which in a year, I would be graduating from.

Another piece of closure I needed was with my grandmother. I wanted to learn more of my grandmother's story and give her a voice to tell it herself. I imagined her on stage and started to write. But something stopped me. Now that I had studied psychology, I found a striking parallel between our stories. My grandmother must have struggled with PTSD as well, although our healing journeys couldn't have been more different. Or were they really?

Once I started to understand Post-Traumatic Stress Syndrome, I learned that the body holds traumatic memories that take a long time to untangle and let go. In my grandma's case, PTSD was not even a word. Thousands of Holocaust survivors came out of the camps, released from an unthinkable hell, and many were met with scorn, misunderstanding, and even disbelief. How did it affect my grandmother to be met with such hurtful reactions?

So many survivors in my grandmother's generation kept their memories bottled up inside. Now, survivors of all sorts of trauma were out in the open talking about their experiences. If my grandmother were living today, how would she be received? More importantly, if the research and understanding was available then, how would it have changed her?

How could I honor the words of my grandmother and continue to make art? That's when I discovered a new course offered that semester: Oral Histories. I enthusiastically enrolled and wrote up a project proposal based on my grandmother's life surviving the Holocaust and coming over to America—an ideal bridge between history, memory, psychology, creating theatre, and performing.

I looked at a glass of water and remembered what it was like to be denied a water bottle for years. Did my grandma look at a glass of water and remember being denied water in the camps? Or maybe she remembered the ocean on a ship coming to America? I went to bed that night, dreaming about water, myself, and her.

Reacting to my "abnormality," society offered their condolences and pity. They would see everything I have accomplished since my coma and still ask, "So how long have you been sick?" Or, "You must be so sorry this happened to you." What happened to me is neither good nor bad. It just is.

I didn't want to share my story for other people to feel badly about themselves. I shared it to show what the human spirit is capable of. What makes my "detour" different from anyone else's and, more importantly, can artistic expression help us come to terms with whatever our detour may be?

According to everyone, my grandmother never spoke much about anything. I almost gave up trying to get her story together. No relative seemed to remember anything.

Mom: She never talked about the atrocities. She would talk pieces of bread people stole from people. She said there were all kinds of people in the camp—good, bad, generous. They lived off of potato peels. I'm sure she felt a lot of guilt.

To fill in the gaps, I read books on history and memory, post-memory, dug through Jewish history databases, called museums, libraries, and old diners in Brooklyn my grandparents had frequented. More facts led to enough questions to create twelve comprehensive oral history guides for family members I hadn't even met. I was determined to follow the trail of memory (or lack thereof) to see where it may lead.

One relative connected me to another, and soon, I was getting emails and Facebook messages from people I didn't even know I was related to. I introduced my quest with one question: "Do you remember my grandma?" Mostly, the answer was, "A bit. She was sweet. Quiet. Great cook." But the more questions I asked, the more discoveries I made, including the deaths of her friends, her oldest brother, and her first husband. How, even with these irreplaceable losses, did she go on to lead such a beautiful, honorable life?

An aunt then warned me as I dared to tread further, "It was kind of an unstated rule when you're with Holocaust survivors that you don't go there. Nobody comes out and says it, but it's true for all of us that are first generation." But I went "there," just to end up in a maze, in search of facts, dates, and places with no "finish line" in sight. Throughout my pursuit, my relatives were sure to constantly remind me that I'd never find enough facts. *"All you'll get is memory. No history."*

What I discovered was an even greater gift than history. I found precious family anecdotes that even my own mother didn't know. Every family member had a personal piece of history and in stringing them together, I was creating the family narrative.

I interviewed nieces, nephews, great aunts, uncles, grandparents, distant cousins, and distant cousins from Belgium, France, Prague, Israel, and San Francisco. I went to research and history archives and uncovered photographs and old documents from my past, including the ship that my grandparents came to America on. I logged hours transcribing tape upon tape and discovered that a single spoken word can become an entire treasure chest, if just listened.

It was my Great Uncle Morris, whom the rest of my family told me was more passionate about playing bridge than telling stories, that finally came to my rescue. I never met him, but through voicemails, I felt closer to him with every message.

Morris: We never thought of the fact of whether or not we would see them again. Every day was a survival day, and we lived for that day. Thank God we all joined up after the war. I never thought to ask Hannah what it was like to be liberated from the camps. I've often felt pain from all of her war years, as the worst possible thing a woman could go through.

Those who argue that oral history is not "reliable" are countered by those who believe the anecdotes of ordinary people about their experiences are truer than written document. Without memory, there are only facts. True stories are what bring the heart to history, to my grandma, and to FIBERS, the play I was now writing. Sewing threads together is what enabled my grandmother to survive, and now, sewing these unfinished stories into a linear narrative, and threading my own story of survival into hers could answer my lingering question: What do we do with the tattered, entangled threads of a life that we are still learning to live again?"

CHAPTER 58

Shaping the Detourist Path

We live in a world of caves, gardens, and underground passageways to no place and everywhere. So, the artist must be the sculptor and the builder, chiseling out those pathways though his craft and illuminating them to the outside world.

THROUGH MY COURSES, I was understanding the process I had used intuitively to survive. I could envision a world where "detours" in life were everyday blessings. Taking a social entrepreneurship course turned this vision into action. "Don't think about what *you* want; think about what problem you can solve," my professor advised me. The problem? Obstacles. So, I formed a singular focus of helping others navigate their detours and turn obstacles into opportunities.

Sharpening my business focus around this "problem" I was trying to solve led to another question: What kind of impact did I want "Detourism" to make? Maybe there was a replicable, sharable business strategy solution to survival. Presenting at conferences was opening up my world. With each one, I was realizing how powerful telling my story could be for others.

Mom: She was the youngest person presenting at the storytelling conference but managed to reach the people with her wit, insight, and honesty. At the end of her talk, I caught a glimpse of Amy and saw she was being embraced by this beautiful woman. Amy called me over, and they told me how she has been following Amy's blog and came hoping she would meet Amy. My daughter the warrior. What greater satisfaction is there than to affect another person's life?

As I saw my honesty impacting others, I realized what I had once called Tiger Lilly's "warrior traits" were now core values of the business that was starting to form.

Success meant taking chances. Taking chances meant making choices.

The more I choices I made and chances I took, the more alive I felt. That was my new personal success.

My grandmother had kept her inner struggles hidden from me as a child. Now I realized that the most important resource I could share with others was compassion.

My grandmother was never bitter after the war. There was sometimes sadness in her eyes, but she was loving, grateful, generous, and happy for as long as I knew her. However, I know she held a lot in that it would sometimes come out in a melancholy gaze or bout of quiet. Was my grandmother unable to live a full life due to the trauma she had suffered, even when she was surrounded by adoring friends and family? Do we really understand someone if we shower them with affection but don't address what they willingly choose to hold in?

Through my play, *Storage*, I explored how each member of my family had been affected by my trauma and how each one was healing from it.

In the meantime, writing *Fibers* was giving me crucial closure with my grandmother. As I wove the threads of each family member's narrative together, I could see the magic of my play take form.

Wounded Amy and Thriving Amy were the two halves of my traumatized protagonist. They learned to forgive each other, and only when they worked together could they move forward.

My two selves had to accept that each was a part of the other. The breakthrough moment had to come when Thriving Amy accepted Wounded Amy as part of her now, not a "mutant" born from disaster, but a woman with wisdom to impart.

CHAPTER 59

Work, Life, and Play

FOR YEARS, I WOULD WAKE UP, jump right to my yoga mat to allay my fear of standing still, frenetically stretch for ninety minutes, then jump right to my laptop after closing the blinds, typing for hours, or for as long as I could manage to stay numb. Now, I was living by my four hardcore resiliency skills, which I had designed for students of all ages and people of all backgrounds, and my speaking gigs were proving that my four hardcore skills could work for everyone. With every interview or presentation, people were delighted by how simple, yet effective these tools were. I was sharing trauma's best kept secret, and it was actually working for other people besides myself! Business was a true reward from the inside out.

My blog had started off about others who had inspired me. Now, bloggers were putting me in a similar light.

Even my high school teacher who had once watched me numb through my abuse, and had visited me in the hospital, was writing to me about my story and the reach I now had.

And I finally had someone to share my heart with. The thing I was most grateful for? I could eat. And boy, was I eating a ton.

I went from painting by accident, to painting for healing, to painting as a profession. Like the hero crossing the final threshold, I had a gift to give society. I was selling my work and teaching my art technique to adults who were surprised how much fun they had in my "anything goes classes." One woman who thought my first class was crazy when I said we were going to "just bang out a lot of canvases, shred a lot of napkins and toilet paper, and rip a bunch of cardboard boxes" later commented that it was the best course she ever took.

I still needed hope, because as my business ventures were finally paying off, my open wound still refused to heal. I still carried my emergency bag with me wherever I went, hoping for the day I could finally pick up and go somewhere without worrying about a precautionary suitcase of equipment. I had to be willing to "create" and visualize everything being okay, even if my mind wasn't giving me a clear picture. Giving others hope was a way I could move forward, too.

For so long, my story had been the centerpiece of my life. But if all we do is share our own experience, soon we run out of it. I had to receive as well as give.

Now, I was posting other people's stories on my blog in a weekly "Why Not? Wednesday #LoveMyDetour" feature and noticing how everyone who submitted a post had somehow been shaped by what happened to them. Detourists from all over were holding up my own story as a model and using that same framework to look ahead.

As I started presenting at health advocacy, education, and social justice conferences, I learned that there was a term for drawing all people together through "Detourism." INCLUSION.

On a whim, I asked Jeff, who I knew had no free hours in his emergency schedule day at Mt. Sinai, to take a "bonding road trip" with me.

Jeff agreed and drove me to Cape Cod to present at the New England Equal Educational Opportunity Association, where I was speaking to higher education professionals on PTSD and maximizing student success. As he helped me finetune my PowerPoint presentation, I couldn't help but look at him with the utmost affection, seeing his newly learned understanding of what I had been through. As we packed up to go, Jeff was still reeling over my talk. "Wow, you really know this stuff, Ames!" We had come full circle. Once I received his compassion and empathy, I was able to heal even more.

Adam, who had the hardest time letting go as the caring oldest brother, put his overprotectiveness to great use by taking on a new role in my life. Now that I was bringing my show everywhere from Minnesota to Washington, DC, big brother Adam became my official *Gutless & Grateful* stage manager. About four states later, he knew every audio cue by heart.

During one conference, "Storytelling in a Changing World," I sat down with my mother and had some bonding time in the brief story-swap exercises we were given. As my mother and I swapped stories, I thought to myself, "How far we have come." We were two married women. But more than that, we were caretakers, survivors, healers, women, learners, and now, Detourists. My mom and I had always traveled this path together, and we were going to come out of this together.

I thought back to when I told my mother my secrets—part of the story I was incorporating into my play. We were telling new secrets, new stories. As she told me of her mother, I knew I would tell my own child one day what a hero my own mother had been to me.

Stories really are a way to pass on our legacy.

As I stepped away from my own story, I looked everywhere for fresh sources of inspiration and new ideas. As I scanned the Internet, I quickly immersed myself in TEDx talks, and watched artists, scientists, kids, teachers, and people with innovative ideas—and all kinds of challenging lives—share what thoughts they felt could change the world...all in ten minutes!

With all the conferences, I was beginning to develop a national persona for myself as a speaker. But I didn't connect the dots until my endless Googling of TEDx talks took me to an actual call for speakers. It turned out that TEDx Syracuse was looking for ideas based on the theme of a glitch. Like a Detour? TEDx Syracuse was a perfect opportunity, so I got to work. The application for TEDx was basically like applying for college, requiring well-crafted essays and a solid "idea worth spreading." *This was not just about being an inspiring motivational speaker.*

My idea worth spreading? That someone who follows life's unexpected detours and searches for the flowers along the way to make their journey meaningful is, in fact, a Detourist. Being a Detourist empowered me with a sense of ownership at a time when life felt very uncertain. I figured it could help other people, too.

I proposed a talk called "Follow Your Road, Find Your Flower," in which I would share how each detour planted the seeds for a new "flower," and by finding those "flowers," we could all be Detourists.

While waiting to hear from TEDx, I was hard at work on my play. I was introduced to Talya, a British dramaturge who was very taken by my play but couldn't get through my script because it was dense as fruitcake. Her first words of advice struck me: don't make it autobiographical.

The day I gave in, my process completely transformed, and by the next week, the script was half the length. All I had to do was trust that the story could stand on its own outside of my own story. Then, I remembered a quote from *The Body Keeps the Score* by Dr. Bessel Van Der Kolk: "The imprints of traumatic experiences are organized not as coherent logical narratives but in fragmented sensory and emotional traces: images, sounds, and physical sensations." That was enough to change the title of my play from *Storage* to *Imprints*.

I had another gap in my play to fill in. How could Pat, the new protagonist of my script, feel whole again?

I wrote a scene where the Patty (Wounded Amy) and Patricia (Thriving Amy) mirrored each other's gestures until their hands eventually touched. It was the perfect way for them to finally face each other and this collaborative "dance" replaced pages of dialogue.

After months of waiting, I finally heard back from TEDx Syracuse—I got the TEDx talk! Standing on that red-circle-carpeted stage opened a whole new world for me and catapulted me into a world of much greater public recognition than I'd ever had before. Being a TEDx speaker opened all sorts of doors for me, but I still hadn't found closure for my wounds—neither my fistula that wouldn't heal or the psychological wounds Blaine had inflicted on me. My trauma had left indelible marks on me, and it was only through completing *Imprints* that I could accept and begin to love my scars.

By the time I took the stage at the International Conference of Diversity and Disability in Honolulu, I had a wedding ring and complications from a surgery I'd expected to be totally done with. But here I was performing my show in an auditorium of 800 people and hearing other speakers talk about inclusion. What a year 2016 had been! My play was done, I was almost through college, after spending a term studying theatre at the at the Eugene O'Neill Theater Center, and my academic, artistic, and business pursuits were starting to finally gel.

I had just done my TEDx talk and was waiting anxiously for the video to come out. I had performed on a stage in Hawaii. And Ryan and I would soon be celebrating our one-year anniversary. Everything was lined up for a season of new beginnings. But life is full of unexpected surprises—and endings you didn't plan for.

CHAPTER 60

Hello and Goodbye

THE TRIUMPHANT ENDING to my talk—and the final flower on my path—was finding my husband as the "beautiful clearing" of my detoured journey. But life is never that neat. The week after my triumphant, married TEDx Talk went live, Ryan texted me—that's right, texted me—that he wanted a divorce. So much for my story. Suddenly, I was forced to practice what I preached, which was harder than I thought.

The dizzying speed with which my marriage was taken away left me in shock. As days passed with every attempt at contact unreturned, I was faced with *yet another detour*. Love was supposed to mean warmth, compassion, and security. So, how could anything be safe anymore? I didn't know *who* I could lean on.

When my TEDx video was finally uploaded and shared on social media, I was afraid to look. It was painful to watch a time when I thought my "detour" had earned me the love of my life. But then I realized that maybe this was a time in my life where I needed to hear this talk more than ever. So, I tried to stick to the words I had uttered with such confidence just a month before.

Cheer up, Amy. Because you have lost, you are working so hard to gain now. Gaining in every way from every angle. You take to life like a bad habit. Life fooled you once and it will fool you again and again. But that's just life. You fall down and you get back up but from a different place and into new, uncharted territory. Just gotta laugh it off, dust yourself off, and start over again.

I wrote these words to myself eight years ago. Before I made a fancy #LoveMyDetour hashtag, I was still reassuring myself that an unexpected path would one day be a reward. Maybe all I needed to do was *trust* my detour. A Detourist knows that no turn is a wrong turn. No matter what, they forge ahead. So, I forced myself to watch my TEDx Talk—post-marriage.

I cried a bit after seeing my wedding photo projected onto the big TEDx screen and thought about what direction I was supposed to take now—one step at a time. The next day, I was supposed to perform at a showcase for women in the arts. But still subject to outbursts of despair at the slightest thought of moving on, I didn't even want to get out of bed, let alone take a few trains down to Delancey Street. But I wasn't going to let one curveball sabotage the rest of my life. I pushed myself to go to the city on my own.

Once I finally navigated the subway system, I faced the empty stage. Another performance of many, but now as a newly, unmarried woman. It was a shift of awareness I was still trying to get used to. It's natural to miss someone you assumed had your back for life. You hear everyone else's online dating horror stories, but you never think they can happen to you...until they do.

But that was no matter now. I had made it, past the TEDx Talk, past the divorce, onto a subway, and now, onto Delancey Street, into a theatre, in front of a mic. I stood on that stage by myself, and I sang. And I smiled, thinking to myself, "By turning things outward, I've built a support system that goes beyond family and friends. A whole network is rooting for me." I pushed past the fear of feeling and I felt deeply.

Learning the importance of self-care and "Detourism" is critical for trauma survivors. This time I knew, even if I didn't know exactly, where it would lead. I was a woman. Regardless of who or what I had. I had myself and my two feet, marching forward and onto an open road.

Ryan was a twist in my life that had illuminated a new part of my awareness. He showed me I was capable of being a real person after illness, capable of caring for someone else, and participating fully and equally in a relationship. More than that, I was likeable and fun to be around. And then, just like I had with Blaine, I had grown so "dependent" on this relationship, that I even started to lose my own sense of ownership and independence. And now, with Ryan out of my life, I was forced to feel comfortable with that again, comfortable that I could take subways on my own, pick which art to display, find good material for my show, and even run a website. I was powerful enough as I was. I needed to be my own best friend, married or not. And I would be okay.

On the train ride home—yes, I even managed to figure out how to get back—I met some other strong, vital, and hopelessly romantic women, and we had a good laugh as we swapped love horror stories—a new chapter to add in my journey.

I felt such power returning home. And the next morning was a new start. Anything was possible. A new friend took me for a hike, and we saw the most exquisite mountain laurels in full blossom. Gazing down on the winding trail, I decided, divorce was just another glitch.

When we can't go in the direction we anticipated, we've got to switch gears and adapt. We have to resource inner strengths that we never knew we were capable of accessing.

Every detour leads somewhere. And I know that one day, I will "Love My Detour." But for now, I "Trust My Detour."

CHAPTER 61

A Detour Within a Detour

I DIDN'T LOVE MY DIVORCE DETOUR, but I didn't have to. My marriage was over, and it was time to pack up and literally create a new start. In my submission-overdrive-frenzy, I had applied to an artist residency, inspired by Judaism—appropriately called Art Kibbutz. The concept sounded wonderful, but as soon as I received my *Welcome Manual*, bringing all of my belongings on a ferry every morning to no running water, and only porta potties available caused my medical limitations-bordering-on-excuses to cloud my head. Maybe this wasn't right for me.

I stopped and asked myself two questions. 1) What am I searching for, and 2) What am I running away from?

What part of me couldn't hold back from constantly searching calls for speakers, applications, submissions, contests, nominations, and awards? Why, when I sternly told myself I would not apply to one more program, did I still manage to throw in an application? Was I bored? Was I making extra work for myself to fill some kind of void? Had I turned yet another healing resource into another coping skill to muddle up my life with noise?

I decided to hop on a train with my art supplies, a few dresses, and a ton of protein bars, and spent two weeks on an Art Kibbutz on Governor's Island, New York.

Art Kibbutz disconnected me from social media, work, and all things familiar, except my trees, nature, and paintbrush. I was with seven other artists from Kansas, Syria, Israel, Brooklyn, South America, and Greece, connecting with a common understanding that we were all there to transform in some way. I had to get used to the idea that now people would know me post-divorce. I was so used to saying "my husband" this or "my husband" that, and now, a new part of my self was forming. With each stroke of my brush, I prayed that each messy glob of paint might form a stronger me.

It was only a matter of time before real life interrupted my painting spree. Because Ryan had been in charge of my website, I had to conference call him and our lawyers for a deposition to persuade him to let me have ownership back of my site. I tried to carry on as "professionally" as I could, speaking with our lawyers and agreeing on how the website was to be transferred over. Suddenly, I felt no breath in my throat and started to sob over my canvas streaked with wet paint.

"I'm sorry, I just can't. I can't keep talking about this."

"Amy, I thought you wanted this website done," his lawyer responded.

"I had an emotional investment in this marriage, and now we're treating everything like a business transaction. I have to go."

I hung up, sobbing as I sprinted to catch the last ferry.

The next day, my lawyer explained that if this was so emotionally difficult for me, I could file for an emotional reconciliation. It would be a way to get some closure, she assured me, if that was something I needed. It might put the divorce on hold, but this way we could have a chance to see a therapist together and talk things out—something that he had refused to do on his own. I jumped at the chance but was unsure of what I wanted. Was this someone I wanted to be with now? Someone who had decided our marriage was over long before he let on?

I had already learned that having a final confrontation is not always the dramatically cleansing tool you'd imagine it to be. A survivor might "need" a final confrontation to validate memories, seek revenge, find clarity, reconciliation, or try to establish a real relationship. What was I hoping to gain? Was it realistic? And where would we go from here? Although now I was hearing from friends and family all of the "red flags" I had apparently missed along the way about Ryan, I decided to go ahead with the motion, in the back of my head, thinking, "Maybe things weren't that bad. Maybe things can work out." In the meantime, I got back into theatre, wrote and directed a short play, and was looking better. I was laughing again.

The day our motion was finally brought up in court, I woke up early and hopped on a train with my mother to the courthouse. I had never been in a court before and was a bit taken aback when the security guard yelled at me for trying to take a bag of cheese up to the court house—even with a medical note! So, while my mother sat outside with my cheese and emergency-bag scissors, I went up three floors and waited with my lawyer, suddenly nervous to see someone I once thought I'd wake up to every day for the rest of my life.

After an hour, Ryan and his lawyer finally came into the tiny waiting room, and our eyes pulled away like oil and water. I couldn't look him in the face, could I? The four of us then laughed and made nice as we discussed the best way to go about this.

My lawyer took me aside as Ryan's lawyer took him for his own private "huddle."

"This is really up to you." she reassured me.

"You don't have to go through with this if you don't want. It's just if you want to say anything to him. We can request that you two go to a court ordered therapist, but that's going to delay the divorce another six months. I say, especially with these short marriages, just rip the band aid off." Was that all it was? After I had anticipated spending a life together with my husband? Just a stubborn Band-Aid with a brief residual sting?

"Okay, let us just talk here."

She left me and Ryan in the room together. It was the first and last time I was with Ryan like this. I realized, as he started arguing, that I didn't have to hear it. He wasn't my problem anymore. I wished him all the best, unplugged my phone charger, and walked into a new life. I had gotten what I needed. I walked out of that courtroom on my own two feet with the confidence and self-love that my grandma was sprinkling over me.

Once I got home, I took a long walk around my neighborhood. Although it was only the day after Labor Day, there was a lovely October dimness in the crisp air, which reminded me of so many Octobers in my past of transitions and new beginnings. I walked for several hours, allowing the wind to blow over my thoughts and let my mind wander into the tender gusts that surrounded me like pillowy light. I was okay. I was here. And I *had* grown from this experience. I was dependent on nothing, connected to everything, trusting in the path ahead, and firm in where I was. As the sun set, I kept walking.

That night, I went to the hospital. For good reason. I had discovered painting at Yale when my wound ruptured. As terrible as that time was, I will always remember the gorgeous art that lined all the hallways. At one of the worst parts of my life, I was saved by a creative marathon. Now, I reconnected with my old friend, "Dancing Girl," the third painting I had ever created.

The paintings hanging at Yale New Haven Hospital were what had given my father and I things to talk about as we pushed my IV pole up and down the marble hallways and stained tiles. The art there was the one marker of sanity as we passed the days arbitrarily marking time in laps, rounds, and shifts.

That year, Yale opened a brand-new oncology center and established an "evidence-based art program expressly for the emotional and physical well-being of patients and their families." A committee of art consultants, patient advisors, and administrators would select over seven hundred pieces of original art to create the third largest permanent art display in Connecticut.

When I heard Yale was looking for art, I submitted my work, not expecting to hear anything. By now, I was used to people admiring my work, but being rejected from fine art galleries because it wasn't "their thing." (Perhaps they weren't so keen on the glue gun strands hanging off the edges?)

I couldn't think of any place else I'd rather sell my artwork to than Yale. I was overjoyed when I received the call from the Yale curator.

"We love your piece, and we'd love to buy it from you, but our curatorial team has asked that you remove the tear. We feel that for an oncology ward, we need something lighter."

"Oh, for me, it was because life is about the joy and the pain—"

"Right, but we just want to keep the mood more uplifting. So, you would be okay with that?"

I thought about it a bit. No, I really wanted to keep the tear.

"Yeah, I guess it's okay."

It was more important that "Dancing Girl" be in the hospital for others. Teardrop or not.

A few weeks later, they called me again.

"Hi Amy, I have good news. We decided to keep the tear."

I went with my mother and father to the grand opening reception at the new hospital.

How strange it was to walk down unit hallways so similar, but now as an artist, and not a patient at all. I was literally unattached to everything and had everything to look forward to.

With my parents at my side, we were led down all of the beautiful sparkling new hallways to see a breathtaking display of art. I trembled with nervous excitement, wondering what corner my *Dancing Girl* would be jumping midair, with her single tear. And she was where I'd hope she'd be. On the wall of a unit, where staff, patients, and family members could see.

After the tour was over, my parents and I strolled around the new Yale Healing Garden, which was a replica of the old healing garden where I had been stuck. We strolled in the pitch dark, with plates of food in our hands from the reception instead of IV wires. There were no ties anywhere, and nothing weighing down on us. And my parents were so proud. We had all come so far. I had never loved my parents as much as I did in that moment. We had all survived together. And now we were here to celebrate it. We had come full circle.

We come into this world as trusting, open vessels, happy and confident that life won't change. Trust is having a confident expectation that circumstances will turn out—or stay—*like we plan them to.* But life happens, and we realize that people, as well as circumstances around us, can detour unexpectedly. We lose trust in what we expected from others, from life, or from ourselves. If I had learned anything, it was to trust that *there would always be detours.*

I opened up, dated, fell in love, and got married. I trusted my marriage— and my friendship with my husband—would last. They didn't. But that's life. Now, as I reflected, I asked myself, "Why do we continue to trust things when they continue to disappoint us? And where do we discover the resilience to try again?" I used theatre to help me map out some "change points" in my life where I'd lost trust:

- I put trust in my voice teacher. I lost trust when he turned into my molester.
- I put trust in healing emotionally. I lost trust when I woke up in an ICU months later.
- I put trust in my physical recovery. I lost trust with every medical setback.
- I put trust in my husband and my marriage...

When I didn't know what else to trust, I put trust in the solid, family foundation that I had growing up. I felt the support of my family around me. I thought of my grandparents and their overflowing love, generosity, and indomitable spirits. Sometimes, the best way to find the inner strength to trust, is to channel the strength of those that came before you.

I looked back to my own journey of survival at eighteen, the same age of my grandmother in Auschwitz. I was in the Columbia ICU then, the same age that my grandmother was in Auschwitz. In the ICU, I had looked to her spirit for inner strength, waiting for the day I could see her again. Thinking of her gave me the courage to trust the world again and look forward to my physical and spiritual recovery. After their deaths, I lost trust in everything again, even in feeling my emotions. It was safer to be numb. Years later, when I finally allowed myself to grieve my grandparents' deaths and feel—however painful it was—I found trust in the world again because in those tears, I found my *self*. I realized true trust *comes from inside*.

I started conducting interviews with my mother on what it was like for her growing up with Holocaust survivor parents. These interviews eventually evolved into a dialogue about womanhood, families, legacy, and our own relationship thus far. Soon, I had almost two hundred pages of interviews with just my mother alone. I was prompted to reflect on our relationship over the years.

My mother, who slept by my side in the ICU, went through this entire journey with me. Just as I had gone from teen to medical patient to survivor to various other roles within ten years, my mother had worn many hats as well.

I combined these mother-daughter interviews with my own journaled narratives of betrayal when I was sexually abused by my voice teacher. Then I interwove my own beautiful family memories with what it was like waking up from a coma and losing trust in everything. And how, just by journeying together, my mother and I regained trust in everything, including ourselves.

In weaving all of these discoveries together, not only was I creating the-atre, I was creating a new definition of trust for myself. And that is how I found my answer to: Why do we keep trusting? And why should we keep trusting? If we want to rediscover trust, we ALL have to become artists and put those shattered pieces back together in a different way. Anyone can be an artist, and everyone deserves to have trust. To trust myself, I went back to creativity, this time in song form.

When I think of October
I think of Fall and Change and Starting Over
Earth debris and colored leaves
In a mist-fumed light
It's the goblins, it's the changing, filling me with fear
But October, I'll be waiting, find me here.

October was always a month of transformation for me, so to find trust again, I started with what I could always count on. Autumn, trees, and change.

CHAPTER 63

The Road and Beyond

TELLING MY STORY WAS ONCE the biggest risk in my life, and it turned out to be the most healing. It took that little gasp, right before your freefall, and then I realized that not only was I safe, but telling my story would, in fact, save me. I realized I existed. And after more than a decade of wrapping myself in the gifts and painful lessons of trauma, I know where my detour is headed next—to more unknowns and uncertainties. I don't consider this book a memoir—being just over thirty—but the end of a few little detours, springboards, and setbacks in my life. As I end this book, I close the chapter on the detours that have made a part of who I am today, so I can start a new journey. Let's say this traveler's passport has expired, and it's time for a new photo ID for more exciting roads ahead.

I'm also leaving behind, yet taking with me, the childhood that I will never get back and the lost innocence that was taken from me at a young age—as we all have to do. Just like my traumas will always be a part of me, my childhood memories will always make me who I am. I will always be that aggressive theatre girl, getting sent to the principal's office for tap dancing on the teacher's desk. My creativity has always been my voice, my lifeline, my greatest ally. No predator, trauma, or detour can take that away from me. In fact, that is my true Detourist passport.

Everything I seek, I have in myself. It's my job to engage with enough un-expected stimuli to bring it out of me, just like sometimes the only way to stop a hiccup is to surprise yourself with a good scare. Together, we all have a story worth sharing. I realized this for myself after a few more detours, including a twenty-eighth surgery following a car accident. As I did during other times of pain, I went back to my grandmother's story. Just two years before my accident, I had taken a picture wearing my grandmother's kitchen robe over my wedding gown. The following year, I had brought it to my college graduation, right after my thirtieth birthday

Now, when I looked past Grandma in the robe, I discovered Hannah, the woman, the friend, to guide me through my own life.

At first, I wondered how I would survive the dozens of surgeries ahead for me and years of being unable to eat or drink anything by mouth. And I began to wonder even more how my grandmother had survived the atrocities she did. How did she "celebrate when the times are good" after her life had been so torn apart? Could I as her granddaughter do the same?

I spoke these words in my third TEDx talk in Jacksonville Florida, shortly after the school shootings. How could we all endure loss and carry on, even make an impact?

For a long time, I thought no one could relate to my story. I felt like a freak; an outcast forever exiled from the world. After another performance of *Gutless & Grateful* in New York in the summer of 2016, I received this note:

"Just want to tell you that I'm happy I saw your show. It's my third time, and I needed to see it tonight. The show I am trying to put up requires me to put the story of my struggles in life in front of the world, although I don't think anyone can relate to it. Again, thank you."

To know that my story, was serving to inspire, motivate, and validate another struggling person meant everything.

I couldn't wait to camouflage back into the world, different, yet the same self I've always been. I had become a Detourist, but I've always been Amy Oestreicher.

And so, as Amy Oestreicher, I sit down at my Passover table again, as we now do every year. We sit with our friends and family, having traveled so far over the course of the year, and having been shaped by our twisted path along the way. The beauty of Passover is that we can come back to the same table and participate in the same rituals, once again feeling like we, too, have escaped from Egypt and achieved liberation. Each year there is another demon to defeat, a lesson to learn, a battle to fight. Life can change gradually or overnight; the only constant is change.

We have to show up for our detours and follow them. We can hate some detours, pause, and doubt them. But maybe those two steps back will give us a larger view of our "big picture." There may not be an answer, but as old leaves die, new buds burgeon.

Tradition and its accompanying rituals connect us to a bigger picture or larger story—we can never feel lost in the traditions that ground us in who we are, bonding us together through a common story. We're all traveling together—whether out of bondage, out of the hospital, or on a detour. A trauma can never "kick" us out of the world.

The rituals of Passover have one purpose: every year, we are given the chance to access the power of all who came before us. This "Festival of Freedom" is ours to celebrate. This journey is so much easier when we travel together. And that is why we don't have one-person Seders. That is why our chairs were left half pulled out of the tables set for thirty people in our Fairfield, Connecticut basement when I was rushed to the emergency room.

Those chairs were waiting to be warmed once again, to be reclined in, slightly to the left, waiting for their occupants to tell their stories together. Stories never die and there is always a chance to write a new ending. Every story is ours to create, tell, and live.

When my family finally sat back down at our Passover table—a different table, with different chairs, in a different home, with different food, and some different guests to celebrate with—everything had changed, but nothing had changed at all. And as we sang Dayenu, poured our wine, and broke our unleavened bread, we liberated ourselves once again. My mother and I looked at each other as we helped ladle boiling soup into bowls, then looked up and over at the window and saw that sky was blue, just as we had repeated to each other almost fifteen years earlier.

Our whole story passed between us in a glance. To tell our story, we don't always have words, or even need them. It doesn't always have to be chronological, and it doesn't always have to make sense. That's how trauma comes together. We take those broken pieces and we turn them into whatever the heck we want.

When someone asked Arthur Miller once if he was working on a new play, he responded, "I don't know. I might be." We are always creating and continuing stories in our heads. Any little speck of a moment might explode into this mountainous idea for a play, mural, song, anything. Whichever way a tree twists, turns, and transforms, it always grows. And so can we. That is what makes living an adventure.

"Fear not, I'll protect you," the tree says. "I am always with you. Dance beneath the clouds with me and let your voice swirl round my branches. And your body and soul will sail through every passageway."

I'm telling my story and sharing what I did as a model open to be interpreted and tailored to each individual. We all need to find our way through healing by the means unique to us. There was no "road map" for my healing, but who really has a set road map in life? What we need, more than anything, is the trust that we ARE capable of setting our own path. It can be terribly intimidating to make that first mark on a blank canvas. It can be terribly scary to make the first mark on a "new" life when you have to start from scratch. But after we make the first mark, all we have to do is take the next step, and then the next...and the next.

That's also why it's important that we all share our unique stories—because there is no single right way to do this. By hearing how everyone else made a plan for themselves when there really was none, perhaps we'll get an idea of how to navigate a detour on our own.

Safe travels, Detourists.

ABOUT THE AUTHOR

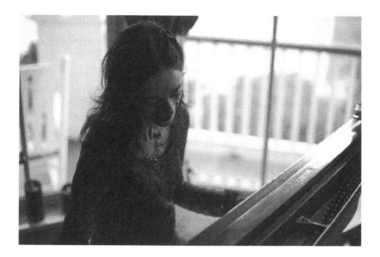

Amy Oestreicher is a songwriter, actress, and Audie-award nominated playwright, mixed media visual artist, author, international keynote, TEDx and RAINN speaker, and award-winning health advocate. She has toured *Gutless & Grateful*, her one-woman musical autobiography, since its NYC debut in 2012, and since its BroadwayWorld nominated debut, to theatres, conferences, and organizations promoting creativity as a path to resilience. Her writings and reviews have appeared in over 70 online and print publications, She's currently touring a mental health advocacy/sexual assault awareness program to colleges nationwide Her newest original works include *Passageways: Songs of Connection, Abnormal & Sublime*, and *More Than Ever Now*, a play based on the life of her grandmother.

To view Amy's 3 TEDx Talks: www.amyoes.com/TEDx

To learn more about Gutless & Grateful: www.amyoes.com/gutless
To view Amy's Art: www.amyoes.com/art-portfolio
For Amy's College Mental Health Program: www.amyoes.com/mental-health-mindset
To see the Frank Cartoon, visit www.amyoes.com/Frank

To learn more about LoveMyDetour, and share your own Detour: https://amyoes.com/lovemydetour/mission

#LoveMyDetour is a campaign inspiring people to flourish because of, rather than in spite of challenges.
#LoveMyDetour aims to encourage growth and healing by sharing our stories; to transform communities by inspiring people to open their minds and reframe their view of "detours" into a new direction for life.
For worksheets on navigating your own detour, visit www.amyoes.com/detourist-workshop

Cover Photos:
Singing Tree, mentioned on page 300 is the painting on the cover image by Amy, her first discovery of making art in Yale Hospital.
The photograph on the cover was taken by Amy while studying at the Eugene O'Neill Center's National Theater Institute.

To keep up with Amy's speaking, performances, music and writing, follow her on:
Facebook @amyoestr
Twitter @amyoes
Instagram @amyoes70